Food Insecurity and Public Health

Edited by
Louise C. Ivers

Associate Professor of Global Health and Social Medicine
Associate Professor of Medicine
Harvard Medical School
Boston, Massachusetts

Associate Physician
Division of Global Health Equity
Brigham and Women's Hospital
Boston, Massachusetts

Senior Health and Policy Advisor
Partners In Health
Boston, Massachusetts

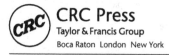

CRC Press
Taylor & Francis Group
Boca Raton London New York

CRC Press is an imprint of the
Taylor & Francis Group, an **informa** business

CRC Press
Taylor & Francis Group
6000 Broken Sound Parkway NW, Suite 300
Boca Raton, FL 33487-2742

First issued in paperback 2021

© 2015 by Taylor & Francis Group, LLC
CRC Press is an imprint of Taylor & Francis Group, an Informa business

No claim to original U.S. Government works

Version Date: 20150318

ISBN 13: 978-1-03-209866-1 (pbk)
ISBN 13: 978-1-4665-9905-5 (hbk)

Visit the Taylor & Francis Web site at
http://www.taylorandfrancis.com

and the CRC Press Web site at
http://www.crcpress.com

For my parents, and for Jeanette, David, George, and Matthew—for supporting me always. And for the people of rural Haiti, who taught me about food insecurity and its devastating impact on their health.

Contents

Foreword

THE FOOD FIGHT

It didn't take the development of what some would term "modern medicine" or "modern nutrition" for our species to learn the significance of proper nutrition to clinical outcomes, including the outcome many of its members agree to be the most important one: sheer survival. There's of course much more debate about when to apply the term "modern" or "scientific" to public health, clinical medicine, and nutrition; ongoing research means that, as in other fields, modernity (and with it, equity of chances of surviving to develop and enjoy one's capabilities and gifts, to paraphrase the great economist of food insecurity, Amartya Sen) is ever a moving target, an aspiration. Significant milestones are known to all historians of these overlapping fields, even if they are forgotten by busy practitioners. Did modern nutrition begin when scurvy among sailors was shown to be prevented by various species of citrus, or when vitamin C was shown to prevent it? Similar stories of discovery abound, from rickets to riboflavin, of the myriad causes of iron-deficiency anemia: daily dietary choices and culturally reinforced preferences, of course (such as the willful avoidance of certain iron-rich foods because of cultural or religious prohibitions, but also because, as they say, there's no accounting for tastes). Or did modern nutrition begin to come into its own when social conditions that have little to do with choice or willfulness or preferences or tastes ("no accounting for it") or that ever-reliable explanatory mechanism, rife ignorance of proper diet and hygiene among the poorly nourished?

When iron deficiency anemia was revealed to be due to (in addition to many dietary deficiencies and several hemoglobinopathies) recurrent hookworm and other helminthiases, especially among the unshod poor; recurrent malaria or other blood parasites; frequent and unplanned pregnancies, and, most of all, the food insecurity that hovers over hundreds of millions of families—when these complex webs of causality are acknowledged by researchers and practitioners, then and only then can we claim to have even the beginnings of a sound analytic purchase on food insecurity. Even more difficult is the simple fact that many of the chief determinants of food insecurity are not even "ethnographically visible" within the clinic or research site, since these determinants are the result of policy decisions (such as "free-trade agreements") made far from the settings in which food insecurity and poor nutrition take their greatest toll. It's *social* medicine, as much as a rapidly expanding understanding of the varied biochemical pathways associated with several nutritional deficiencies, which underpins accurate analysis of food insecurity.

So do those who wish to understand—much less lessen—such a rapidly changing and complex topic as food insecurity throw their hands in the air or hunker down for years of reading and reflection? Not at all. These complexities are the subject of this superb and comprehensive and scholarly book, *Food Insecurity and Public Health,* which is the first volume I've seen that is willing to take on these complexities and move them front and center in an effort to change the paradigm away from a search for analytic simplifications and minimalist and local interventions (whether agricultural or cultural or programmatic or clinical or policies changes) that amount to our understandable desire for "magic bullets."

No Magic Bullet was the title of the historian Allan Brandt's classic study of venereal disease between the widespread uptake, in medical circles, of what was termed "the germ theory of disease"—this occurred in the latter half of the nineteenth century and the close of the pre-antibiotic era in the third and fourth decades of the twentieth century. As lives ravaged by syphilis (and other sexually transmitted diseases) were damaged, and sometimes saved, by new and often toxic agents, there was also a growing awareness of the importance of social conditions, including housing, nutrition, and joblessness. The same was true, many historians have noted, among those who cared for or sought to prevent tuberculosis, or epidemic typhoid and cholera, in these same decades. The great split between social medicine and public health had not yet come to pass, and though claims of causality are always suspect—because numerous and often contradictory, with a strong tendency throughout these centuries to blame the chief victims of these ills, always the poor—there were some who argued that the quest for magic bullets, which seemed to come along as penicillin or sulfa drugs—hastened this split.

It is more likely that growing sub-specialization, in the laboratory and in the clinic, led to a great and creative burst of discovery and that clinical medicine and public health were both given a great push forward by such careful focus on specific topics. This was true in nutritional science as well. But social medicine, the glue that bound together the lab and the clinic and the hospital and the living conditions of the poor and otherwise marginalized, too often faded as a relic of a bygone era. And as the world's population grew, and famines and other extreme manifestations of food insecurity (or lack of food sovereignty) grew, so did, in this same world, epidemics of obesity and diabetes and heart disease.

These topics are and will remain the subject of debates by medical historians and others who seek to "resocialize" our understandings of the impact of diet and nutrition and food insecurity in past decades. Many of these "food fights," though readily encountered in the closing decades of the past century, are discussed, if they are discussed at all, as if they are relics from a distant past, and linked to pre-modern debates about miasmas and ill-humors and the evil eye. And, as ever, the failure to assess what Amartya Sen and others, including the political economists of the nineteenth century, termed *agency*—the ability to choose freely and to have choices and to live up to one's capabilities—was profound in modern clinical medicine, epidemiology, and nutritional science. Adequate nutrition itself—the amount of protein and calories required for health even in the absence of serious co-morbid disease, much of it consumptive, and some of it caused by chronic infections—was too often asserted, in academic subspecialist literature as in popular discourse about topics ranging from malnutrition and stunting to a growing wave of obesity, all occurring at the same time if in different places in a given city or state or nation, was assumed to be a matter of individual family choice, prudent stewardship of readily available resources, and smart decisions by heads of households, especially those who are women.

This book, like many by Amartya Sen and Jean Dreze, debunks these myths. But *Food Insecurity and Public Health* does so for a very different, and too often neglected, audience: clinicians (nurses, doctors, dieticians), public health authorities (regional and national and international), and those who plan and implement programs to prevent or alleviate the impacts of food insecurity in settings of surfeit (too much of the wrong kinds of food) and crass want (not enough calories and protein to keep a poor family alive and healthy, much less to set a sick family member on the road to recovery). Nor is this a book looking back as a medical historian would. For the time in question is *right now*. The book is edited by Louise Ivers, an infectious disease physician from Harvard Medical School, who has worked in highly food insecure Haiti, with Partners In Health and its sister organization Zanmi Lasante, for over a decade. Dr. Ivers has weathered and written about calamities ranging from earthquakes to cholera epidemics and she has conducted novel research about the use of oral cholera vaccine from the midst of what became the world's largest epidemic. But Ivers has also spent patient years in the study and remediation of rural Haiti's calamitous food insecurity, and this volume springs from her passion, and that of many others whose work is gathered here, about the injustice of food insecurity, and about its origins and remedies, in the twenty-first century.

Accordingly, *Food Insecurity and Public Health* draws on, and vibrates with, current research and urgent lessons from Haiti, from central and eastern Africa, to the Navajo Nation, and beyond, even to the settings in which policies are crafted and disseminated, with varying degrees of success at the level of delivery to those enduring food insecurity; it also takes on the implications of this work for specific pathologies, such as AIDS and tuberculosis and diabetes, that are encountered by clinicians, and endured by patients and their primary caregivers (their families), across the world. It even includes a comprehensive review of how poverty and gender inequality conspire to put women at highest risk of direct experience of food insecurity even as they are called to address it through actions (often, changes in their own "knowledge, attitudes, beliefs, and practices") that will have little impact on the larger-scale forces that determine, all too often, their families' risk of malnutrition of one sort or another.

THREE RECENT CASES FROM THE FIELD

I said above that this book is not a history of food insecurity but rather an up-to-date analysis of it. In the past two months alone, I've been reminded that the food fight continues in every setting to which I've traveled in the course of work with Partners In Health. Allow me to mention three patients from two different countries, all of them encountered as this book was going to press and as I was holding it up by failing to submit this foreword on time. Most of the delay may be attributed to my own failings, but part of it may be attributed to the ongoing debate, and great confusion, concerning the social determinants of health and illness (and of course "outcomes" in the clinical sense) and the need for nutritional supplementation to be seen as part of proper medical care. Conversely, the absence of such supplementation can fairly enough be seen as medical malpractice.

Each of these patients are children, and each had at least three *concomitant and life-threatening* pathologies at once: extreme poverty, malnutrition, and one infectious disease (Ebola or tuberculosis or HIV disease). And I will wager that each of these patients might survive, indeed flourish, if the aggressive (and cheap!) interventions advocated in *Food Security and Public Health* become standard practice in both public health and clinical medicine.

None of these children was of the traditional age when kwashiorkor or marasmus strike most commonly: between the age of one, when mixed feeding is all beleaguered and working mothers can offer their infants, and the age of two, when another infant is on the way and the child is weaned altogether. Two of these patients were nine years old; the other was seven.

Aminata (I've changed the names) was one of the nine-year-olds. She is from a small village in a district of Sierra Leone called Port Loko, to the north of its capital city, Freetown. She was febrile and vomiting, and with severe diarrhea, on December 28, 2014, the day she was admitted to an Ebola treatment unit run by Partners In Health. She'd just seen her mother and sister die of Ebola, and was saved from that fate by fluid resuscitation. But she never bounced back. One of the nurses told me that Aminata didn't speak, or eat, during her time in the Ebola unit. Having survived Ebola, she now lay dying of malnutrition in the general hospital's pediatrics ward. By the time she was discharged from the Ebola unit, she weighed a skeletal 27 pounds. A PIH doctor working in the ward, tried feeding her through a nasogastric tube. But Aminata, still mute, pulled it out. Her father had come to see her, but to little effect. He left convinced another of his daughters was sure to die, a view the nurses seemed to share. Another Ebola survivor, older than most—I'd guess she was in her late 50s—was assigned to sit with Aminata and encourage her to eat a high-protein, high calorie paste called RUTF, or ready-to-use-therapeutic food, which had often worked wonders with younger children (and is the subject of discussion in *Food Insecurity and Public Health*). But the older woman too had failed to convince the girl to eat.

In the third week of January 2015, I was asked to see Aminata because she had a fever, and her continued decline led some of the clinicians to think she might have another infection. "We think she's also suffered brain damage," added another of the nurses. "She almost never speaks, and makes no sense when she does." Aminata lay alone in the bed furthest from the door, her face to the wall, as motionless as she was silent. When I spoke to her, she barely glanced at me with what looked like fear followed by disinterest, and turned her eyes back to the wall. I reviewed her medical record, where I could find no documentation of a recent fever (and no evidence that she'd ever been weighed). Re-insert the feeding tube was my only (and wholly unoriginal) suggestion, get basic lab tests (which hadn't been available in November), weight and height.

What turned Aminata around was pairing her with a sympathetic young Ebola survivor, one who listened to her and would take her preferences into account (her first intelligible words to him were "I'd like a special kind of cookies, and some juice") and *then* she would consider the RUTF and rehabilitation that eventually got her back on her feet. The food fight, in this instance: almost all of the survivors were discharged from the Ebola units severely malnourished if they couldn't feed themselves: placing nasogastric tubes and even intravenous lines was considered too dangerous to the staff.

The second patient, Jonas, was also nine. He is from a small village not far from the town in which Dr. Ivers began working over a dozen years ago; indeed, we were together on the day we first saw him, also in January 2015: a small boy, who looked half his age and silent and frightened. He was being bathed by his stout grandmother; others in the household also looked well-nourished. But this boy was marked by anasarca, his legs and abdomen and cheeks looking like those of a two-year-old with severe kwashiorkor. His arms were tiny sticks; he could barely stand, or speak. The story, as we heard it, was that in the course of the past two years, Jonas had had two bouts with a chronic enteropathy—weeks and weeks of loose stools—and loss of appetite and an intermittent fever. He had been admitted, last year, to a nearby hospital, one built by Partners In Health, so we hoped to find his medical records when we clambered down from his family's hilltop perch. Jonas was functionally an orphan; his mother was dead and his father unaccounted for, said to be working in the Dominican Republic. But his grandmother had a chest x-ray at hand, right there: it looked free of tuberculosis—in the lungs, at least. We had been introduced to Jonas by the nurse in charge of the nutritional rehabilitation program, because of the food fight: he didn't fit conventional criteria for traditional nutritional supplements—he didn't have a known diagnosis, nor did he match the age of her other patients—and so had just been started on RUTF, locally made by Partners In Health and its Haitian sister organization, Zanmi Lasante. We did find the medical record, and readmitted him for treatment for extrapulmonary tuberculosis (tuberculous enteropathy) and he has just begun to recover. The food fight: even in a program with its own locally manufactured RUTF, the enrollment criteria were too stringent. A negative chest x-ray and anergia on a TB skin test do not mean a child cannot die of both of these pathologies, and of the third, which so often accompanies being an orphan.

The third, Isabelle, the seven year old, was well known to me, since I had seen her in consultation twice before. She was born with HIV, and had been on antiretroviral therapy ever since. But unlike many other children, she had failed to thrive; her CD4 count waned, and she became progressively ill with opportunistic infections, including tuberculosis (which she survived, in part because of the food supplementation she and her family received). But when this supplementation was cut back—it had been linked to her diagnosis of tuberculosis—she fell ill again.

In each of these three examples, it's possible to parse the social determinants of disease, with which most clinicians do not concern themselves in the course of daily practice, and the improvement of clinical outcomes—significantly, the decrease in case-fatality rate or permanent sequelae—about which doctors and nurses and other clinicians are quite passionate. It's not that failure to understand the social determinants of health and disease constitutes malpractice—if such a criterion were used, most of the most talented and committed clinicians I know would be banned from practice—but rather that excellent clinical outcomes, especially in settings of poverty and food insecurity, are not possible (or, at least, unlikely) unless clinicians understand that even tardy interventions can make the difference between life and death after they have accepted patients into their care. Thus, the material covered in this much-needed book should be part of the shared corpus of knowledge of *all* clinicians and of those who design and implement and evaluate programs to prevent ill health and to improve ill health when it occurs. In other words, this book may be seen as a revelatory compendium of innovation relevant for improving cure rates and diminishing adverse sequelae that could easily have been prevented.

WHY THIS BOOK?

There are at least three reasons why I would hope that *Food Insecurity and Public Health* finds a wider audience than its editor and authors suppose.

First, it's a veritable trove of up-to-date information about food insecurity and its variable and adverse impacts, a sort of handbook and instructional manual for the fight against it, and also a superb reference book. And although I've repeated that this is not a book of medical history, but rather reviews recent developments, most of its chapters are accountable to literature reaching back into the decades when the impact of nutrition, and especially malnutrition, were among the central topics of both medicine and public health. A couple of chapters—and the one on the travails of the Navajo nation stands out as beautifully written, elegiac, and yet pragmatic— are in fact historical overviews of the rise of food insecurity, almost always a result of mean-spirited or uninformed policy decisions in recent decades, and downright violent ones in the more distant, but still remembered, past.

Second, this volume, on the whole, avoids the reductionist tendencies of international health, pitting prevention against care, the quest for the "minimum" package. But the chapters here suggest that there will be no magic bullet, not zinc, not vitamin A, not plumpy-nut—patients with consumptive disease need both increased calories and protein too.

In food-insecure households, patients who are hospitalized gain more weight than at home—if, of course, the hospitals in which they receive care actually serve food at all. Imagine my shock upon first reaching Haiti and seeing that patients admitted to hospitals were fed, if they were fed at all, by their own family members; the same was true in prisons. In one hospital, having patients (many of them malnourished) bring in their own meals was justified as "community participation." This would have been sinister (or at least cynical) had I not known, as I did, that the justifications were spurred by the inability of physicians and nurses to address food insecurity, whether at the "level" of the family, the neighborhood, the region, the nation. In a globalized economy, food security is of course almost never a local issue.

This leads to the third issue, the one clinicians shy away from, either out of modesty or ignorance. And that is the link not only between disease and nutritional status, but also that between food insecurity at the household level and policies made far away. Another tour de force in *Food Insecurity and Public Health* is Gene Bukhman's overview of the ways in which an obsessive focus with "individual risk factors" and "lifestyle choices" (as well as a worthy effort to reduce the impact of modern food processing in spurring obesity and diabetes and heart disease) has obscured the "noncommunicable diseases," some of them in fact infectious in origin, that continue to kill among the world's poorest. This is not only an excellent overview, but the beginnings of a critical sociology of how health policy is formed, and sometimes hijacked, by narrowly focused views of what an agenda should be and how it should be made palatable to those best in a position to move from policy to implementation.

ONE WORLD, NOT THREE

Although this volume is aimed primarily at the pragmatists involved in addressing, directly, the everyday dilemmas encountered in settings of food insecurity, *Food Insecurity and Public Health* is sure to appeal to a broader audience. I wish I could say, for example, "required reading for *every* medical student," since I know, from reviewing these chapters, that the findings, summaries, and syntheses of this book are relevant in every-day clinical practice. The same holds true, of course, for nurses and social workers and other front-line clinical workers, including community-health workers. But at the very least, I hope to join others in insisting on the following: this volume is the ideal reference for clinicians and program managers in such settings, and should be readily available to them. *Food Insecurity and Public Health* is heavy in more ways than one. But it's certainly the best carry-on luggage I could imagine for those heading for many of the places in which we work.

Paul Farmer, MD, PhD
Chief of the Division of Global Health Equity, Brigham and Women's Hospital, Boston;
Kolokotrones University Professor,
Chair of the Department of Global Health and Social Medicine, Harvard Medical School, Boston;
Co-founder and Chief Strategist of Partners In Health (PIH), Boston; and Special Adviser to the United Nations Secretary-General on Community Based Medicine and Lessons from Haiti, New York

Preface

As a physician in a small rural hospital in Boucan Carre, Haiti, I became very aware of the terrible impact of food insecurity on my patients' health. Despite the advent of antiretroviral treatment and comprehensive HIV care in the area, in our clinic (run by Partners In Health and the Haitian Ministry of Health), patients living with HIV who should have been doing medically well, came to their monthly visits with a chief complaint of hunger pains. Despite our efforts to treat their medical issues, the pervasiveness of hunger in the community was evident in the clinic. On home visits accompanied by our social worker, I soon bore witness to what my Haitian colleagues had known for a long time—that the living situation of our patients in the mountains of central Haiti was dire. Our patients' inability to have stable access to food for themselves and their children preoccupied their daily actions and thoughts, and was completely impossible to separate from their health.

Through a variety of mechanisms, food insecurity has a substantial negative impact on health, and in return, through pathways like loss of ability to work, and expenditures on medical costs or transportation, poor health can contribute to food insecurity. This book aims to review the concepts and impacts of food insecurity through the lens of public health. The first three chapters focus on concepts, frameworks, and measures of food insecurity, and Chapter 1 also discusses integration of food security interventions into development programs. Subsequent chapters review in detail the evidence regarding food insecurity's interaction with specific health issues that are of global importance. Each chapter also considers programs or interventions that have been used to attempt to address the issue, including a discussion of U.S. federal food stamps program as part of Chapter 7. In truth, however, there continues to be a dearth of data on the ways in which programs can effectively address the problem of food insecurity at the household, community, or district level in either the short or long term—beyond, of course, the elimination of poverty, which is no doubt a root cause of the problem.

But despite the enormity of that problem—1.2 billion people live in extreme poverty—considering integrated approaches to health and food security in policy and programming at the individual, community, and health systems levels offers the opportunity to make a positive impact in both arenas. The final three chapters of the book are cases that aim to provide further context for the material presented, including a discussion of food insecurity in Navajo Nation, a description of an ambitious project to evaluate the financial cost of hunger in Africa, and a case study of a successful food security intervention undertaken in the context of HIV treatment and care in Kenya.

The book is not intended to be an exhaustive review of nutrition because a number of excellent volumes already exist in this realm (including, e.g., *Nutrition and Health in Developing Countries*, edited by Richard Semba and Martin Bloem, Humana Press), and because nutrition is just one of the pathways by which food insecurity affects health.

In considering the development agenda in the after the Millennium Development Goals—the so-called post-2015 development agenda—the Secretary-General of the United Nations High-Level Panel of Eminent Persons called eradicating extreme poverty by 2030 a central issue. In an illustrative goal, the panel suggested a global call to "ensure food security and good nutrition." In looking toward this goal, it will be critical for health professionals, program managers, policy experts, agronomists, economists, and nutritionists to consider the links between food insecurity and health, and to seek integrated solutions to both problems.

This book has benefited greatly from the contributions of many people, and I thank them all for their dedication, hard work, and support of the project. The expertise of the authors brings a variety of perspectives, knowledge, and experiences that are humbling. I thank the National Institute of Child Health and Human Development for their support of our research in Haiti on addressing food insecurity and HIV infection (R01HD057627). Many thanks are due to Jessica Teng and Hannah Hughes for their invaluable reviews and copyediting of chapters. I am also profoundly grateful for the opportunity to have worked with Partners In Health since 2003, and to have learned so much from the collaboration, mentorship, and support of my tireless colleagues in that organization—there are too many to mention in detail, but it is certain that without Paul Farmer, Joia Mukherkee, Loune Viaud, and Fernet Leandre, I would never have been inspired to be a part of this book—thank you all.

Editor

Dr. Louise C. Ivers, MB, BCh, BAO, MPH, DTM&H is a medical doctor, and senior health and policy advisor for Partners In Health (PIH), an international non-profit organization that provides direct health care and social services to poor communities around the world. She is trained in infectious diseases, tropical medicine, and public health and is also associate professor of global health and social medicine, and associate professor of medicine at Harvard Medical School in Boston. Dr. Ivers has spent her medical career to date implementing health programs and working to improve the delivery of health care in resource-poor settings through service and research. In addition to implementing primary health care, HIV, TB, and cholera programs, she has significant experience in coordination and implementation of disaster relief efforts. Based in Haiti from 2003 to 2012, she led the Partners In Health responses to hurricane-related flooding in 2008, a major earthquake in 2010, and an ongoing cholera epidemic in Haiti. Dr. Ivers has contributed to published articles on HIV/AIDS, food insecurity, post-disaster humanitarian response, and cholera treatment and prevention. She has served as a technical advisor to the World Health Organization and mentors Haitian and American physicians. She was previously clinical director and chief of mission for Partners In Health in Haiti. Through her decade of experience in Haiti, she gained programmatic and academic insights into the impact of food insecurity on health, and leads NIH-funded research on the topic.

Contributors

Jonathan Abeita
Crownpoint Service Unit Community
   Health Representative Program
Crownpoint, New Mexico

Mae-Gilene Begay
Navajo Nation Community Health
   Representative Outreach Program
Window Rock, Arizona

Sherry Begaye
Crownpoint Service Unit Community
   Health Representative Program
Crownpoint, New Mexico

Gilles Bergeron
Food and Nutrition Technical
   Assistance (FANTA)
Washington, DC

Martin W. Bloem
Friedman School of Nutrition Science
   and Policy
Tufts University
Boston, Massachusetts

and

Bloomberg School of Public Health
Johns Hopkins University
Baltimore, Maryland

and

United Nations World Food Programme
Rome, Italy

Paula Braitstein
School of Medicine
Indiana University
Bloomington, Indianapolis

Gene Bukhman
Harvard Medical School
and
Division of Global Health Equity
Brigham and Women's Hospital
Boston, Massachusetts

Maxine Castillo
Crownpoint Service Unit
   Community Health
   Representative Program
Crownpoint, New Mexico

Tony Castleman
George Washington University
Washington, DC

Cleophas Wanyonyi Chesoli
Jomo Kenyatta University of
   Agriculture and Technology
Nairobi, Kenya

and

Academic Model Providing Access to
   Healthcare Program
Moi University
Moi, Kenya

Jennifer Coates
Friedman School of Nutrition Science
   and Policy
Tufts University
Boston, Massachusetts

Kimberly A. Cullen
University of Massachusetts Medical
   School
Worcester, Massachusetts

LaJuanna Daye
Crownpoint Service Unit Community
    Health Representative
    Program
Crownpoint, New Mexico

Robert Einterz
School of Medicine
Indiana University
Bloomington, Indianapolis

Dana Eldridge
Diné Policy Institute
Tsaile, Arizona

Edward A. Frongillo
Arnold School of Public Health
University of South Carolina
Columbia, South Carolina

Catherine Gichunge
School of Medicine
Moi University
Eldoret, Kenya

Cara S. Guenther
Partners In Health
Boston, Massachusetts

Abigail M. Hatcher
Division of HIV/AIDS
San Francisco General Hospital
and
Department of Medicine
University of California,
    San Francisco
San Francisco, California

and

Wits Reproductive Health and HIV
    Institute
University of the Witwatersrand
Johannesburg, South Africa

Louise C. Ivers
Harvard Medical School
and
Division of Global Health Equity
Brigham and Women's Hospital
and
Partners In Health
Boston, Massachusetts

Robyn Jackson
Diné Policy Institute
Tsaile, Arizona

Fanice Komen Jerop
Moi Teaching and Referral Hospital
Eldoret, Kenya

Jacque Jim
Crownpoint Service Unit
    Community Health
    Representative Program
Crownpoint, New Mexico

Leroy Joe
Crownpoint Service Unit Community
    Health Representative Program
Crownpoint, New Mexico

Sylvester Kimaiyo
School of Medicine
Moi University
Eldoret, Kenya

Barbara Laraia
School of Public Health
University of California, Berkeley
Berkeley, California

Stephen Lewis
Appropriate Grass Roots Initiative
Eldoret, Kenya

Joseph Mamlin
School of Medicine
Indiana University
Bloomington, Indianapolis

Divya Mehra
United Nations World Food
    Programme
Rome, Italy

Meria Miller-Castillo
Crownpoint Service Unit Community
    Health Representative Program
Crownpoint, New Mexico

Kartika Palar
Division of HIV/AIDS
San Francisco General Hospital
and
Department of Medicine
University of California,
    San Francisco
San Francisco, California

Saskia de Pee
Friedman School of Nutrition Science
    and Policy
Tufts University
Boston, Massachusetts

and

United Nations World Food Programme
Rome, Italy

Tomeka Petersen
School of Medicine
Indiana University
Bloomington, Indianapolis

Emily Piltch
Agriculture, Food and Environment
    Program
Friedman School of Nutrition Science
    and Policy
Tufts University
Boston, Massachusetts

Shruthi Rajashekra
Harvard Medical School
Boston, Massachusetts

and

COPE Project
Gallup, New Mexico

Sonya Shin
Harvard Medical School
and
Division of Global Health Equity
and
Division of Infectious Diseases
Brigham and Women's Hospital
Boston, Massachusetts

and

COPE Project
Gallup, New Mexico

Hannah Tadayo
Ministry of Health
Nairobi, Kenya

Jessica E. Teng
Division of Global Health Equity
Brigham and Women's Hospital
and
Partners In Health
Boston, Massachusetts

Vangie Tully
Crownpoint Service Unit Community
    Health Representative Program
Crownpoint, New Mexico

Joan VanWassenhove
COPE Project
Gallup, New Mexico

and

Friedman School of Nutrition
    Science and Policy
Tufts University
Boston, Massachusetts

Sheri D. Weiser
Division of HIV/AIDS
San Francisco General Hospital
and
Department of Medicine
University of California, San Francisco
San Francisco, California

Martha Williams
Crownpoint Service Unit Community
    Health Representative Program
Crownpoint, New Mexico

Yuehwern Yih
Purdue University
Lafayette, Indiana

Sera Young
Department of Nutritional
    Sciences
Cornell University
Ithaca, New York

INSTITUTIONAL CONTRIBUTORS

African Union Commission

AMPATH—The Academic Model Providing Access to Healthcare: Moi University, Moi Teaching and Referral Hospital and a consortium of North American academic health centers led by Indiana University working in partnership with the Government of Kenya.

New Partnership of Africa's Development Planning and Coordinating Agency

United Nations Economic Commission for Africa

United Nations World Food Programme

1 Food Security and Program Integration
An Overview

Tony Castleman and Gilles Bergeron

CONTENTS

> The quest for food security can be the common thread that links the different challenges we face and helps build a sustainable future.
>
> **José Graziano da Silva**
> *United Nations Food and Agriculture Organization (FAO) Director-General*

INTRODUCTION

As the quotation above suggests, food security is increasingly recognized as integral not only to reducing hunger and malnutrition but also to broader development goals. Public health programs and policies often consider underlying social, economic, and environmental factors that influence health, and in many contexts, food security emerges as a prominent factor. Direct effects of food security on health occur through nutritional status, itself a critical component of an individual's health. For example, child malnutrition is a significant source of child mortality (Black et al. 2013). But in addition to this direct effect, food security also affects health through constraints to accessing health care, expenditure decisions, mental health, and other pathways described in further detail in Chapter 2.

Given the relationship between food security and health, understanding the different dimensions of food security and the program approaches used to reduce food insecurity can inform and enhance the design and implementation of public health programs. Varying degrees of integration between food security and health services are called for in different contexts. Programs aimed at improving food security often use different structures, partners, and implementation approaches than public health programs do, and understanding these differences can assist in the planning of when, and how, to integrate food security and health services.

This chapter provides an overview of the concept of food security, related concepts, threats to food security, programmatic approaches, and options and considerations for integrated programming. The overview presented here sets the stage for the remaining chapters of the book, which examine specific aspects of food security and its relationship to health in greater depth.

DIMENSIONS OF FOOD SECURITY

There are several definitions of food security to be found in the literature. This is because the concept has evolved over time and because different agencies emphasize different aspects of food security. One widely used definition is the United Nations (UN) definition that was developed at the 1996 United Nations World Food Summit:

> When all people, at all times, have physical, social and economic access to sufficient, safe and nutritious food which meets their dietary needs and food preferences for an active and healthy life (Food and Agriculture Organization 1996).

There are four dimensions of food security: food availability, food access, food utilization, and stability. These four dimensions are widely used in programs, policies, and research. (Previously, USAID [United States Agency for International Development] did not include stability in its food security framework, but it has now been incorporated into the framework for Feed the Future, the U.S. Government's Global Hunger and Food Security Initiative [Feed the Future 2013].) The definition of each dimension is presented in Figure 1.1. The dimensions can be seen as sequentially conditional on each other, with availability necessary but not sufficient to access, and access necessary but not sufficient to utilization. As Pinstup-Andersen (2009, p. 5) puts it, "...availability does not assure access, and enough calories do not assure a healthy and nutritional diet."

Note that both the UN and USAID definitions of food security focus on *access* to food, though both the UN and USAID conceptions of food security include multiple

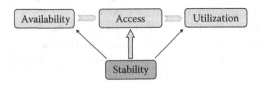

FIGURE 1.1   Dimensions of food security.

dimensions of food security, only one of which is access. The term "food security" is sometimes used colloquially to refer to access to food. For example, health service providers may refer to their clients' food security constraints, meaning poor household access to food. In other contexts, the term "food security" is used to encompass aspects that are broader than the four dimensions presented above. For example, Feed the Future states that "a family is considered food-secure when its members do not live in hunger or fear of hunger" (Feed the Future 2013, p. 5). This notion of food security includes anxiety and uncertainty about access to food.

Figure 1.1 is a diagram of the four dimensions and the interactions among them. Horizontal arrows represent the relationship described above, in which availability is necessary for access, and access for utilization. Arrows from stability to the other dimensions signify that the stability dimension means the stability of the other three dimensions. That is, while availability, access, and utilization refer to food availability, food access, and food utilization, stability refers to the stability of food availability, food access, and food utilization. Although the FAO description of stability points out that it can refer to both availability and access, the thick vertical arrow signifies that in programmatic contexts, stability often refers to stable access to food.

Figure 1.1 is a highly stylized, simple diagram of the relationship between the dimensions. Figure 1.2 offers a more detailed conceptual framework that was developed as part of the recent Food Aid and Food Security Assessment of USAID food aid programs. This framework depicts the sources and determinants of three dimensions of food security (not including stability), the pathways by which these factors influence the different dimensions of food security, and the pathways by which these dimensions influence each other.

Figure 1.2 also presents the levels at which each of these three food security dimensions most commonly operate. Food availability is generally applied at the national—or in some cases subnational—level, as implied by the mention of domestic production and imports in FAO's definition. Certainly, it is also possible to consider availability at the household level, for example, the sufficiency of food physically available to a household irrespective of whether the household has the means to access it. But in general, food availability is examined and measured at the national level.

The access dimension is generally applied at the household level, referring to the extent to which households have the means to access food using their income, own production, food assistance, bartering, and other sources. In some contexts, consideration of food access at the individual level is valuable in order to account for intrahousehold distribution of food or resources, heterogeneous nutritional needs across household members, and contexts where individuals such as inpatients or street children are not part of households. However, because income and food production are usually pooled within domestic units, food access is most often applied at the household level.

Given its biological nature, the dimension of food utilization applies at the individual level. It is possible to examine utilization outcomes at the household level, such as the presence of malnutrition. However, food utilization is inherently an individual concept and is widely applied and measured at the individual level. The health and sanitation determinants of utilization make this dimension of food security particularly relevant to public health programs and services. (Note that while the figure shows knowledge, culture, and workload influencing food utilization through

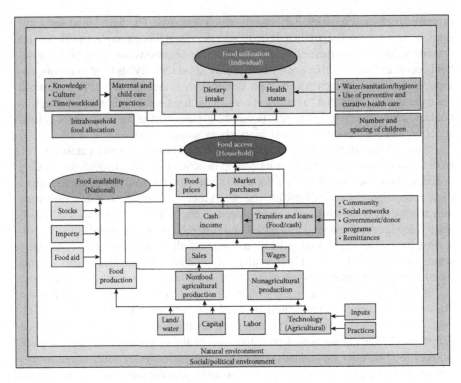

FIGURE 1.2 Relationships among the dimensions of food security. (Adapted from van Haeften, R., M. A. Anderson, H. Caudill, and E. Kilmartin. 2013. *Second Food Aid and Food Security Assessment (FAFSA-2).* Washington, DC: FHI 360/FANTA; Riely, F. et al. 1999. *Food Security Indicators and Framework for Use in the Monitoring and Evaluation of Food Aid Programs.* Arlington, VA: Food Security and Nutrition Monitoring Project (IMPACT), ISTI, Inc.; UNICEF. 1990. *Strategy for Improved Nutrition of Children and Women in Developing Countries.* New York: UNICEF.)

maternal and child care practices, these factors can also influence malnutrition among populations other than mothers and children.)

The descending levels at which the food security dimensions apply—from national to individual level—reinforce the sequential conditionality described above, with availability at the national level necessary (though not sufficient) for household access to food, which is necessary (though not sufficient) for healthy food utilization outcomes at the individual level.

While these are the established dimensions along which food security is commonly organized, other approaches also exist for classifying and analyzing food security. The UN definition cited above is composed of three attributes of food required for food security to exist: sufficiency, quality, and safety of food. Using these attributes to analyze food security and identify programming needs can add value to—though not substitute for—the conventional dimensions. Food security can also be classified along various axes, such as temporal incidence, which distinguishes between temporary and chronic food insecurity, or such as severity, which distinguishes among depths of food deprivation. Temporal categorizations are often applied to household food access, and severity can be applied to household food access as well as to food utilization because standard cutoffs exist for severe, moderate, and mild malnutrition of various types, for example, stunting, wasting, and anemia.

MEASUREMENT OF FOOD SECURITY

The dimensions of food security provide a framework for measuring food security. While scope exists for multidimensional measures of food security, most food security indicators measure one of these dimensions, or a component of the dimension. Furthermore, since availability, access, and utilization generally correspond to the national, household, and individual levels, respectively, each dimension is usually measured at its corresponding level. For instance, programs aiming to address food utilization use measures such as the rate of stunting (low height-for-age) among children under the age of five as outcome indicators. Programs aiming to address access to food use measures such as the Household Dietary Diversity Scale or the Household Hunger Scale, both of which use households as the units. Programs aiming to address availability use measures at the national level, such as FAO's undernourishment indicator. Chapter 3 of this book provides a more detailed discussion of measurement of food security.

RELATED CONCEPTS

There are a number of concepts that are related to, but distinct from, food security. Examining these concepts helps elucidate how they influence food security and how food security is situated among related constructs.

Food sovereignty, a concept that has gained attention over the past two decades, emphasizes food producers' rights and the need for greater local control over policies affecting food security. The concept emerged in 1996 when an international farmers movement called La Via Campesina issued a document titled "Food Sovereignty: A Future without Hunger" (Via Campesina 1996, Beuchelt and Virchow 2012). Definitions of food sovereignty vary, but Beuchelt and Virchow (2012) offer a helpful overarching definition: "The right of communities, peoples and states to independently determine their own food and agricultural policies."

Proponents of food sovereignty apply a rights-based approach, citing food and food production as basic human rights. Elements of food sovereignty that civil society groups advocate for include decentralization of the governance of agriculture, increased self-sufficiency in food production at community or subnational levels, improved access to productive resources by marginalized farmers, prohibition of export subsidies, and prioritization of national food needs over exports in trade policies (Beauregard and Gottlieb 2009, Kerr 2011, Beuchelt and Virchow 2012). The food price crisis in 2007–2008 spurred the food sovereignty movement to call for alternative approaches to food and agriculture governance and policies (for instance, see Holt-Giménez 2009, Wittman et al. 2010). A number of countries have incorporated food sovereignty and its principles into their constitutions and policies, including Bolivia, Ecuador, Mali, Nepal, Senegal, and Venezuela (Beauregard and Gottlieb 2009).

As the discussion above suggests, food sovereignty is distinct from food security, but is part of the social and policy environment depicted in Figure 1.2 that affects food security. Food sovereignty influences several of the determinants of food availability and food access identified in the figure, including land, water, capital, wages, imports, and food aid. Hence, while food sovereignty may support food security, it is preferable, for conceptual clarity, to keep the two constructs separate.

The term *nutrition security* is also germane to, but distinct from, food security. It specifically refers to the presence of conditions that ensure healthy nutritional status. Definitions by the International Food Policy Research Institute (IFPRI) (Benson 2004), the World Bank (von Braun et al. 2006), and the Road Map for Scaling-Up Nutrition (Scaling Up Nutrition 2010) all frame food security—or at least food access—as being necessary but not sufficient for nutrition security. The three definitions are quite similar; the World Bank definition is given here: "Nutrition security is achieved for a household when secure access to food is coupled with a sanitary environment, adequate health services, and knowledgeable care to ensure a healthy life for all household members." The attributes of nutrition security thus point squarely at food utilization—in a sense pulling out food utilization as its own construct, separate from food security. Nutrition security emphasizes the stability of food utilization and the extent to which nutrition outcomes can be assured within households. Herein lies a difference between nutrition security and food utilization, namely, that nutrition security occurs at the household level, whereas food utilization generally applies at the individual level.

The emergence of the concept of nutrition security reflects the tendency to view food security to mean food availability and access, not encompassing nutrition. For example, in many contexts "food security and nutrition" is used, implying the two are distinct. Practically speaking, while the concept of food security does include food utilization, food security programs generally refer to programs addressing food access, while nutrition programs address food utilization. The Committee on World Food Security (2012) tried to clarify the conceptual and terminology issues and recommends use of the term *food and nutrition security* to combine both concepts.

Another concept that has informed food security analysis and programming recently is *resilience*. Resilience refers to the capacity to effectively cope with negative shocks that affect income, food production, or other sources of livelihood. In addition to natural disasters and conflict, such shocks can include events such as disease or significant price changes. The U.K. Department for International Development (DFID) defines resilience as "the ability of countries, communities, and households to manage change by maintaining or transforming living standards in the face of shocks or stresses—such as earthquakes, drought or violent conflict—without compromising their long-term prospects" (Department for International Development 2011, p. 6). Resilience is often applied at the household level to describe the extent to which households can continue to meet their food and other basic needs in the face of shocks. As the DFID definition indicates, the concept is also applied to larger units than the household, such as community resilience and even food system resilience (see, e.g., Pingali et al. 2005). Resilience to climate change has also become a prominent topic of interest.

The concept of resilience encompasses a broader set of sectors and outcomes than food security. But food is an essential need, and ensuring continued access to food is often the highest priority for households facing shocks in resource-poor settings.

Therefore, resilience is a highly relevant determinant of food security, and efforts to strengthen household or community resilience are critical to reducing food insecurity among vulnerable populations.

While food sovereignty, nutrition security, and resilience have all entered the discourse relatively recently, *hunger* is among the oldest concepts, predating the notion of food security by millennia. Hunger is sometimes used as a more colloquial term for food insecurity, and more precisely it is used for the physical impact that food insecurity has on individuals. The Committee on World Food Security (Committee on World Food Security 2012, p. 12) report on terminology states, "When people do not have access to the amount of dietary energy needed for their normal level of activity, they feel hungry." While this statement refers to access, hunger is more directly the result of not *consuming* adequate energy. Holben makes the useful distinction between the narrower definition of hunger as "the physical feeling caused by lack of food" and the broader concept of "resource-constrained hunger [which] is involuntary and recurrent, chronic or prolonged physiological hunger due to resource constraints that negatively impact access to food" (Holben 2005). The latter use of hunger refers to food deprivation caused by poor food access.

For advocacy purposes, hunger is a more compelling concept with greater public resonance than the more technical term of food security. Hunger is widely used in advocacy campaigns and policies ranging from the first Millennium Development Goal to eradicate hunger and extreme poverty, to national policies such as Brazil's Zero Hunger Program, to local campaigns such as Walk for Hunger in the United States. For programmatic purposes, however, the concept of food security is more heuristic and flexible.

THREATS TO FOOD SECURITY

A range of factors threaten food security by negatively affecting the determinants depicted in Figure 1.2. Program responses to these threats include efforts to influence the threats themselves, such as preventing environmental degradation or treating disease; efforts to strengthen specific determinants of food security affected by the threats or minimize the threats' impact on these determinants, such as strengthening alternative livelihood sources to cope with income shocks; and efforts to directly address food security crises brought about by the threats, such as food assistance or other social safety net services. Program responses are described in more detail in the following section.

Threats can be organized into various categories. For instance, Webb and Rogers categorize risks to food security into natural risks, economic risks, and social and health risks (Webb and Rogers 2003). Seven primary threats to food security are described below.

Poverty is a dominant, long-term source of food insecurity. Lack of resources directly inhibits access to food and indirectly affects other dimensions and determinants of food security. Poverty threatens food security at various levels. At the national level, poverty can limit food production and food imports and can prevent the development of the physical and human infrastructure needed to facilitate household access to sufficient, diverse, and safe foods. At the subnational level, low resource levels can similarly affect food availability, roads, and markets. At the household and individual levels, poverty can prevent adequate access to food and can lead to poor food choices and unhealthy diets. Poverty at the household or individual level can also affect other determinants of food utilization, such as sanitation and health care. Within a given country, poverty can affect food security at one level but not at another, such as when poor households experience food insecurity in countries that have adequate food availability at the national level, or conversely when food-secure households and well-nourished individuals exist in countries with low food availability.

Given the central role that poverty plays in threatening food security, long-term solutions to reducing food insecurity invariably involve poverty reduction. For example, eradicating extreme poverty and hunger are combined into a single Millennium Development Goal; and decreases in country poverty rates is one of the two highest-level indicators of Feed the Future (Feed the Future 2013). However, reducing poverty does not necessarily improve food utilization; for example, the "silent hunger" of micronutrient undernutrition can persist even in affluent households (von Braun et al. 1989, Herforth et al. 2012).

While poverty is a major source of chronic food insecurity, *conflict* can cause periods of acute food insecurity. There are several channels by which conflict affects food security. It can dramatically reduce food production—and threaten food availability—through destruction of land or inputs, removal of agricultural labor due to combat, or safety and security concerns that inhibit cultivation. Conflict can also destroy food stocks, either through deliberate military action or as an unintentional casualty. It can disrupt transportation and communication, preventing communities from accessing food markets or preventing markets from generating income with which to purchase food. More broadly, conflict can drastically reduce livelihood opportunities, negatively affecting the functioning of markets and/or the ability to purchase food. In some conflicts, certain populations are deliberately prevented from accessing food for political or military reasons. The 1984–1985 famine in Ethiopia is a well-known example of this, with the foreign minister explicitly stating, "Food is a major element of our strategy against the secessionists" (De Waal 1997, Marcus 2003).

The impact of conflict on food security does not end when the conflict ends. In post conflict settings, many of the same factors such as lost food stocks and destroyed land persist, as well as issues specific to post conflict periods; such as land disputes arising from the return of internally displaced people, changes in the availability of arable land, or reintegration of soldiers into communities and households.

The relationship between conflict and food insecurity can be bidirectional. In addition to the negative impacts conflict has on food security, food insecurity itself can contribute to civil unrest, revolt against the government, or conflict between competing groups for food, water, land, and other resources (Messer et al. 2001, Messer and Cohen 2006, Bora et al. 2011). Examples from the 1970s include famines in Upper Volta and Niger that contributed to coups there and food shortages in Ethiopia that helped to incite revolt against the government (Messer et al. 2001). More recent examples include cases in which factors underlying food insecurity have contributed to conflict, such as the finding by Miguel et al. (2004) in several African countries that rainfall shocks significantly increase the likelihood of civil war.

Natural disasters such as droughts, floods, and earthquakes can impede all four dimensions of food security. Food availability is directly affected when droughts or floods lead to lower production of food. By reducing livelihood opportunities and income, destroying or forcing the sale of productive assets, and reducing own production of food, natural disasters diminish household access to food. Disasters negatively affect food utilization through several channels: poor sanitation following floods and earthquakes and in internally displaced person camps; illness and infections that may be prevalent in camps and reduced access to health care services due to the disasters; consumption of less diverse or nutritious foods due to reduced food access; and poorer infant and young child care and feeding practices when parents, especially mothers, are killed or injured by the disaster. Natural disasters are a source of poor food stability; when they affect food availability, access, or utilization through the channels described above, the stability of food security is disrupted.

In recent years, increasing attention has been paid to the impacts of *environmental degradation* on food security, particularly degradation caused by climate change. Climate change can threaten food availability when changes in temperature, rainfall, or the growing season reduce crop production. These changes can have wider impacts than just the directly affected crops through effects on food prices and markets (Gregory et al. 2005). The impact of climate change on food security varies across geographic regions, depending on biophysical factors and national and local capacity to adapt to changes (Gregory et al. 2005).

Efforts to identify and quantify the impact of climate change on food security often rely on projections or simulations because the magnitude of climate change is expected to increase in coming years. Pointing out that most simulations have focused on food availability, Schmidhuber and Tubiello identify how climate change affects all four dimensions: food availability through agro-ecological changes that influence agricultural production; food access through slower income growth from agriculture, especially in sub-Saharan Africa, and possibly increased food prices; food utilization through increases in water and food-borne diseases due to higher temperatures and increased incidence of extreme rainfall events; and stability through greater climate fluctuations and more frequent extreme weather events such as droughts and floods (Schmidhuber and Tubiello 2007).

In addition to climate change, other sources and types of environmental degradation can also negatively impact food security, such as falling water tables (Rosegrant et al. 2002) and soil degradation (Scherr 1999). Studies have indicated that changes in ozone concentrations can also pose a threat to food production (Morgan et al. 2006, Rai et al. 2010). Conversely, food security needs can lead to environmental degradation in some contexts. The clearing of primary forest land using slash and burn methods by forest dwellers in order to secure food is a well-known example (Freudenberger and Freudenberger 2002).

Adaptation by farmers to climate change and other forms of environmental degradation can help to reduce the impact on food security. For example, a study in Ethiopia found that adaptations such as changing crop varieties, soil and water conservation, and tree planting by farmers increased productivity of food crops. Farmers with access to credit, agricultural extension services, and other information were most likely to adapt to climate change (Di Falco et al. 2011).

Food price increases, especially rapid spikes in food prices such as occurred in 2007–2008, can significantly threaten food security. While some farmers producing food can benefit from the higher incomes generated by higher food prices, price increases can have grave effects on food security for net purchasers of food. Poor urban populations, in particular, are severely affected by food price spikes because food purchases are a significant portion of their expenditures and they often depend primarily or entirely on cash food purchases in markets, as opposed to their own production (Cohen and Garrett 2010, Ruel et al. 2010). However, members of the rural poor, especially the landless and other net purchasers of food, can also be vulnerable to food insecurity as a result of food price increases (Ruel et al. 2010).

These effects operate largely through the dimension of food access, with increased prices leading to poorer access to food for a given income and resources available to households. As households respond to the poorer access by reducing the quantity and diversity of food consumed, food utilization is also affected; evidence suggests the 2007–2008 food price increase led to lower quantity, frequency, and diversity of food consumption in several countries (Brinkman et al. 2010). Policy responses to food price spikes—and to drops in food prices—play a key role in the food security impacts of these price changes (Webb 2010).

In the context of threats to food security, it is worth noting here that *disease* threatens food security through various pathways. Chapter 2 provides an in-depth analysis of the conceptual framework that defines the relationship between food security and health and disease. Most directly, in many contexts, disease impairs nutritional status, especially for infants and young children, HIV-infected individuals, and other populations vulnerable to malnutrition.

In addition to its effect on food utilization, disease can threaten food security through food access and stability, and in rare cases of widespread disease, through availability as well. By decreasing available household labor—due to physical impairment (or death) of a household member, or due to increased caregiving responsibilities of other productive members—disease can reduce household income available for food purchases. Prolonged periods of lost income from disease, such as HIV, can lead households to deplete assets, including productive assets, in order to meet basic needs, thereby limiting long-term livelihood prospects (Barnett and Rugalema 2001, De Waal and Whiteside 2003). The cost of health care thereby competes with food for scarce household resources. In addition, intergenerational transfer of knowledge and skills is lost to adult illness or death (De Waal and Whiteside 2003). Furthermore, when diseases such as HIV affect many members of a community, it can weaken community and social safety nets that would otherwise be able to support households experiencing food shortfalls. In discussing the impacts of HIV in Malawi, Mtika (2001) refers to weakened "social immunity" to describe how erosion of social capital compromises food security.

Because of HIV's pervasiveness in certain areas of east and southern Africa, and because of its impact on working-age adults and on household food security, the relationship between the disease and food security has been well studied. This relationship can be bidirectional, such as when food insecurity leads to coping strategies that increase risk of infection (Weiser et al. 2007, 2011, Miller et al. 2011). Other diseases such as tuberculosis and malaria can also threaten household food security for reasons similar to those mentioned above, though the wider impacts on community support systems may be less for these diseases than it is for HIV.

Knowledge and appropriate practices can contribute to food security, and conversely poor *knowledge and practices* can threaten food security. Care and feeding practices are a critical factor in child nutrition, and poor care and feeding practices can contribute to chronic malnutrition among children. For example, Ruel and Menon (2002) offer evidence of this from Latin America; Baig-Ansari et al. (2006) analyze evidence from Pakistan; and Ruel et al. (1998) review evidence from urban settings. Gaps in agricultural knowledge and practices can threaten food availability and access by constraining food production. Lack of knowledge about storage technologies contributes to food waste, negatively affecting both food availability and stability (Godfray et al. 2010).

Extending knowledge and practices to the national level, effective *policies* can strengthen food security, but poor—or deliberately harmful—policies can threaten food security. As mentioned in the discussion of conflict, one type of policy that threatens food security is a government policy that deliberately or negligently prevents food from reaching a group of its citizens, such as the grain quotas instituted by the Soviet Union that led to famine in the Ukraine in 1932 (Marcus 2003). Other policies, such as land reform policies in Zimbabwe, did not aim to inhibit food access for the country's population, but significantly worsened food security throughout the country (Clover 2003).

Some analysts point out that international trade agreements, such as the WTO Agreement on Agriculture provisions on agriculture subsidies, have favored agricultural production in developed countries over developing countries, negatively impacting food security in developing countries (Gonzalez 2002, Clover 2003). Given the important role that women play in agriculture and household food security, insufficient policies—as well as legal and social institutions—to support women farmers are cited as contributing factors in food insecurity in southern Africa (Quisumbing 2000, Gawaya 2008). More broadly, Clover (2003) points to insufficient public investment in agriculture as a factor in food insecurity in Africa, though such investment will likely increase through the Comprehensive Africa Agriculture Development Programme (CAADP) process led by the New Partnership for Africa's Development (NEPAD), and through increased focus on agricultural development by donors such as the World Bank and the U.S. Government's Feed the Future initiative.

FOOD SECURITY PROGRAMS AND INTEGRATION

FOOD SECURITY PROGRAM APPROACHES

Given the complex, multidimensional, and often context-specific nature of food security, programs apply a wide range of approaches to address food insecurity. Table 1.1 summarizes approaches commonly used to address each dimension of food insecurity.

As reflected in the table, program approaches to address food insecurity focus on different objectives, depending on what dimension and domain are prioritized. Accordingly, while some programmatic actions, such as income generation or gender empowerment, cut across domains, there may be considerable variation in how

TABLE 1.1
Program Approaches to Address Food Insecurity

Dimension	Domain of Intervention	Objective	Programmatic Actions
Availability	Food imports	Supplement national food availability	Maintain terms of trade in international markets, food aid
	National food production	Support agricultural research and extension	Technological intensification, agriculture extension interventions
		Expand internal markets	Develop national value chains, market infrastructure
Access	Household incomes	Increase opportunities for income generation	Microcredit, enterprise development, skills and capacity building, women's empowerment, participation in value chain
		Control the impact of food prices on consumers	
			Subsidies, vouchers
	Household food production	Increase food production	Agriculture extension for technological intensification; reduce postharvest losses, empowerment of women in agriculture
		Expand other sources of household food	
			Conditional, nonconditional food assistance
Utilization	Malnutrition prevention	Prevent macro/ micronutrient malnutrition	Food supplementation, fortification, dietary diversification, health care, hygiene services, PM2A
	Malnutrition treatment	Treat acute malnutrition	CMAM[a], NACS[b]
		Treat chronic malnutrition	Targeted recuperation programs, NACS
Stability	Risk management	Reduce likelihoods of shocks	Environmental protection, peacekeeping
		Reduce vulnerability to shocks	Social/economic structures, income generation
	Coping ability	Build and consolidate assets	Savings programs, social networking, environmental protection actions

[a] CMAM: Community-Based Management of Acute Malnutrition (Deconinck et al. 2008).
[b] NACS: Nutrition Assessment, Counseling and Support (FANTA 2012).

food security is concretely pursued, depending on the dimension and objectives at stake. It is an arena where the dictum "Think globally, act sectorally" (World Bank 2013) applies with particular force.

Food security programs are often designed to address a particular dimension, or even one component of a dimension. For example, programs aimed at addressing chronic malnutrition among infants and young children, such as USAID's Preventing Malnutrition in Children under Two Years of Age (PM2A) program, are designed to address the dimension of food utilization (FANTA-2 2010). Access to food is a determinant of chronic malnutrition among the program's target population, and program design therefore considers access issues. But activities are not designed to improve household food access, although it would be natural and feasible, if resources are available, to add such a component to PM2A programs. Similarly, programs aimed at acute malnutrition, micronutrient malnutrition, maternal and child health, and water and sanitation, also focus on utilization. Other programs, such as those supported by the World Food Program (WFP), aim to improve household access to food by providing household food rations, or in some cases, by strengthening livelihoods. Such programs may positively influence food utilization because of improved access, but may not produce measurable impacts on nutrition outcomes because they focus on increasing incomes or food production capacity and not on other components of utilization like health, sanitation, and feeding practices.

In some cases, programs do aim to directly improve multiple dimensions of food security through integrated programming. For example, some USAID Title II food aid programs address maternal and child health and nutrition, as well as household food access through multiple activities occurring in the same geographic area.

Types of Program Integration

Because of the range of approaches, sectors, and types of services entailed in food security programs, food security efforts often integrate program services. Program integration refers to linking different services together. In their examination of integrated health interventions, Atun et al. (2010) point out that "there is no commonly accepted definition of 'integration.'" Indeed, the term is used to describe a wide range of intensities of integration. Different intensities of integration are appropriate depending on the context, the interventions, and the needs of program participants.

In the context of food security, the lightest intensity of integration involves sharing information about the availability of other services, such as when providers of child nutrition services inform clients about livelihood strengthening services or other programs that help strengthen household food access. The next level of integration involves active referral systems between different food security services. An example would be if the child nutrition and livelihood strengthening services each screen clients for potential eligibility for the other service and provide referrals to clients accordingly. A further level of integration involves coordinating between distinct services for planning, targeting, supervision, and/or monitoring.

More intensive integration entails coordinated *delivery* of services or commodities, such that multiple types of services are planned and delivered as part of a package. The next, and perhaps final, level of integration entails joint delivery of services at the same delivery point and time. Following the earlier example, this could involve providing education about infant and young child feeding and other nutrition services as part of women's microfinance groups that strengthen household food access. Leatherman et al. (2011), Hamad et al. (2011), and Smith (2002) all study examples of integrating health education into women's microfinance groups. Harris and Drimie (2012) present a useful graphic depiction of the various intensities of coordination among sectoral services and reserve the term "integration" for only the most intensive stage of integrated services.

In addition to the various intensities of integration, there are also various sets of domains across which program integration can occur. In the context of food security, program integration occurs across three different (though related) sets of domains.

The first set of domains is the four dimensions of food security. As Table 1.1 illustrates, program services aimed at addressing one dimension of food insecurity are often quite distinct from services aimed at addressing another dimension. Given that populations often experience deprivations in multiple dimensions of food security at the same time and given the sequential conditionality among the dimensions described earlier, some food security programs take a comprehensive approach by addressing multiple dimensions. For example, some Feed the Future country programs link agricultural production interventions with nutrition services and education interventions to improve dietary diversity.

Sectors are the second set of domains for program integration; the multidimensionality of food security calls for multisectoral programming in some settings. The most relevant sectors for food security are agriculture, health, microenterprise, microfinance, humanitarian assistance, and water and sanitation. Social protection, which in some contexts is considered a sector, is also closely related to food security. Multisectoral programming involves integrating services from different sectors together in the same geographic area, usually managed by the same implementing agency, which may be a government or private organization. Multisectoral programming may involve delivering the services to the same populations at the same delivery points, or may just involve coordination between the services. USAID Title II food security programs often employ multisectoral approaches, such as maternal and child health and nutrition (MCHN) services (targeting food utilization) operating together with agriculture services (targeting food access). The Millennium Villages Project operating in several African countries is an example of a program that is highly multisectoral, with coordinated interventions—several of which are designed to address food security—across a wide range of sectors including agriculture, maternal and child health and nutrition, education, and microfinance.

In considering how sectoral programs influence food security, it is worth noting that in many cases there is significant scope for sectoral programs to address food security even if it is not the program's primary objective. For example, Ruel and Alderman (2013) point to the potential that agriculture, social safety nets, early child development, and education have to be "nutrition-sensitive." While nutrition is generally not the main objective of programs in these sectors, considering the pathways to nutrition outcomes in the program design can help generate positive nutrition impacts.

A third, related type of integration involves incorporating specific food security services into a larger sectoral program. This type of integration is particularly relevant to the health sector because health programs are often the platform into which nutrition services are incorporated. For example, nutrition assessment, counseling and support (NACS), supported by the U.S. Government's President's Emergency Plan for AIDS Relief (PEPFAR) in several countries, incorporate a set of nutrition care services into the larger health system, often as part of HIV care services (FANTA 2012). In some cases, food access services are incorporated into a health program. The program described in Chapter 10 includes interventions to improve access to food as part of clinic-based services.

While this discussion of integration has focused on programs with specific activities that target households or clients, it is important to recognize that some of the sectors and players that most powerfully affect food security are not involved in the delivery of conventional food security programs. For example, food markets and prices affect food availability and access; private sector behavior and investments influence employment and livelihood opportunities, which in turn affect food access; and as discussed above, political and military actors in conflict can influence all dimensions of food security. In general, the relationship between food security programs and these forces has been less about integration and more about considering these characteristics of the environment in program design, and, where possible, leveraging actions by broader sets of stakeholders to promote food security and advance program objectives. This relationship is evolving, and some elements of the food industry are becoming more directly involved in food security efforts, both through philanthropic initiatives and through integration of food security concerns into their business strategies and orientations.

BENEFITS, CHALLENGES, AND CONSIDERATIONS OF PROGRAM INTEGRATION

Effective integration of food security programs can result in a number of benefits. The primary benefit stems from the primary rationale for integration: since food-insecure populations often experience deprivations in multiple dimensions of food security, integrated programming can help ensure that all of the deprivations are addressed. Integrated programming can also more effectively address long-term, underlying sources of food insecurity. To use a simple example, managing individuals' malnutrition while also strengthening household food access may be more sustainable than addressing malnutrition in isolation. Similarly, meeting immediate food access needs without reducing longer-term instability of access will not be as sustainable as an integrated program that addresses both access and stability.

Integrated programming can also yield efficiencies in targeting, management, supervision, and monitoring by reducing the need for parallel systems that exist in separate, stand-alone programs. Another benefit of integrated programming is that it offers opportunities for information sharing and learning across program areas. For example, nutrition service providers who learn from clients about specific household constraints affecting their diets can advise program staff managing food access components of the program. This currently occurs in Guatemala (Woldt and Bergeron 2013). Similarly, awareness of the agricultural products supported by a program's agriculture component can enhance nutrition education and counseling by focusing on the use of these products.

While integration of food security services often makes sense in principle, in practice integrated programs often face operational challenges. The different sectors and dimensions of food security are often addressed by different stakeholders with divergent orientations. For example, stakeholders addressing food availability may be agronomists focused on agricultural production; those addressing food access may be economists focused on employment and income generation; and those addressing food utilization may be nutritionists who approach the program with a medical or public health perspective. Forging a cohesive program from these varied orientations can be challenging, and in some contexts may not be the best approach.

Coordination can be time and resource intensive. Program implementers for specific areas or sectors can have specialized skills for specialized functions, and in some situations too great a focus on integration can risk compromising quality. In particular, frontline workers are often already stretched in many directions; requiring community health workers to learn and engage with their communities about nutrition is itself often a challenge, and introducing agricultural functions may be unrealistic in many situations.

Another challenge of integration is the different levels at which the dimensions of food security are addressed. Programs aimed at improving food availability often operate at the national or subnational level, strengthening agricultural production, trade, markets, and value chains. Programs aimed at improving food access often target households with livelihood strengthening and other interventions. Programs targeting food utilization focus on individuals, though interventions can be targeted to households as well. These different levels can complicate efforts to integrate programs across dimensions of food security, though it can also offer opportunities for well-designed programs to address different levels simultaneously.

Even within organizations, program imperatives may vary across levels of management. In Feed the Future programs, for instance, top-level management may be chiefly concerned with avoiding a repeat of the 2008 food crisis, while field implementers are mandated to improve the food access and nutrition of producer households. While these goals are not necessarily at odds, they imply tensions in how resource allocation is prioritized.

Given the challenges that program integration can face, the different intensities of integration, and the different domains across which integration can occur, there are a number of factors that program designers and implementers can consider in deciding whether and how to integrate program services:

- *Objectives of the program.* Programs with broad objectives, such as reducing multiple types of food insecurity or sustainably addressing the underlying factors of food insecurity for a population, may be more inclined to integrate across sectors or across types of food security services than programs with narrower objectives. For programs with broader objectives, the benefits of a more comprehensive program may be worth the costs and challenges of integration. On the other hand, programs designed to narrowly address a specific component of one dimension of food security, such as a fortification program to address micronutrient deficiencies, may find it more efficient to avoid extensive integration.
- *Sources of food insecurity in program areas.* The sources of food insecurity drive the types of activities that a program implements, and therefore determine the options and opportunities for integration. If a program identifies factors that negatively affect the food security of its participants, but it is not addressing these factors, it may consider integrating with other services that do address these factors if such services exist. If a primary source of food insecurity cannot be addressed by services, as in the case of conflict, then integration may be of more limited utility, at

least insofar as addressing the source of food insecurity. Understanding the factors contributing to food insecurity enables program teams to assess whether and what sort of integration will help achieve program objectives.

- *Existing services in the program areas.* While in some cases it is possible to initiate and incorporate services from another sector into a program "from scratch," more often integration involves linking services that already exist. Therefore, which services exist in a program's geographic area is clearly a central factor in determining what type of integration is possible.

- *Demand and interest from program participants and community members.* As with any aspect of a program, integrated services will be more effective if there is demand from participants for the services being integrated. In the case of integration, an added consideration is whether participants prefer services to be delivered in an integrated fashion, or separately. Delivering services together may save transportation and other transaction costs for participants. On the other hand, in cases where different household members access the different services, or in contexts where stigma is present, such as among HIV clients in some settings, participants may prefer services not to be closely integrated.

- *Stakeholders involved in program services and their compatibility.* Since integration requires coordination and communication among the institutions and stakeholders that provide the various services, the compatibility of these actors should be considered in integration decisions. In cases where organizational orientations significantly diverge or where there is a history of competition or strained relations, integration may be less successful than in cases where the groups have similar values and priorities or have a history of collaboration. See Garrett and Natalicchio (2011) for more details on this issue.

- *Available resources.* Integration can require additional resources to manage coordination, establish referral mechanisms, or expand service delivery points to house additional services. Consideration of available financial and human resources—as well as the relative value of competing priorities for these resources—can inform decisions about whether, and to what extent, to integrate services.

Some program leaders may determine that it is most efficient and effective not to integrate a program with other services. This may be decided for a variety of reasons, such as limited management capacity to handle the necessary coordination, challenging relations with institutions operating other services, prioritization of the efficiencies of specialization over broadening of services, or a desire to protect frontline workers from additional responsibilities. For example, some agricultural extension programs focused on improving productivity in a targeted area are not integrated with other food security services (though other extension programs may find it beneficial to integrate with livelihood or nutrition services).

In some cases, program managers choose not to integrate with other food security services but to integrate their services into a larger sectoral set of services. This is the case for management of acute malnutrition services, which are often integrated into the larger health system but not necessarily with other food security services.

The example of management of acute malnutrition points to the relevance for health programs of integrating food security services. Health programs that include nutrition components are, in a sense, already integrating a type of food security service (nutrition) into a broader health program. Managers of such programs may also consider whether there is value in integrating with other food security services, especially if these services address food security constraints that underlie health or nutrition problems faced by the health program's clients. Such integration may range from light linkages and referrals to more intensive joint service delivery.

Decisions about whether and to what extent to integrate health programs with food access services depend on some of the benefits and challenges discussed above. Integrated approaches can more comprehensively address health and nutrition problems. At the same time, consideration should be given to the physical and human resource capacity of the health facilities or community structures involved, including the workload of health care workers. Where capacity may be overstretched, lighter linkages to existing services may be more feasible. The AMPATH program described in Chapter 10 is an example of a health program that has integrated food access services directly into its program.

CONCLUSION

This chapter has provided an overview of food security, related concepts, threats to food security, and program responses with an emphasis on integration of services. As the diagram of determinants of food security and the discussion of threats both indicate, food security is closely bound up with several other critical elements of social and economic development, including health, sanitation, income poverty, conflict and security, women's empowerment, and technology. The close links between food security and other components and outcomes of development lend support to the idea articulated by the FAO Director-General in the opening quotation—that food security can serve as a common thread linking various development objectives and can thereby play a central role in sustainable development.

As the remaining chapters of this book elucidate, food security has particular relevance to programs and services that aim to improve health conditions. The bidirectional relationship between health and food security, described in greater detail in the next chapter, highlights the importance of supporting health care managers and service providers to understand client populations' food security situation.

REFERENCES

Atun, R., T. De Jongh, F. Secci, K. Ohiri, and O. Adeyi. 2010. Integration of targeted health interventions into health systems: A conceptual framework for analysis. *Health Policy Planning* 25 (2):104–111.

Baig-Ansari, N., M. H. Rahbar, Z. A. Bhutta, and S. H. Badruddin. 2006. Child's gender and household food insecurity are associated with stunting among young Pakistani children residing in urban squatter settlements. *Food and Nutrition Bulletin* 27:114–127.

Barnett, T. and G. Rugalema. 2001. HIV/AIDS: A critical health and development issue. In *The Unfinished Agenda: Perspectives on Overcoming Hunger, Poverty, and Environmental Degradation*, 43–47. Washington, DC: International Food Policy Research Institute.

Beauregard, S. and R. Gottlieb. 2009. Food policy for people: Incorporating food sovereignty principles into State governance. In *Senior Comprehensive Report*. Occidental College, Los Angeles: Urban and Environmental Policy Institute.

Benson, T. 2004. *Assessing Africa's Food Nutrition Security Situation: 2020 Africa Conference Brief I*. International Food Policy Research Institute Conference, Washington, DC.

Beuchelt, T. D. and D. Virchow. 2012. Food sovereignty or the human right to adequate food: Which concept serves better as international development policy for global hunger and poverty reduction? *Agricultural and Human Values* 29 (2):259–273.

Black, R. E., C. G. Victora, S. P. Walker, Z. A. Bhutta, P. Christian, M. de Onis, and R. Martorell. 2013. Maternal and child undernutrition and overweight in low-income and middle-income countries. *Lancet* 382 (9890):427–451.

Bora, S., I. Ceccacci, C. Delgado, and R. Townsend. 2011. *Food Security and Conflict, World Development Report 2011*. World Bank. Washington, DC.

Brinkman, H. J., S. De Pee, I. Sanago, L. Subran, and M. W. Bloem. 2010. High food prices and the global financial crisis have reduced access to nutritious food and worsened nutritional status and health. *Journal of Nutrition* 140:153S–161S.

Clover, J. 2003. Food security in Sub-Saharan Africa. *African Security Review* 12 (1):5–15.

Cohen, M. J. and J. L. Garrett. 2010. The food price crisis and urban food (In) security. *Environment and Urbanization* 22 (2):467–482.

Committee on World Food Security. 2012. Coming to terms with terminology.

De Waal, A. 1997. *Famine Crimes: Politics and the Disaster Relief Industry in Africa*. Bloomington, IN: Indiana University Press.

De Waal, A. and A. Whiteside. 2003. New variant famine: AIDS and food crisis in southern Africa. *Lancet* 362 (9391):1234–1237.

Deconinck, H., A. Swindale, F. Grant, and C. Navarro-Colorado. 2008. Review of Community-based Management of Acute Malnutrition (CMAM) in the Post-Emergency Context: Synthesis of Lessons on Integration of CMAM into National Health Systems. Ethiopia, Malawi and Niger, April–June 2007. Washington, DC: FANTA, FHI 360.

Department for International Development. 2011. Defining Disaster Resilience: A DFID Approach Paper.

Di Falco, S., M. Veronesi, and M. Yesuf. 2011. Di & Does adaptation to climate change provide food security? A micro-perspective from Ethiopia. *American Journal of Agricultural Economics* 93 (3):829–846.

FANTA-2. 2010. TRM-01: Preventing Malnutrition in Children Under 2 Approach (PM2A): A Food-Assisted Approach. [Title II Technical Reference Materials]. Food and Nutrition Technical Assistance II Project (FANTA-2)/FHI 360. Accessed September 3, 2014. http://www.fantaproject.org/sites/default/files/resources/TRM_PM2A_RevisedNov2010_ENGLISH.pdf.

FANTA. 2012. Defining Nutrition Assessment, Counseling, and Support (NACS). [Technical Note No. 13]. FHI 360/FANTA. Accessed September 3, 2014. http://www.fhi360.org/sites/default/files/media/documents/FANTA-NACS-TechNote-Jul2012.pdf.

Feed the Future. 2013. Feed the Future Progress Scorecard. Accessed September 3, 2014. http://feedthefuture.gov/resource/feed-future-progress-scorecard-2013.

Food and Agriculture Organization. 1996. *Rome Declaration on World Food Security, World Food Summit*. Food and Agriculture Organization, Rome. http://www.fao.org/docrep/003/w3613e/w3613e00.HTM

Freudenberger, M. S. and K. S. Freudenberger. 2002. Contradictions in agricultural intensifica-
tion and improved natural resource management: Issues in the Fianarantsoa Forest Corridor
of Madagascar. *In* C.B. Barret and A.A. Aboud (eds.) *Natural Resource Management in
African Agriculture Understanding and Improving Current Practices* 181–192.

Garrett, J. and M. Natalicchio. 2011. *Working Multisectorally in Nutrition: Principles,
Practices, and Case Studies.* doi:http://dx.doi.org/10.2499/9780896291812.

Gawaya, R. 2008. Investing in women farmers to eliminate food insecurity in southern Africa:
Policy-related research from Mozambique. *Gender Development* 16 (1):147–159.

Godfray, H. C. J., J. R. Beddington, I. R. Crute, L. Haddad, D. Lawrence, J. F. Muir, and C.
Toulmin. 2010. Food security: The challenge of feeding 9 billion people. *Science* 327
(5967):812–818.

Gonzalez, C. G. 2002. Institutionalizing inequality: The WTO agreement on agriculture, food,
security, and developing countries. *Columbia Journal of Environmental Law* 27:433–489.

Gregory, P. J., J. S. I. Ingram, and M. Brklacich. 2005. Climate change and food security.
*Philosophical Transactions of the Royal Society of London. Series B, Biological
Sciences* 360 (1463):2139–2148.

Hamad, R., L. C. Fernald, and D. S. Karlan. 2011. Health education for microcredit clients in
Peru, a randomized controlled trial. *BMC Public Health* 11 (51):1–10.

Harris, J. and S. Drimie. 2012. Toward an integrated approach for addressing malnutrition
in Zambia: A literature review and institutional analysis. International Food Policy
Research Institute. Accessed September 3, 2014. http://www.ifpri.org/sites/default/files/
publications/ifpridp01200.pdf.

Herforth, A., A. Jones, and P. Pinstrup-Andersen. 2012. *Prioritizing Nutrition in Agriculture and
Rural Development: Guiding Principles for Operational Investments.* Washington, DC:
The World Bank.

Holben, D. H. 2005. The concept and definition of hunger and its relationship to food insecurity. Washington, DC: National Academies of Science.

Holt-Giménez, E. 2009. From food crisis to food sovereignty. *Monthly Review* 61 (3):142–156.

Kerr, W. A. 2011. Food sovereignty: Old protectionism in somewhat recycled bottles. *ATDF
Journal* 8: 1–2.

Leatherman, S., M. Metcalfe, K. Geissler, and C. Dunford. 2011. Integrating microfinance and
health strategies: Examining the evidence to inform policy and practice. *Health Policy
Planning* 201 (1):1–17.

Marcus, D. 2003. Famine crimes in international law. *American Journal of International Law*
97 (2 SRC - GoogleScholar):245–281.

Messer, E. and M. J. Cohen. 2006. Conflict, Food Security, and Globalization. [FCND
Discussion Paper 206]. International Food Policy Research Institute. Accessed
September 3, 2014. http://www.ifpri.org/sites/default/files/publications/fcndp206.pdf.

Messer, E., M. J. Cohen, and T. Marchione. 2001. Conflict: A cause and effect of hunger. In
Environmental Change and Security Program Report 7. http://www.wilsoncenter.org/
publication/conflict-cause-and-effect-hunger (accessed September 3, 2014).

Miguel, E., S. Satyanath, and E. Sergenti. 2004. Economic shocks and civil conflict: An instrumental variables approach. *Journal of Political Economy* 112 (4 SRC - GoogleScholar):
725–753.

Miller, C. L., D. R. Bangsberg, D. M. Tuller, J. Senkungu, A. Kawuma, E. A. Frongillo, and
S. D. Weiser. 2011. Food insecurity and sexual risk in an HIV endemic community in
Uganda. *AIDS and Behavior* 15 (7):1512–1519.

Morgan, P. B., T. A. Mies, G. A. Bollero, R. L. Nelson, and S. P. Long. 2006. Season-long
elevation of ozone concentration to projected 2050 levels under fully open-air conditions substantially decreases the growth and production of soybean. *New Phytologist*
170 (2):333–343.

Mtika, M. M. 2001. The AIDS epidemic in Malawi and its threat to household food security. *Human Organization* 60 (2):178–188.

Pingali, P., L. Alinovi, and J. Sutton. 2005. Food security in complex emergencies: Enhancing food system resilience. *Disasters* 29 (Suppl 1):S5–24.

Pinstrup-Andersen, P. 2009. Food security: Definition and measurement. *Food Security* 1 (1):5–7. doi: 10.1007/s12571-008-0002-y.

Quisumbing, A. 2000. Women: The Key to Food Security. International Food Policy Research Institute. Accessed September 3, 2014. http://www.ifpri.org/sites/default/files/pubs/pubs/ib/ib3.pdf.

Rai, R., M. Argrawal, and S. B. Argrawal. 2010. Threat to food security under current levels of ground level ozone: A case study for Indian cultivars of rice. *Atmospheric Environment* 44 (34):4272–4282.

Riely, F., N. Mock, B. Cogill, L. Bailey, and E. Kenefick. 1999. *Food Security Indicators and Framework for Use in the Monitoring and Evaluation of Food Aid Programs*. Arlington, VA: Food Security and Nutrition Monitoring Project (IMPACT), ISTI, Inc.

Rosegrant, M. W., X. Cai, and S. A. Cline. 2002. Global Water Outlook to 2025: Averting an Impending Crisis. International Food Policy Research Institute. Accessed September 3, 2014. http://www.ifpri.org/sites/default/files/pubs/pubs/fpr/fprwater2025.pdf.

Ruel, M. T. and H. Alderman. 2013. Nutrition-sensitive interventions and programmes: How can they help to accelerate progress in improving maternal and child nutrition? *Lancet* 382 (9891):536–551.

Ruel, M. T., J. L. Garrett, C. Hawkes, and M. J. Cohen. 2010. The food, fuel, and financial crisis affect the urban and rural poor disproportionately: A review of evidence. *Journal of Nutrition* 140:170S–176S.

Ruel, M. T., J. L. Garrett, S. S. Morris, D. G. Maxwell, A. Oshaug, P. L. Engle, and L. J. Haddad. 1998. Urban challenges to food and nutrition security: A review of food security, health, and caregiving in the cities. International Food Policy Research Institute. Accessed September 3, 2014. http://www.ifpri.org/publication/urban-challenges-food-and-nutrition-security.

Ruel, M. T. and P. Menon. 2002. Child feeding practices are associated with child nutritional status in Latin America: Innovative uses of the demographic and health surveys. *Journal of Nutrition* 132 (6):1180–1187.

Scaling Up Nutrition. 2010. Scaling up nutrition movement. *Scaling Up Nutrition Road Map* 1.

Scherr, S. J. 1999. *Soil Degradation: A Threat to Developing-Country Food Security by 2010?* [Food, Agriculture, and Environment Discussion Paper No. 27]. International Food Policy Research Institute.

Schmidhuber, J. and F. N. Tubiello. 2007. Global food security under climate change. *Proceedings of the National Academy of Sciences of the United States of America* 104 (50):19703–19708.

Smith, S. 2002. Village banking and maternal and child health: Evidence from Ecuador and Honduras. *World Development* 30 (4):707–723.

UNICEF. 1990. *Strategy for Improved Nutrition of Children and Women in Developing Countries*. New York: UNICEF.

Via Campesina. 1996. Tlaxcala Declaration of the Via Campesina (Declaration of the Second International Conference of Via Campesina, Tlaxcala, Mexico).

van Haeften, R., M. A. Anderson, H. Caudill, and E. Kilmartin. 2013. *Second Food Aid and Food Security Assessment (FAFSA-2)*. Washington, DC: FHI 360/FANTA.

von Braun, J., D. Hotchkiss, and M. Imminck. 1989. Nontraditional Export Crops in Guatemala: Effects on Production, Income, and Nutrition. [Research Report]. International Food Policy Research Institute. Accessed September 3, 2014. http://www.ifpri.org/sites/default/files/pubs/pubs/abstract/73/rr73.pdf.

von Braun, J., M.S. Swaminathan, M. W. Rosegrant, M. M. Santiago, L. J. Stone, J. Church, and J. Piaget. 2006. *Repositioning nutrition as central to development: A strategy for large scale action. Directions in Development.* Washington, DC: World Bank.

Webb, P. 2010. Medium- to long-run implications of high food prices for global nutrition. *Journal of Nutrition* 140 (1):143S–147S.

Webb, P. and B. Rogers. 2003. Addressing the "In" in Food Insecurity. Food and Nutrition Technical Assistance Project, Academy for Educational Development.

Weiser, S. D., K. Leiter, D. R. Bangsberg, L. M. Butler, F. Percy-de Korte, Z. Hlanze, and M. Heisler. 2007. Food insufficiency is associated with high-risk sexual behavior among women in Botswana and Swaziland. *PLOS Medicine* 4 (10):1589–1597; discussion 1598. doi: 10.1371/journal.pmed.0040260.

Weiser, S. D., S. L. Young, C. R. Cohen, M. B. Kushel, A. C. Tsai, P. C. Tien, and D. R. Bangsberg. 2011. Conceptual framework for understanding the bidirectional links between food insecurity and HIV/AIDS. *American Journal of Clinical Nutrition* 94 (6): 1729S–1739S.

Wittman, H., A. Desmarais, and N. Wiebe. 2010. The origins and potential of food sovereignty. In H. Wittman (ed.) *Food Sovereignty: Reconnecting Food, Nature and Community,* 1–14. Halifax: Fernwood Publishers.

Woldt, M. and G. Bergeron. 2013. Title. http://blog.usaid.gov/2013/09/optifood-to-improve-diets-and-prevent-child-malnutrition-in-guatemala/.

World Bank. 2013. Improving Nutrition through Multisectoral Approaches. [Social Protection Brief 75105]. World Bank. Accessed September 3, 2014. http://www-wds.worldbank.org/external/default/WDSContentServer/WDSP/IB/2013/02/05/000333037_20130205111223/Rendered/PDF/751050BRI0Impr00Box374299B00PUBLIC0.pdf.

2 Food Insecurity and Health

A Conceptual Framework

*Sheri D. Weiser, Kartika Palar, Abigail M. Hatcher,
Sera Young, Edward A. Frongillo, and
Barbara Laraia*

CONTENTS

INTRODUCTION

Food insecurity is a leading cause of morbidity and mortality worldwide. Food insecurity is defined as having uncertain or limited availability of nutritionally adequate or safe food, or the inability to acquire personally acceptable foods in socially acceptable ways (Radimer et al. 1992). The essential components of food insecurity, according to the U.S. Department of Agriculture (USDA) (see Figure 2.1) include

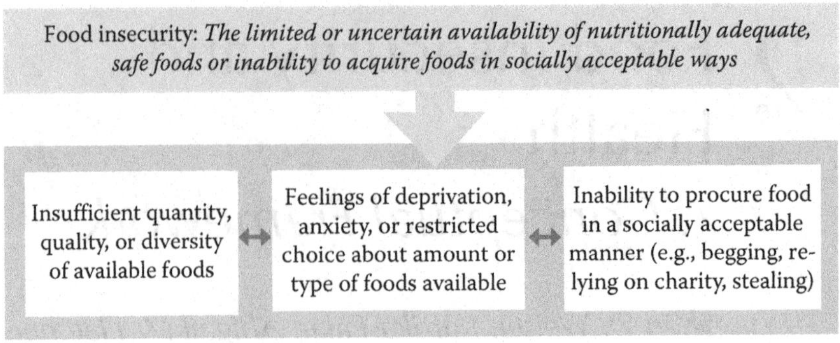

Food insecurity: *The limited or uncertain availability of nutritionally adequate, safe foods or inability to acquire foods in socially acceptable ways*

| Insufficient quantity, quality, or diversity of available foods | Feelings of deprivation, anxiety, or restricted choice about amount or type of foods available | Inability to procure food in a socially acceptable manner (e.g., begging, relying on charity, stealing) |

FIGURE 2.1   Definition of food insecurity.

insufficient food intake, inability to access foods of sufficient dietary quality, worry or anxiety over food supplies, and having to acquire food in socially unacceptable ways (Bickel et al. 2000). Protein–energy malnutrition, stunting, and wasting are some of the more obvious sequelae of severe food insecurity (Food and Agriculture Organization 2012). As of 2012, 870 million people worldwide were estimated to be undernourished, many of these in sub-Saharan Africa, south and southeast Asia, and parts of Latin America and the Caribbean (Food and Agriculture Organization 2012). Additionally, many more individuals suffer from mild, moderate, or severe food insecurity. Food insecurity is also prevalent in resource-rich settings. For example, in 2011, approximately 15% of households in the United States—or 17.9 million households—were food-insecure (Coleman-Jensen et al. 2012).

A consistent theme that has emerged in both resource-rich and resource-limited settings is that women bear an inequitable burden of food insecurity (Weiser et al. 2007). Female-headed households experience more food insecurity than male-headed ones (Nord et al. 2010) and women in relationships are often more food-insecure than their male partners. These inequalities result from a variety of causes, including unequal control over resources and household food allocation. Furthermore, women often leave work to serve as caregivers, and are therefore constrained in their abilities to make further investments in their own skills and education, increasing their susceptibility to food insecurity (Taylor et al. 1996).

Food insecurity has a wide range of negative health impacts beyond undernutrition. Studies among adults from resource-rich settings have shown that food insecurity is associated with poor self-reported health status (Stuff et al. 2004) and chronic disease risk factors, such as obesity (Dinour et al. 2007), and abnormal blood lipids (Seligman et al. 2010). Food insecurity has also been linked to high blood pressure (Seligman et al. 2010), increased rates of diabetes and poor diabetes outcomes (Seligman et al. 2007, 2010), and developing gestational diabetes mellitus (Laraia et al. 2010). Household food insecurity has consistently been associated with higher levels of perceived stress, depression, and anxiety among women (Laraia et al. 2006, Whitaker et al. 2006). Across resource-poor and resource-rich settings, food insecurity has been associated with HIV acquisition risk (Miller et al. 2011, Tsai et al. 2012, Vogenthaler et al. 2013), and poor HIV-related health (Weiser, Palar et al. 2014, Weiser, Yuan et al. 2013). Among children in resource-poor settings, food insecurity has been documented as a risk factor for childhood stunting (Baig-Ansari et al. 2006), while among children in resource-rich settings, it has been linked with delayed development (Rose-Jacobs et al. 2008), decreased health care access (Ma et al. 2008), poor health (Gundersen and Kreider 2009), and subsequent mental health and behavioral problems (Whitaker et al. 2006). Undernutrition directly contributes to 45% of all child deaths (Black et al. 2013).

A sound understanding of the complex linkages between food insecurity and health outcomes is critical if we are to provide empirical evidence to guide the integration of food programs and health programs to prevent disease, optimize disease treatment outcomes, and improve quality of life for people living with chronic diseases and their households. In this chapter, we propose a conceptual framework to explain the vicious cycle of food insecurity and poor health, informed by the literature and previous frameworks describing the relationship between food insecurity and health (Weiser et al. 2011). After describing an overview of our framework, we then illustrate its utility using HIV and chronic noncommunicable diseases (NCD) (with a focus on diabetes and cardiovascular disease risk factors) as examples. Together, HIV and cardiovascular disease account for 17% of disability-adjusted life years worldwide (Lim et al. 2013). For each example, we discuss the pathways through which food insecurity can result in negative health outcomes, and then conclude by discussing how disease states contribute to food insecurity. We consider implications of this framework for policy and practice. This information can be used to better understand the relationships between food insecurity and poor health, to inform research priorities, and to contribute toward the development of effective interventions.

OVERVIEW OF CONCEPTUAL FRAMEWORK

Food insecurity and health are intertwined in a vicious cycle through nutritional, mental health, and behavioral pathways (Figure 2.2). Our conceptual framework spans three levels of determinants (i.e., community, household, and individual) and expands upon an existing framework that describes the linkages between food security and health (Weiser et al. 2011).

Broader structural factors influence food security at the community level. These include climactic features (e.g., drought, flooding), socioeconomic factors (poverty, access to education), social factors (gender inequality, health-related stigma), and local food availability. Numerous studies have explored how neighborhood environments impact the availability and consumption of healthy foods (Larson et al. 2009), and ultimately may play a role in chronic disease (Brown et al. 2007). Food insecurity typically operates at the level of the household, and is also influenced by other household-level factors, such as family structure and social support. Food insecurity, in turn, shapes individual behaviors and health outcomes through nutritional, mental health, and behavioral pathways.

This framework also portrays the reciprocal relationship between food insecurity and poor health. For example, when a family member dies, becomes ill, or loses employment, the household may face economic shocks that increase the risk of food insecurity, such as loss of income, high funeral costs, or needing to sell off household

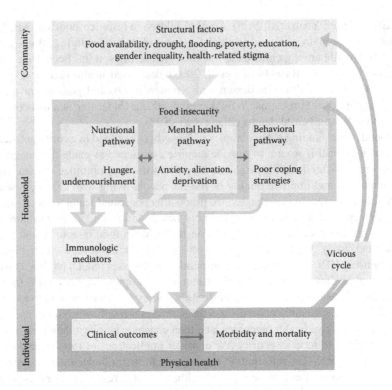

FIGURE 2.2   Conceptual framework of food insecurity and health.

assets for additional income. With fewer assets, surviving household members may fall into behavioral patterns that increase the risk of disease, reinitiating the cycle of food insecurity and poor health.

The nutritional, mental health, and behavioral pathways through which food insecurity negatively affects disease acquisition and progression emerge directly from the definition of food insecurity described in Figure 2.1 above. Insufficient quality and quantity of food can lead to macronutrient and micronutrient deficiencies, which can affect both acquisition of HIV and chronic diseases and health outcomes among people with those conditions. Feelings of deprivation or anxiety about food supply can have mental health consequences, such as depression and anxiety, which can contribute to acquisition and progression of HIV and NCDs. The inability to procure food in socially or personally acceptable ways can lead to non adherence with treatment and care recommendations and other adverse health behaviors, which can contribute to increased morbidity and mortality. We explore each of these pathways in more detail below.

NUTRITIONAL PATHWAY

Food insecurity affects total caloric intake as well as diet quality (i.e., macro- and micronutrient intake) and nutritional status (Dixon et al. 2001, Kirkpatrick and Tarasuk 2008, Rose 1999). Nationally, representative studies of adults in the United States (Dixon et al. 2001, Rose 1999) and Canada (Kirkpatrick and Tarasuk 2008) have linked food insecurity to inadequate dietary intakes and serum nutrient levels. When food quantity is limited, hunger and undernutrition can arise, which can eventually lead to wasting, stunting, and immune deficiency (Schaible and Stefan 2007). On the other hand, food insecurity also exerts negative impacts on health through effects on obesity, disordered eating behaviors among women (Laraia et al. 2013), and poor diet quality (Seligman et al. 2007). Researchers have hypothesized that these associations are driven by substitutions to cheaper, energy-dense foods (Drewnowski and Darmon 2005), overconsumption during periods of food availability (Wilde and Ranney 2000), and compensatory changes in metabolism. These nutritional abnormalities can also lead to subsequent potential for inflammation and gut abnormalities that can in turn lead to greater risk of disease.

MENTAL HEALTH PATHWAY

Qualitative studies conducted in diverse cultural contexts have identified feelings of helplessness, shame, and humiliation as central to the experience of food insecurity (Coates et al. 2006, Hamelin et al. 2002). Food insecurity has been found to be associated with poor mental health status independent of other indicators of low socioeconomic status, in both resource-rich (Alaimo et al. 2002) and resource-poor (Cole and Tembo 2011) settings. Specifically, it has been associated with anxiety (Hadley et al. 2008), depression (Alaimo et al. 2002), and stress (Belle Doucet 2003, Hadley et al. 2008). The mental health consequences of food insecurity can contribute both to disease acquisition as well as worse health outcomes among ill persons. For example, food insecurity and mental health are strongly associated with drug, alcohol use, and tobacco dependence (Weiser, Bangsberg et al. 2009), which is one pathway to disease acquisition.

Negative impacts of food insecurity on mental health have been documented primarily among women (Heflin et al. 2005), with less evidence of a relationship among men. One possible explanation is that women go to significant lengths to provide adequate food for their families, particularly their children, even if this means sacrificing their own needs (Martin and Lippert 2012). Research on poverty also indicates that apart from caregiving roles, having insufficient food can undermine social relationships and lead to feelings of low self-efficacy among women (Belle Doucet 2003). Food insecurity may thus trigger a particularly deep sense of helplessness among women, leading to mental and emotional distress (Belle Doucet 2003, Heflin et al. 2005).

BEHAVIORAL PATHWAY

Food insecurity is also linked to health behaviors affecting the prevention, management, and treatment of disease. An inability to fulfill subsistence needs, including household food needs, can lead people to make unhealthy decisions that may increase their risk of illness, such as engaging in risky sexual behaviors in exchange for food, or overreliance on cheap, calorically dense nutrient-poor foods. Once ill, food insecurity and other competing subsistence needs (e.g., unstable housing) are associated with worsened access and adherence to general medical care among low-income adults (Bengle et al. 2010, Cunningham et al. 1999, Kushel et al. 2006,

Weiser et al. 2010). For example, in research among a national survey of low-income adults from the general U.S. population, food insecurity was associated with postponing needed medications and care, and with increased emergency-department use and hospitalizations (Kushel et al. 2006).

POSSIBLE IMMUNE PATHWAYS

Immunologic consequences arising from the nutritional and mental health pathways may further mediate the effect of food insecurity on health. In animal studies, obesity has been found to be associated with microbial translocation of gut-derived endotoxin in mice (Erridge 2008). In human studies, obesity has been associated with a chronic inflammatory state among women (Womack et al. 2007), while consumption of high-fat meals has been shown to negatively impact the composition of gut microbiota (Erridge et al. 2007, Maslowski and Mackay 2011). Gut microbial translocation, in turn, leads to persistent immune activation and chronic inflammation, which can contribute to higher morbidity and mortality in certain conditions. Stress, an important consequence of food insecurity, has also been linked to chronic inflammation (Black and Garbutt 2002), which is closely tied to cardiovascular disease and diabetes.

PATHWAYS LINKING FOOD INSECURITY TO DIABETES AND CARDIOVASCULAR RISK

Noncommunicable chronic diseases (NCDs) are the leading cause of death in all regions of the world except for Africa. NCDs kill roughly 35 million people each year (Lozano et al. 2013), 25% of whom are under the age of 60, and significantly increase morbidity and decrease quality of life (Lim et al. 2013). Cardiovascular diseases, such as heart disease, stroke, and diabetes accounted for over half of NCD deaths annually, or approximately 14.2 million deaths (Lozano et al. 2013). Although these diseases are often thought of as primarily affecting high-income countries, 80% of all NCD deaths occur in low- or middle-income countries (World Health Organization 2013). Even in resource-rich settings, NCD rates are higher in disadvantaged communities than in better-off groups (Dalstra et al. 2005).

Previous studies have shown associations between food insecurity and chronic disease risk and prevalence (Laraia 2013), including abnormal blood lipid levels (dyslipidemia) (Seligman et al. 2010, Stuff et al. 2007), high blood pressure (hypertension) (Seligman et al. 2010, Stuff et al. 2007), heart disease (Stuff et al. 2007), type II diabetes (Seligman et al. 2007), and gestational diabetes (Laraia et al. 2010) in resource-rich settings. Fetal exposure to diabetes disrupts metabolic pathways and is associated with increased risk for obesity and type II diabetes (Battista et al. 2011). Poor diets have been identified as a major risk factor in morbidity and mortality from NCDs (Lim et al. 2013). Figure 2.3 depicts the pathways through which food insecurity negatively impacts health for NCDs.

NUTRITIONAL PATHWAY

Obesity is a major risk factor for diabetes and cardiovascular diseases (Must et al. 1999), and studies have suggested that food insecurity and overweight or

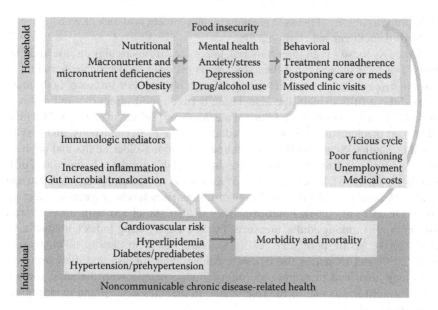

FIGURE 2.3 Food insecurity and cardiovascular health.

obesity coexist among low-income individuals. Both food insecurity and obesity are consequences of social disadvantage (Walsemann et al. 2012). Despite close associations between food insecurity and obesity among certain populations and in some settings (Dinour et al. 2007, Larson and Story 2011), the literature is inconsistent about the relationship between food insecurity and weight status. Most consistently, studies have found that food insecurity is associated with overweight and obesity in women, especially among women of color (Larson and Story 2011). Because maternal nutritional status is one of the most important predictors of infant health, this nutritional pathway also has marked impacts on infant and child health, including obstetric outcomes (Leddy et al. 2008), child growth (Whitaker 2004), development, and neurocognitive outcomes (Herman et al. 2014). There is almost no evidence on associations between food insecurity and overweight or obesity in men, although some studies have found associations between food insecurity and obesity and weight gain in adults more generally (Wilde and Peterman 2006).

Food insecurity may lead to obesity, in part, due to the greater affordability of energy-dense, high-fat foods (Drewnowski and Darmon 2005). Furthermore, models of animal response suggest stress triggered by food scarcity can modify metabolic processes and lead to overconsumption of high-fat, high-sugar foods (Dallman et al. 2003). This biologically driven learned behavior then activates overeating as a coping mechanism for future episodes of scarcity, even at much lower levels of stress (Dallman et al. 2005). Other mechanisms linking food insecurity to obesity have also been hypothesized, including that food scarcity may create a biological disposition to store extra energy as fat (Neel 1962), or developmental pathways whereby children born to mothers who experienced food deprivation while pregnant may be more prone to obesity if the post pregnancy environment is abundant with highcalo-rie foods (Gluckman and Hanson 2008).

Although obesity is an important risk factor for cardiovascular disease and dia-betes, evidence suggests that the associations between food insecurity and these chronic diseases do not operate solely through obesity. For instance, body mass index did not fully explain the association between food insecurity and diabetes in a recent study, suggesting additional mechanisms (Seligman et al. 2007). These additional mechanisms may include reduced intake of key nutrients, and overall low diet quality. Some studies have found that among older adults and women, food insecurity is linked to lower fruit and vegetable intake (Dixon et al. 2001, Kendall et al. 1996), lower fiber intake (Kendall et al. 1996), lower micronutrient intakes (Dixon et al. 2001), and lower serum nutrient levels (Bhattacharya et al. 2004, Dixon et al. 2001). Food insecurity is also associated with lower overall dietary quality among adults, measured by the Health Eating Index (Bhattacharya et al. 2004). While poor diet quality is associated with obesity (Wolongevicz et al. 2010) and increases the risk of cardiovascular disease and diabetes, poor diets may also lead to greater morbidity among people with diabetes, regard-less of weight status due to the role of diet in diabetes control and management (Seligman et al. 2012).

MENTAL HEALTH PATHWAY

As described above, food insecurity is associated with stress, depression, and anxiety (Whitaker et al. 2006), which have also been linked with obesity and cardiovascular risk (Black and Garbutt 2002). Studies in animal models have shown that stress trig-gered by food scarcity activates the thalamic–pituitary–adrenal systems and stimu-lates the release of cortisol, which can alter metabolism (Dallman et al. 2003). At the same time, food scarcity also activates the reward pathway and memory (Dallman et al. 2003), which together with the stress pathway, may explain observations that animals are drawn to "comfort foods"—that is, high-fat, high-sugar foods—that alleviate scarcity-related stress (Dallman et al. 2003). Applied to humans, these ani-mal models suggest that chronic psychosocial stress may increase the risk for obesity by increasing the relative consumption of energy-dense foods. Increases in cortisol levels due to stress also increase blood glucose and insulin levels, which play critical roles in diabetes, implying a pathway to chronic disease that is independent of diet and weight status (Rosmond et al. 1998).

The impact of mental health on chronic disease risk may be particularly detri-mental for women and children. Food insecurity has been associated with greater changes in cortisol in poor women (Frith 2006) and with higher perceived stress, anxiety, and depression, as well as lower levels of self-esteem and mastery among pregnant women (Laraia et al. 2006). Two studies have also shown that the interac-tion of maternal stress and food insecurity are associated with elevated weight gain among children (Gundersen et al. 2008). Maternal food insecurity was also linked to childhood behavioral problems, an association that strengthened after adjusting for maternal anxiety and depression (Whitaker et al. 2006).

BEHAVIORAL PATHWAYS

Food insecurity is linked with poor adherence to health care recommendations, which may be particularly harmful to those with cardiovascular and metabolic problems. For example, food-insecure patients are more likely to report cost-related non adherence behaviors for prescription medications in general (Bengle et al. 2010), and less likely to be adherent to blood glucose monitoring for diabetes (Seligman et al. 2010), which in turn negatively impacts disease outcomes. Among people with hypertension, non adherence to prescribed antihypertensive treatment increases the risk of acute cardiovascular events (Mazzaglia et al. 2009). Among patients who develop type II diabetes (for which food insecurity is a risk factor) (Seligman et al. 2007), missed appointments and medication non adherence are predictors of uncontrolled disease and disease complications in both resource-rich and resource-poor settings (Gibson et al. 2010; Schectman et al. 2002).

Associations between household food insecurity and markers of diabetes management have been documented in several scientific studies. The strongest associations between food insecurity and poor diabetes management have been found in studies using clinic-based samples where the prevalence of diabetes is higher (between 14% and 51%) compared to population-based studies (between 6% and 15.5%). For example, an early observational study in 1998 identified a strong link between food insecurity and poor diabetes management. The authors found that 61% of adults receiving insulin to treat diabetes in an urban county hospital reported hypoglycemic reactions, indicating poor diabetes management, and one-third of these reported the cause to be the inability to afford food (Nelson et al. 1998). Other studies using clinic-based samples have repeatedly reported an association between household food insecurity and hypoglycemic events (Seligman et al. 2010) and poor glycemic control among adults (Seligman et al. 2012) and children with diabetes (Marjerrison et al. 2011).

Results from population-based studies have been less consistent. In two studies, using data from the National Health and Nutrition Examination Survey, Seligman et al. found food that insecurity was significantly associated with poor glycemic control among adults meeting diagnostic criteria for diabetes (Seligman et al. 2007), and in a follow-up study found that household food insecurity was associated with indicators of poor diabetes self-management (Seligman et al. 2010). However, a Canadian population-based study found no association between household food insecurity and poor diabetes management (Gucciardi et al. 2009). Other studies have also found food insecurity to be associated with behavioral factors that can potentially affect diabetes control and management, including challenges with maintaining a nutritionally adequate diet, lower self-efficacy, and higher emotional distress related to diabetes management (Seligman et al. 2012).

PATHWAYS LINKING FOOD INSECURITY TO HIV ACQUISITION AND DISEASE PROGRESSION

The prevalence of food insecurity is particularly high among people living with HIV (PLHIV) in both resource-rich and resource-poor settings. For example, studies from Kenya and Uganda have found that the vast majority of PLHIV are moderately or severely food-insecure (Mbugua et al. 2008, Weiser, Tsai et al. 2012). Nearly half of low-income PLHIV patients on antiretroviral therapy (ART) in urban resource-rich settings have been estimated to be food-insecure (Weiser, Bangsberg et al. 2009, Weiser, Frongillo et al. 2009). Women are, again, the most affected by the parallel epidemics of HIV and food insecurity. Similar to food insecurity, HIV disproportionately impacts poor women (Farmer et al. 1993) due to gender inequalities, poverty, and absence of support as head of household, among other reasons (Farmer et al. 1993, Weiser et al. 2007).

Food insecurity contributes to both HIV acquisition risk and worse HIV health outcomes among people already living with HIV. Food insecurity increases the likelihood of risky sexual practices, exacerbating the horizontal spread of HIV (Weiser et al. 2007), and can also increase the likelihood of vertical transmission through risky infant feeding practices (Young et al. 2011) and poorer maternal health status (Mehta et al. 2008). Among PLHIV, food insecurity has been associated with lower antiretroviral (ARV) adherence (Weiser, Frongillo et al. 2009), declines in physical health status (Weiser, Bangsberg et al. 2009), decreased viral suppression (Kalichman et al. 2010, Weiser, Frongillo et al. 2009), worse immunologic status (Weiser, Bangsberg et al. 2009), increased incidence of serious illness (Weiser, Tsai et al. 2012), and increased mortality (Weiser, Fernandes et al. 2009). As shown in Figure 2.4, food insecurity is linked with HIV acquisition risk and worse HIV health outcomes through nutritional, mental health, and behavioral pathways.

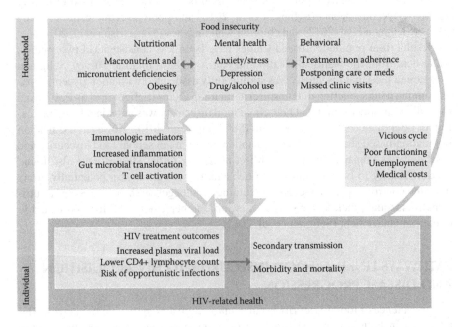

FIGURE 2.4   Food insecurity and HIV-related health.

Nutritional Pathway

Micronutrient deficiencies in uninfected, HIV-exposed individuals can impair the integrity of the gut and genital epithelial lining and the differentiation of target cells, as well as cripple other host defense mechanisms, which could, in turn, increase susceptibility to infection for both other adults and infants (Friis 2005). In individuals living with HIV, oxidative stress caused by micronutrient deficiencies may cause HIV viral loads to increase (Schreck et al. 1991), thereby increasing an individual's infectiousness and likelihood of transmitting HIV to others (Royce et al. 1997). In terms of macronutrient deficiencies and infectivity, wasting and low weight gain during pregnancy have been associated with increased mother-to-child transmission (MTCT) in one prospective study in Tanzania (Mehta et al. 2008). Food insecurity can also increase vertical transmission of HIV by increasing the prevalence of mixed formula and breast-feeding, a practice that has been shown to increase risk of MTCT fourfold compared to exclusive breastfeeding (Iliff et al. 2005). In Malawi, for example, women experiencing food insecurity felt that their breast milk production was inadequate and were more likely to supplement with other non-breast milk sources of nutrition prior to 6 months of age (Kerr et al. 2007). Similarly, Kenyan and Ugandan HIV-infected mothers experiencing food insecurity felt they were unable to exclusively breastfeed for 6 months (Webb-Girard et al. 2012).

Nutritional pathways also mediate impacts of food insecurity on HIV outcomes among people already living with HIV through a number of mechanisms. Among PLHIV, food insecurity is associated with undernutrition, micronutrient deficiencies, and HIV wasting (Campa et al. 2005). Protein and energy undernutrition and micronutrient deficiencies, in turn, are associated with higher risk of disease progression and mortality in PLHIV (Friis 2005, Zachariah et al. 2006). Specifically, weight loss, low body mass index (BMI), low albumin, and micronutrient deficiencies have been shown to predict opportunistic infections, immunologic decline, and shorter survival time in both untreated and ART-treated individuals (Macallan et al. 1995, van der Sande et al. 2004). HIV increases metabolic requirements (Babameto and Kotler 1997, Macallan et al. 1995) and is associated with diarrhea and malabsorption of fat and carbohydrates (Babameto and Kotler 1997), which further compounds the links between malnutrition and disease progression. Finally, lack of food may impede optimal absorption of certain ARV medications (Bardsley-Elliot and Plosker 2000, Gustavson et al. 2000), which may, in turn, contribute to treatment failure. Several protease inhibitors (PIs), such as nelfinavir and ritonavir, require food for maximal absorption, and the absence of food may negatively affect the pharmacokinetics of these drugs (Bardsley-Elliot and Plosker 2000).

Undernutrition is not the only pathway through which food insecurity negatively impacts health outcomes. For example, a study among ART-treated patients in Vancouver found that while the impact of food insecurity on mortality was most pronounced among malnourished individuals (Adjusted Hazard Ratio [AHR] = 1.94, 95% CI 1.10–3.40), individuals who were normal weight but food-insecure also had a trend toward increased morality (AHR = 1.40, 95% CI = 0.91–2.05), while individuals who were food-secure but malnourished did not have increased mortality risk (Weiser, Fernandes, et al. 2009). This suggests that under nutrition is not the only pathway through which food insecurity negatively impacts health outcomes.

Another nutritional pathway toward worse HIV outcomes pertains to the close relationship between food insecurity, obesity, and other metabolic abnormalities (discussed above), which may be particularly detrimental for people with HIV. Treatment with certain ARV medications has been linked to metabolic abnormalities, including endothelial dysfunction, atherogenic dyslipidemia, and abnormal glucose metabolism (Friis-Møller et al. 2003). Excess weight can exacerbate metabolic syndrome, including central fat accumulation, insulin resistance, lipid abnormalities, and hypertension (Friis-Møller et al. 2003) and is associated with increased risk of cardiovascular disease and type 2 diabetes mellitus (Alberti et al. 2005), including among PLHIV. Furthermore, obesity is associated with poorer immunologic response to ART (Crum-Cianflone et al. 2010). Metabolic abnormalities, together with the rising prevalence of obesity among PLHIV (Crum-Cianflone et al. 2010), underscore the need to better understand the relationships between food insecurity and metabolic outcomes among PLHIV.

Mental Health Pathway

Among PLHIV, several studies have reported that food insecurity is associated with depression (Vogenthaler et al. 2011) and worse overall mental health status (Weiser, Bangsberg, et al. 2009). At least one study has shown that the effects of food security on depression were most pronounced among women (Tsai et al. 2012). Worse mental health, in turn, is strongly associated with HIV transmission risk behaviors (Carey 1997). For example, an early review of mental illness and HIV risk behaviors found that in studies among the seriously mentally ill, 20%–40% had multiple partners compared to 17% of the general population, and 7%–28% reported trading sex for material gain (e.g., drugs and food) (Carey 1997). Only about one-quarter of sexual encounters were protected using condoms. There has, however, been little study of the role of mental illness in mediating HIV transmission risk among food-insecure individuals. Food insecurity has also been associated with drug abuse among PLHIV in resource-rich settings (Anema et al. 2010), which in turn is well known to contribute to HIV transmission risk.

Food insecurity can also negatively impact HIV health outcomes through worsened mental health. Depression and anxiety disorders (which are more prevalent among food-insecure individuals), have been shown to predict reduced uptake of and non adherence to ART (Kacanek et al. 2010, Tegger et al. 2008), as well as higher viral loads and higher activated CD8+ cell counts (Evans et al. 2002). Impacts of depression on HIV treatment outcomes are not fully explained via impacts on ART adherence. Even after adjusting for ART adherence, depression has been associated with worsened HIV treatment outcomes, including CD4+ T-lymphocyte count decline (Ickovics et al. 2001), increased probability of AIDS-defining illness (Anastos et al. 2005), and AIDS-related mortality (Ickovics et al. 2001). The role of depression in accelerating disease progression is strengthened by the fact that the treatment of depression has been demonstrated to improve ART adherence and viral suppression (Tsai et al. 2010). Decreased adherence and worse HIV health outcomes have also been linked to increased drug and alcohol use and tobacco dependence (Tucker et al. 2003), which can be exacerbated by food insecurity.

Behavioral Pathway

Studies from resource-rich and resource-poor settings have found that individuals may engage in high-risk sexual behaviors as a means of coping with food insecurity, which may in turn contribute to increased HIV transmission. In Botswana and Swaziland, food insufficiency was independently associated with inconsistent condom use with a non-primary partner, sex exchange, intergenerational sexual relationships, and lack of control in sexual relationships among women (Weiser et al. 2007). In a study among sex workers in Lagos, Nigeria, 35% of respondents said that poverty and lack of other means to get food were responsible for their decision to join the sex trade industry (Oyefara 2007). Among sexually active women in Brazil, food insecurity was associated with lower odds of consistent condom use and condom use during the last sexual encounter, and higher odds of symptoms of a sexually transmitted infection (Tsai et al. 2012). Qualitative studies conducted in Botswana, Swaziland, and Uganda showed that women's control over sexual decision-making is severely constrained as a result of their dependence on men for food and other resources (Miller et al. 2011, Physicians for Human Rights 2007). Women in these settings often feel that they have to engage in unsafe sex to negotiate their subsistence needs, and food insecurity can contribute to sex exchange in situations where women feel they had no other options for feeding themselves and their children. Links between food insecurity and sexual risk-taking have also been shown in resource-rich settings. In San Francisco, food insecurity was associated with inconsistent condom use and multiple sexual partnerships in a longitudinal study among a population of predominately male homeless and marginally housed PLHIV (Vogenthaler et al. 2013). In a longitudinal study in Vancouver among injection drug users with HIV, severe food insecurity was associated with unprotected sex in adjusted analyses (Shannon et al. 2011).

Food insecurity has also been shown to contribute to sexual victimization in sub-Saharan Africa. In Botswana, food insufficiency was associated with over 2 times higher odds of sexual violence among women (Tsai, Leiter, et al. 2011). In qualitative studies from Uganda, Botswana, and Swaziland, women said that they were compelled to remain in abusive relationships as a result of food insecurity and poverty (Miller et al. 2011, Physicians for Human Rights 2007).

For men and women in resource-poor settings, another possible mechanism through which food insecurity may lead to increased sexual risk-taking is that lack of food often leads to migration for work (Singh 2003). Migration, in turn, has been found to be associated with increased sexual risk-taking and HIV prevalence for both men and women in multiple studies (Lagarde et al. 2003, Sopheab et al. 2006).

Behavioral pathways also link food insecurity with HIV health outcomes. Both cross-sectional quantitative and qualitative studies have documented strong links between food insecurity and ART non adherence among PLHIV (Young et al. 2014), one of the key predictors of morbidity and mortality among HIV-infected individuals (Bangsberg et al. 2001). In cross-sectional studies among urban poor PLHIV in North America, food insecurity has been associated with ART non adherence as measured by both unannounced pill counts and pharmacy refill (Kalichman et al. 2010, Weiser, Frongillo et al. 2009). In Atlanta, food insecurity was also associated with common barriers to adherence, such as lack of social support, drug use, and not being able to afford medications (Kalichman et al. 2010). In a large, nationally representative sample of nearly 5000 PLHIV in France, food privation was associated with increased odds of self-reported ART non adherence among heterosexual men and a trend toward increased odds of non adherence among heterosexual women (Peretti-Watel et al. 2006). Qualitative studies in Kenya, Uganda, Botswana, and Swaziland found that food insecurity is one of the most commonly cited barriers to ART treatment adherence (Physicians for Human Rights 2007, Weiser et al. 2010). Longitudinal studies in San Francisco (Weiser, Yuan et al. 2013) and Uganda (Weiser, Palar et al. 2014) found food insecurity to be associated with low ART adherence (<90%), low CD4 counts, and unsuppressed viral loads. When adherence was included in models of CD4 count and viral non suppression, it explained the association between food insecurity and viral non suppression in Uganda but not in San Francisco, and did not explain associations between food insecurity and low CD4 count in either setting. Since food insecurity is associated with unsuppressed viral loads (Weiser, Frongillo et al. 2009, Weiser, Palar et al. 2014, Weiser, Yuan et al. 2013), it may also heighten risk of HIV transmission via vertical, sexual, and drug-using routes.

In addition to ART non adherence and treatment interruptions, food-insecure individuals often miss scheduled clinic visits, and may have decreased uptake of ART as a result of competing demands between food and other resources (Weiser et al. 2010). One United States-based study found that competing subsistence needs were associated with worse access to health care among PLHIV (Cunningham et al. 1999). In rural Uganda, severe food insecurity was associated with decreased outpatient clinic visits, and many participants had forgone ART (15%), other medications (22%), outpatient care (28%), and inpatient care (28%) in order to secure food (Weiser, Tsai et al. 2012). A greater proportion of study participants reported that they had prioritized medical care; participants had forgone food to obtain ART (83%), access outpatient care (76%), and access inpatient care (44%). This suggests that the relatively high levels of adherence reported among ART-treated individuals in resource-poor settings (Mills et al. 2006) may not be sustainable in the long term unless food insecurity and poverty reduction become essential components of comprehensive HIV care programs.

IMMUNOLOGIC PATHWAYS RELATED TO CARDIOVASCULAR DISEASE AND HIV

Increased inflammation and immune activation is another potential pathway linking food insecurity to worse health outcomes for both HIV and cardiovascular disease. Obesity, a key consequence of food insecurity as described above, has been found to be associated with microbial translocation (MT) of gut-derived endotoxin in mice (Erridge 2008). Data from the Women's Interagency HIV study suggest that obesity may result in a chronic inflammatory state due to increased cytokine production by adipose tissue (Womack et al. 2007). Consumption of a single high-fat meal has been associated with increased endotoxin concentrations in human subjects (Erridge et al. 2007). Low-fiber, high-fat, high-sugar diets (typical among food-insecure individuals) have also been shown to negatively impact the composition of gut microbiota (Maslowski and Mackay 2011).

Gut MT is a leading cause of persistent immune activation in HIV, and T-cell activation is a well-known mediator of HIV pathogenesis, contributing both to more rapid progression to AIDS and death, and decreased immunologic recovery on HAART (Hunt 2007). Food insecurity also results in worse virologic control, which in turn has been associated with higher levels of inflammation and T-cell activation (Nixon and Landay 2010). Recent animal and human studies have also shown a link between microbial translocation and insulin resistance and diabetes (Erridge 2008). Immune activation and inflammation are also thought to contribute to the development of cardiovascular disease among PLHIV (Kuller et al. 2008).

Food insecurity has also been linked with inflammation in general population studies. Using data from the National Health and Examination Survey, Gowda et al. found that food insecurity was associated with 20% higher odds of being in the upper quartile of C-reactive protein, a biomarker of systemic inflammation (Gowda et al. 2012). Furthermore, this relationship was partially mediated by high white blood cell counts indicating immune activation and potential infection. The relationship between food insecurity and inflammation may also be mediated by stress, which has been tied to food insecurity (Whitaker et al. 2006) and which leads to an inflammatory response linked to cardiovascular disease and diabetes (Black and Garbutt 2002).

POOR HEALTH CONTRIBUTES TO FOOD INSECURITY

The previous sections have focused on how food insecurity may lead to poor health. However, the relationship between food security and health outcomes is bi directional, causing households and individuals to be caught in a "vicious cycle" of poor outcomes. Poor physical health is associated with higher food insecurity (Tarasuk et al. 2013). Health problems such as HIV and chronic diseases worsen family food insecurity due to the debilitation of the most productive household members, decreased individual and household economic capacity, and increased caregiver burden (McIntyre et al. 2006). When working-age adults fall ill, their households lose income, assets, labor, and skills, and must cope with potentially catastrophic treatment and funeral costs (McIntyre et al. 2006). For example, national survey data from Kenya indicate that the net value of household crop production declined by 68% following the death of a male head of household, and that affected households adopted short-term survival strategies (such as selling off productive assets and shifting from high-value to subsistence crops) that impaired financial viability in the long term (Yamano and Jayne 2004). Furthermore, intergenerational transmission of poverty and food insecurity occur when children are withdrawn from school to provide informal care, to compensate for lost adult labor, or because school fees become unaffordable (Yamano and Jayne 2005). Having fewer assets (especially arable land) lowers household earning potential, lessens the potential for education, increases household expenses and, in turn, worsens food insecurity. Similarly, mental health problems have been shown to impede sustained food security because these problems can interfere with finding lasting employment (Lent et al. 2009).

The impacts of poor health on food insecurity are compounded for PLHIV, in part, due to stigma and discrimination. HIV continues to be heavily stigmatized in much of sub-Saharan Africa, which can prevent HIV-affected households from drawing upon informal support needed to ensure food security (Danziger 1994). For example, among ART-treated PLHIV in rural Uganda, both internalized HIV stigma (internalizing negative views about HIV by PLHIV) and enacted HIV stigma (experiences of discrimination related to HIV status) were strongly associated with food insecurity in a longitudinal study (Tsai, Bangsberg et al. 2011).

Conversely, improvements in physical and mental health can lead to improvements in food security. For example, in Uganda, food insecurity decreased and nutritional status improved over time for PLHIV after initiation of ART (Weiser, Gupta et al. 2012, Palar et al. 2012). Changes in food insecurity were partially explained by improvements in physical health status (Weiser, Gupta et al. 2012) and mental health (Palar et al. 2012).

IMPLICATIONS FOR RESEARCH AND POLICY

We have suggested that nutritional, mental health, behavioral, and immunologic pathways explain how food insecurity may impact disease prevention and health outcomes. The next step is to better understand how these pathways operate across different settings and what the relative importance of each pathway is. Here, we identify specific priorities for future research and suggest lessons for both practitioners and policy-makers working in related fields.

Despite the rich body of literature in support of our conceptual model, few studies to date have confirmed these links, nor specifically assessed the relative importance of each causal pathway between food insecurity and poor health outcomes. Longitudinal studies based on larger, more representative samples are therefore needed to further assess the relative importance of each mechanism underlying the relationships between food insecurity and health. We also need to understand whether the mechanisms for how food insecurity adversely impacts health outcomes and prevention differ between resource-rich and resource-poor settings. Further clarification of these mechanisms can have important policy and programmatic implications. Understanding the relative importance of the different pathways will help in choosing among the various programmatic and policy options to improve food security such as income transfer for food, provision of prepared meals (e.g., soup kitchens, warm meal delivery), augmenting food supply (e.g., food pantries and food packages given out in clinics), and livelihood and vocational training programs, while considering challenges such as dependency, anxiety, and stigma. As shown in Table 2.1, programmatic options can be tailored to different pathways.

If, for example, *nutritional* pathways predominate, then providing food or food coupons may be a necessary intervention. However, in light of studies showing that participation in food programs may worsen obesity in women (Leroy et al. 2013), information on the nutritional pathway—whether it be for obesity or undernutrition—may guide the type of food support or counseling offered. Dietary counseling has been shown to be an effective approach to increasing fruit and vegetable consumption among low-income adults (Steptoe et al. 2003), and improving food security among recipients of supplemental nutrition benefits (aka food stamps) (Eicher-Miller et al. 2009) in the United States.

TABLE 2.1
Intervention Options

Structural Programs

• Household income transfers	• Livelihoods interventions (e.g., job skills,
• Improved access to food support (e.g.,	vocational training, microsavings/credit)
added locations, facilitated enrolment)	• Agricultural training/community gardens

Nutritional Programs

Obesity	Undernutrition	Behavioral Programs	Mental Health Programs
• Food provision (e.g., food banks; fruits and vegetables)	• Prepared meal delivery, soup kitchen, food bank	• Social work case management	• Mental health counseling and referral
• Diet counseling	• Diet counseling	• Transportation vouchers	• Substance abuse counseling and referral
• Exercise for weight loss	• Nutrient-rich foods	• Medication adherence counseling	
		• Comprehensive medical care	
		• Support groups	

Immunologic Programs

• Pre or probiotics

• Nutritional supplementation

• Earlier medication initiation

If either *behavioral or mental health* pathways are critical, income transfers for food may better target ongoing anxiety about the food supply or procuring food in socially unacceptable ways compared with provision of prepared meals or food banks. Likewise, skills or vocational training programs could address upstream determinants of food insecurity and lead to cost savings in the long term by decreasing dependence on food assistance. Should *behavioral pathway* mediators prove to have the largest impacts, this may strengthen the rationale for social services to be paired with clinical services. For example, food-insecure households often make trade-offs in order to buy food (Kushel et al. 2006) (e.g., buying less medicine, visiting clinics less often), suggesting that vouchers for services like transportation may be useful. If *mental health pathways* are central, food support programs should be accompanied by mental health screening and referral in order to maximally improve health outcomes. If *immunologic factors* are critical mediators, future interventions would need to focus on decreasing inflammation and immune activation, for example, by using pre- and probiotics and other nutritional supplements, interventions that may be particularly useful among food-insecure individuals (Maslowski and Mackay 2011). Regardless of the specific intervention recommendations, a stronger scientific understanding of food insecurity pathways will marshal attention and resources to solve this pervasive epidemic.

Policy-makers have long acknowledged the potential for food security interventions to positively impact health (WHO 2003). Despite these recommendations, little research exists to document the efficacy, effectiveness, or cost-effectiveness of food-security interventions on NCD or HIV-related health outcomes (Mahlungulu et al. 2007). Such research is critical if we are to provide empirical evidence to guide policies to integrate structural interventions into the expansion of HIV care, treatment, and prevention programs.

Existing intervention approaches to improve HIV treatment outcomes via food security (such as Food by Prescription Programs) are limited in their scalability and sustainability (Sztam et al. 2010). Most interventions in resource-rich settings are focused on nutritional education, with the assumption that food insecurity is a product of poor or limited food choices. This individualistic approach fails to address the social and environmental factors that drive nutrition and food insecurity. In resource-poor settings, most intervention studies have focused on macronutrient supplementation as the food security intervention, and have demonstrated the potential for macronutrient supplementation to affect health outcomes among PLHIV (Koethe et al. 2009). Macronutrient supplementation, while providing critical nutritional support, tends to focus on short-term dietary needs and does not address all of the downstream health consequences of food insecurity, potentially causing dependency on health programs for receipt of food aid. Moreover, relying on health programs for food may be socially unacceptable or may contribute to ongoing anxiety and uncertainty about food supply and feelings of deprivation and alienation. Finally, providing clinic- or pantry-based food supplementation is costly, and may be difficult to scale up in a variety of settings (Sztam et al. 2010).

Domestic and global policy institutions have begun to shift their attention from short-term food-supplementation programs to longer-range strategies to improve food security and health. Livelihood and economic interventions target some of the root causes of food insecurity and have the potential to address numerous pathways—nutritional, mental health, and behavioral—through which food insecurity negatively impacts health. For example, conditional cash transfer programs in Mexico and Brazil have shown robust evidence to suggest that social protection may be an effective way to improve child nutritional outcomes (Fernald et al. 2008, Paes-Sousa et al. 2011). Based on the South American success, cash transfer programs in multiple sub-Saharan African settings are currently being evaluated and may show an impact on nutritional and health outcomes (Food and Agriculture Organization 2013).

CONCLUSION

The relationship between food security and health outcomes is bi directional, causing households and individuals to be caught in a "vicious cycle" of poor outcomes. Food insecurity negatively impacts health outcomes across a range of diseases, and operates through nutritional, mental health, and behavioral pathways. Creative solutions will be required to best meet the food needs of impoverished populations in different parts of the world to improve their health and well-being. While food security has garnered increased attention in the public health field, several crucial questions remain unanswered. What are the relative importance of the different pathways linking food insecurity to increased morbidity and mortality? Which interventions have the greatest ability to address food insecurity and the pathways through which food insecurity negatively impacts health? Does this vary across country and context? And, how might successful interventions be rapidly scaled up to reach the growing population of food-insecure households in the coming years? Our ability to answer these pressing questions and to translate findings into impactful programs will have benefits, not only for the public health system—as costs associated with treating concomitant morbidity decline—but also for the health and well-being of the billions of persons across the globe who are food-insecure.

REFERENCES

Alaimo, K., C. M. Olson, and E. A. Frongillo. 2002. Family food insufficiency, but not low family income, is positively associated with dysthymia and suicide symptoms in adolescents. *Journal of Nutrition* 132 (4):719–25.

Alberti, K. G., P. Zimmet, and J. Shaw. 2005. The metabolic syndrome—A new worldwide definition. *Lancet* 366 (9491):1059.

Anastos, K., M. F. Schneider, S. J. Gange, H. Minkoff, R. M. Greenblatt, J. Feldman, and M. Cohen. 2005. The association of race, sociodemographic, and behavioral characteristics with response to highly active antiretroviral therapy in women. *JAIDS Journal of Acquired Immune Deficiency Syndromes* 39 (5):537–44. doi: 00126334-200508150-00005 [pii].

Anema, A., E. Wood, S. D. Weiser, J. Q., Julio, S. G. Montaner, and T. Kerr. 2010. Hunger and associated harms among injection drug users in an urban Canadian setting. *Substance Abuse Treatment, Prevention, and Policy* 5:20–20.

Babameto, G. and D. P. Kotler. 1997. Malnutrition in HIV infection. *Gastroenterology Clinics of North America* 26 (2):393–415.

Baig-Ansari, N., M. H. Rahbar, Z. A. Bhutta, and S. H. Badruddin. 2006. Child's gender and household food insecurity are associated with stunting among young Pakistani children residing in urban squatter settlements. *Food and Nutrition Bulletin* 27:114–27.

Bangsberg, D. R., S. Perry, E. D. Charlebois, R. A. Clark, M. Roberston, A. R. Zolopa, and A. Moss. 2001. Non-adherence to highly active antiretroviral therapy predicts progression to AIDS. *AIDS* 15 (9):1181–3.

Bardsley-Elliot, A. and G. L. Plosker. 2000. Nelfinavir: An update on its use in HIV infection. *Drugs* 59 (3):581–620.

Battista, M.-C., M.-F. Hivert, K. Duval, and J.-P. Baillargeon. 2011. Intergenerational cycle of obesity and diabetes: How can we reduce the burdens of these conditions on the health of future generations? *Experimental Diabetes Research* 2011:1–9.

Belle Doucet, D. 2003. Poverty, inequality, and discrimination as sources of depression among US women. *Psychology of Women Quarterly* 27 (2):101–13.

Bengle, R., S. Sinnett, T. Johnson, M. A. Johnson, A. Brown, and J. S. Lee. 2010. Food insecurity is associated with cost-related medication non-adherence in community-dwelling, low-income older adults in Georgia. *Journal of Nutrition for the Elderly* 29 (2):170–91. doi: 10.1080/01639361003772400.

Bhattacharya, J., J. Currie, and S. Haider. 2004. Poverty, food insecurity, and nutritional outcomes in children and adults. *Journal of Health Economics* 23 (4):839–62.

Bickel, G., M. Nord, C. Price, W. Hamilton, and J. Cook. 2000. *Guide to Measuring Household Food Security, Revised 2000.* Alexandria, VA: U.S. Department of Agriculture, Food and Nutrition Service.

Black, P. H. and L. D. Garbutt. 2002. Stress, inflammation and cardiovascular disease. *Journal of Psychosomatic Research* 52 (1):1–23.

Black, R. E., C. G. Victora, S. P. Walker, Z. A. Bhutta, P. Christian, M. de Onis, and R. Martorell. 2013. Maternal and child undernutrition and overweight in low-income and middle-income countries. *Lancet* 382 (9890):427–51. doi: 10.1016/S0140-6736(13) 60937-X.

Brown, A. F., A. Ang, and A. R. Pebley. 2007. The relationship between neighborhood characteristics and self-rated health for adults with chronic conditions. *American Journal of Public Health* 97 (5):926–32.

Campa, A., Z. Yang, S. Lai, L. Xue, J. C. Phillips, S. Sales, and M. K. Baum. 2005. HIV-related wasting in HIV-infected drug users in the era of highly active antiretroviral therapy. *Clinical Infectious Diseases* 41 (8):1179–85. doi: 10.1086/444499.

Carey, M. P., K. B. Carey, and S. C. Kalichman. 1997. Risk for human immunodeficiency virus (HIV) infection among persons with severe mental illnesses. *Clinical Psychology Review* 17 (3):271–91. doi: S0272-7358(97)00019-6 [pii].

Coates, J., E. A. Frongillo, B. L. Rogers, P. Webb, P. E. Wilde, and R. Houser. 2006. Commonalities in the experience of household food insecurity across cultures: What are measures missing? *Journal of Nutrition* 136 (5):1438S–48S.

Cole, S. M. and G. Tembo. 2011. The effect of food insecurity on mental health: Panel evidence from rural Zambia. *Social Science & Medicine* 73 (7):1071–79.

Coleman-Jensen, A., M. Nord, M. Andrews, and S. Carlson. 2012. Household food security in the United States in 2011. *USDA-ERS Economic Research Report*.

Crum-Cianflone, N., M. P. Roediger, L. Eberly, M. Headd, V. Marconi, A. Ganesan, and B. K. Agan. 2010. Increasing rates of obesity among HIV-infected persons during the HIV epidemic. *PLOS ONE* 5 (4):e10106.

Crum-Cianflone, N. F., M. Roediger, L. E. Eberly, K. Vyas, M. L. Landrum, A. Ganesan, and B. K. Agan. 2010. Obesity among HIV-infected persons: Impact of weight on CD4 cell count. *AIDS* 24 (7):1069.

Cunningham, W. E., R. M. Andersen, M. H. Katz, M. D. Stein, B. J. Turner, S. Crystal, and M. F. Shapiro. 1999. The impact of competing subsistence needs and barriers on access to medical care for persons with human immunodeficiency virus receiving care in the United States. *Medical Care* 37 (12):1270–81.

Dallman, M. F., N. C. Pecoraro, and S. E. la Fleur. 2005. Chronic stress and comfort foods: Self-medication and abdominal obesity. *Brain, Behavior, and Immunity* 19 (4):275–80.

Dallman, M. F., N. Pecoraro, S. F. Akana, S. E. La Fleur, F. Gomez, H. Houshyar, and S. Manalo. 2003. Chronic stress and obesity: A new view of "comfort food". *Proceedings of the National Academy of Sciences* 100 (20):11696–701.

Dalstra, J. A. A., A. E. Kunst, C. Borrell, E. Breeze, E. Cambois, G. Costa, and N. K. Rasmussen. 2005. Socioeconomic differences in the prevalence of common chronic diseases: An overview of eight European countries. *International Journal of Epidemiology* 34 (2):316–26.

Danziger, R. 1994. The social impact of HIV/AIDS in developing countries. *Social Science & Medicine* 39 (7):905–17.

Dinour, L. M., D. Bergen, and M.-C. Yeh. 2007. The food insecurity-obesity paradox: A review of the literature and the role food stamps may play. *Journal of the American Dietetic Association* 107 (11):1952–61.

Dixon, L. B., M. A. Winkleby, and K. L. Radimer. 2001. Dietary intakes and serum nutrients differ between adults from food-insufficient and food-sufficient families: Third National Health and Nutrition Examination Survey, 1988–1994. *Journal of Nutrition* 131 (4):1232–46.

Drewnowski, A. and N. Darmon. 2005. The economics of obesity: Dietary energy density and energy cost. *American Journal of Clinical Nutrition* 82 (1 Suppl):265S–73S.

Eicher-Miller, H. A., A. C. Mason, A. R. Abbott, G. P. McCabe, and C. J. Boushey. 2009. The effect of Food Stamp Nutrition Education on the food insecurity of low-income women participants. *Journal of Nutrition Education and Behavior* 41 (3):161–8.

Erridge, C. 2008. The roles of pathogen-associated molecular patterns in atherosclerosis. *Trends in Cardiovascular Medicine* 18 (2):52–6.

Erridge, C., T. Attina, C. M. Spickett, and D. J. Webb. 2007. A high-fat meal induces low-grade endotoxemia: Evidence of a novel mechanism of postprandial inflammation. *American Journal of Clinical Nutrition* 86 (5):1286–92. doi: 86/5/1286 [pii].

Evans, D. L., T. R. Ten Have, S. D. Douglas, D. R. Gettes, M. Morrison, M. S. Chiappini, and J. M. Petitto. 2002. Association of depression with viral load, CD8 T lymphocytes, and natural killer cells in women with HIV infection. *American Journal of Psychiatry* 159 (10):1752–9.

Farmer, P., S. Lindenbaum, and M. Good. 1993. Women, poverty and AIDS: An introduction. *Culture, Medicine and Psychiatry* 17:387–97.

Fernald, L. C., P. J. Gertler, and L. M. Neufeld. 2008. Role of cash in conditional cash transfer programmes for child health, growth, and development: An analysis of Mexico's Oportunidades. *Lancet* 371 (9615):828–37. doi: 10.1016/S0140-6736(08)60382-7.

Food and Agriculture Organization. 2012. *The State of Food Insecurity in the World 2012* http://www.fao.org/publications/sofi/en/. Rome: FAO.

Food and Agriculture Organization. 2013. From Protection to Production: The role of cash transfer programmes in fostering broad-based economic development in sub-Saharan Africa. [Project Brief]. Food and Agriculture Organization. Accessed September 10, 2014. http://www.fao.org/fileadmin/user_upload/p2p/Documents/flyer_PtoP_bassa-bis.pdf.

Friis, H. 2005. *Micronutrients and HIV Infection: A Review of Current Evidence*. Durban, South Africa: World Health Organization.

Friis-Møller, N., R. Weber, P. Reiss, R. Thiébaut, O. Kirk, A. A. Monforte, and M. Law. 2003. Cardiovascular disease risk factors in HIV patients-association with antiretroviral therapy. Results from the DAD study. *AIDS* 17 (8):1179.

Frith, A. L. 2006. The Influence of Maternal Nutritional and Support Interventions and Stress on Maternal-Infant Feeding Interaction in Bangladesh. Doctoral thesis, Division of Nutritional Sciences, Cornell University.

Gibson, T. B., X. Song, B. Alemayehu, S. S. Wang, J. L. Waddell, J. R. Bouchard, and F. Forma. 2010. Cost sharing, adherence, and health outcomes in patients with diabetes. *American Journal of Managed Care* 16 (8):589–600.

Gluckman, P. D. and M. A. Hanson. 2008. Developmental and epigenetic pathways to obesity: An evolutionary-developmental perspective. *International Journal of Obesity* 32:S62–71.

Gowda, C., C. Hadley, and A. E. Aiello. 2012. The association between food insecurity and inflammation in the US adult population. *American Journal of Public Health* 102 (8):1579–86.

Gucciardi, E., J. A. Vogt, M. DeMelo, and D. E. Stewart. 2009. Exploration of the relationship between household food insecurity and diabetes in Canada. *Diabetes Care* 32 (12):2218–24.

Gundersen, C., B. J. Lohman, S. Garasky, S. Stewart, and J. Eisenmann. 2008. Food security, maternal stressors, and overweight among low-income US children: Results from the national health and nutrition examination survey (1999–2002). *Pediatrics* 122 (3): e529–40.

Gundersen, C. and B. Kreider. 2009. Bounding the effects of food insecurity on children's health outcomes. *Journal of Health Economics* 28 (5):971–83. doi: 10.1016/j.jhealeco.2009.06.012.

Gustavson, L., W. Lam, R. Bertz, A. Hsu, K. Rynkiewicz, Q. Ji, and E. Sun. 2000. Assessment of the bioequivalence and food effects for liquid and soft gelatin capsule co-formulations of ABT-378/ritonavir (ABT-378/r) in healthy subjects. *40th Interscience Conference on Antimicrobial Agents and Chemotherapy*, Toronto, Canada.

Hadley, C., A. Tegegn, F. Tessema, J. A. Cowan, M. Asefa, and S. Galea. 2008. Food insecurity, stressful life events and symptoms of anxiety and depression in east Africa: Evidence from the Gilgel Gibe growth and development study. *Journal of Epidemiology and Community Health* 62 (11):980–6.

Hamelin, A. M., M. Beaudry, and J. P. Habicht. 2002. Characterization of household food insecurity in Quebec: Food and feelings. *Social Science & Medicine* 54 (1):119–32.

Heflin, C. M., K. Siefert, and D. R. Williams. 2005. Food insufficiency and women's mental health: Findings from a 3-year panel of welfare recipients. *Social Science & Medicine* 61 (9):1971–82.

Herman, D. R., M. Taylor Baer, E. Adams, L. Cunningham-Sabo, N. Duran, D. B. Johnson, and E. Yakes. 2014. Life course perspective: Evidence for the role of nutrition. *Maternal and Child Health Journal.* 18(2):450–61. doi: 10.1007/s10995-013-1280-3.

Hunt, P. W. 2007. Role of immune activation in HIV pathogenesis. *Current HIV/AIDS Reports* 4 (1):42–7.

Ickovics, J. R., M. E. Hamburger, D. Vlahov, E. E. Schoenbaum, P. Schuman, R. J. Boland, and J. Moore. 2001. Mortality, CD4 cell count decline, and depressive symptoms among HIV-seropositive women: Longitudinal analysis from the HIV Epidemiology Research Study. *JAMA* 285 (11):1466–74. doi: joc01588 [pii].

Iliff, P. J., E. G. Piwoz, N. V. Tavengwa, C. D. Zunguza, E. T. Marinda, K. J. Nathoo, and J. H. Humphrey. 2005. Early exclusive breastfeeding reduces the risk of postnatal HIV-1 transmission and increases HIV-free survival. *AIDS* 19 (7):699–708. doi: 00002030-200504290-00007 [pii].

Kacanek, D., D. L. Jacobson, D. Spiegelman, C. Wanke, R. Isaac, and I. B. Wilson. 2010. Incident depression symptoms are associated with poorer HAART adherence: A longitudinal analysis from the Nutrition for Healthy Living Study. *JAIDS Journal of Acquired Immune Deficiency Syndromes* 53 (2):266–72. doi: 10.1097/QAI.0b013e3181b720e7.

Kalichman, S. C., C. Cherry, C. Amaral, D. White, M. O. Kalichman, H. Pope, and R. Macy. 2010. Health and treatment implications of food insufficiency among people living with HIV/AIDS, Atlanta, Georgia. *Journal of Urban Health* 87 (4):631–41. doi: 10.1007/s11524-010-9446-4.

Kendall, A., C. M. Olson, and E. A. Frongillo Jr. 1996. Relationship of hunger and food insecurity to food availability and consumption. *Journal of the American Dietetic Association* 96 (10):1019–24.

Kerr, R. B., P. R. Berti, and M. Chirwa. 2007. Breastfeeding and mixed feeding practices in Malawi: Timing, reasons, decision makers, and child health consequences. *Food and Nutrition Bulletin* 28 (1):90–9.

Kirkpatrick, S. I. and V. Tarasuk. 2008. Food insecurity is associated with nutrient inadequacies among Canadian adults and adolescents. *Journal of Nutrition* 138 (3):604–12.

Koethe, J. R., B. H. Chi, K. M. Megazzini, D. C. Heimburger, and J. S. Stringer. 2009. Macronutrient supplementation for malnourished HIV-infected adults: A review of the evidence in resource-adequate and resource-constrained settings. *Clinical Infectious Diseases* 49 (5):787–98.

Kuller, L. H., R. Tracy, W. Belloso, S. De Wit, F. Drummond, H. C. Lane, and J. D. Neaton. 2008. Inflammatory and coagulation biomarkers and mortality in patients with HIV infection. *PLOS Medicine* 5 (10):e203. doi: 10.1371/journal.pmed.0050203.

Kushel, M. B., R. Gupta, L. Gee, and J. S. Haas. 2006. Housing instability and food insecurity as barriers to health care among low-income Americans. *Journal of General Internal Medicine* 21 (1):71–7.

Lagarde, E., M. Schim van der Loeff, C. Enel, B. Holmgren, R. Dray-Spira, G. Pison, and P. Aaby. 2003. Mobility and the spread of human immunodeficiency virus into rural areas of West Africa. *International Journal of Epidemiology* 32 (5):744–52.

Laraia, B. A. 2013. Food insecurity and chronic disease. *Advances in Nutrition: An International Review Journal* 4 (2):203–12.

Laraia, B. A., A. M. Siega-Riz, and C. Gundersen. 2010. Household food insecurity is associated with self-reported pregravid weight status, gestational weight gain, and pregnancy complications. *Journal of the American Dietetic Association* 110 (5):692–701.

Laraia, B. A., A. M. Siega-Riz, C. Gundersen, and N. Dole. 2006. Psychosocial factors and socioeconomic indicators are associated with household food insecurity among pregnant women. *Journal of Nutrition* 136 (1):177–82.

Laraia, B., E. Epel, and A. M. Siega-Riz. 2013. Food insecurity with past experience of restrained eating is a recipe for increased gestational weight gain. *Appetite* 65:187–84. doi: 10.1016/j.appet.2013.01.018.

Larson, N. I. and M. T. Story. 2011. Food insecurity and weight status among US children and families: A review of the literature. *American Journal of Preventive Medicine* 40 (2):166–73.

Larson, N. I., M. T. Story, and M. C. Nelson. 2009. Neighborhood environments: Disparities in access to healthy foods in the US. *American Journal of Preventive Medicine* 36 (1): 74–81. e10.

Leddy, M. A., M. L. Power, and J. Schulkin. 2008. The impact of maternal obesity on maternal and fetal health. *Reviews in Obstetrics and Gynecology* 1 (4):170.

Lent, M. D., L. E. Petrovic, J. A. Swanson, and C. M. Olson. 2009. Maternal mental health and the persistence of food insecurity in poor rural families. *Journal of Health Care for the Poor and Underserved* 20 (3):645–61. doi: 10.1353/hpu.0.0182.

Leroy, J. L., P. Gadsden, T. González de Cossío, and P. Gertler. 2013. Cash and in-kind transfers lead to excess weight gain in a population of women with a high prevalence of overweight in rural Mexico. *Journal of Nutrition* 143 (3):378–83.

Lim, S. S., T. Vos, A. D. Flaxman, G. Danaei, K. Shibuya, H. Adair-Rohani, and Z. A. Memish. 2013. A comparative risk assessment of burden of disease and injury attributable to 67 risk factors and risk factor clusters in 21 regions, 1990–2010: A systematic analysis for the Global Burden of Disease Study 2010. *Lancet* 380 (9859):2224–60. doi: 10.1016/S0140-6736(12)61766-8.

Lozano, R., M. Naghavi, K. Foreman, S. Lim, K. Shibuya, V. Aboyans, and St. Y. Ahn. 2013. Global and regional mortality from 235 causes of death for 20 age groups in 1990 and 2010: A systematic analysis for the Global Burden of Disease Study 2010. *Lancet* 380 (9859):2095–128.

Ma, C. T., L. Gee, and M. B. Kushel. 2008. Associations between housing instability and food insecurity with health care access in low-income children. *Ambulatory Pediatrics* 8 (1):50–7. doi: 10.1016/j.ambp.2007.08.004.

Macallan, D. C., C. Noble, C. Baldwin, S. A. Jebb, A. M. Prentice, W. A. Coward, and G. E. Griffin. 1995. Energy expenditure and wasting in human immunodeficiency virus infection. *New England Journal of Medicine* 333 (2):83–8.

Mahlungulu, S., L. A. Grobler, M. E. Visser, and J. Volmink. 2007. Nutritional interventions for reducing morbidity and mortality in people with HIV. *Cochrane Database of Systematic Reviews* (3):CD004536. doi: 10.1002/14651858.CD004536.pub2.

Marjerrison, S., E. A. Cummings, N. T. Glanville, S. F. L. Kirk, and M. Ledwell. 2011. Prevalance and associations of food insecurity in children with diabetes mellitus. *Journal of Pediatrics* 158 (4):607–11.

Martin, M. A. and A. M. Lippert. 2012. Feeding her children, but risking her health: The intersection of gender, household food insecurity and obesity. *Social Science & Medicine* 74 (11):1754–64. doi: 10.1016/j.socscimed.2011.11.013.

Maslowski, K. M. and C. R. Mackay. 2011. Diet, gut microbiota and immune responses. *Nature Immunology* 12 (1):5–9. doi: 10.1038/ni0111-5.

Mazzaglia, G., E. Ambrosioni, M. Alacqua, A. Filippi, E. Sessa, V. Immordino, and L. G. Mantovani. 2009. Adherence to antihypertensive medications and cardiovascular morbidity among newly diagnosed hypertensive patients. *Circulation* 120 (16):1598–605.

Mbugua, S., N. Andersen, P. Tuitoek, F. Yeudall, D. Sellen, N. Karanja, and G. Prain. 2008. Assessment of food security and nutrition status among households affected by HIV/AIDS in Nakuru Municipality, Kenya. *XVII International AIDS Conference*, Mexico City, August 3–8, 2008.

McIntyre, D., M. Thiede, G. Dahlgren, and M. Whitehead. 2006. What are the economic consequences for households of illness and of paying for health care in low- and middle-income country contexts? *Social Science & Medicine* 62 (4):858–65.

Mehta, S., K. P. Manji, A. M. Young, E. R. Brown, C. Chasela, T. E. Taha, and W. W. Fawzi. 2008. Nutritional indicators of adverse pregnancy outcomes and mother-to-child transmission of HIV among HIV-infected women. *American Journal of Clinical Nutrition* 87 (6):1639–49. doi: 87/6/1639 [pii].

Miller, C. L., D. R. Bangsberg, D. M. Tuller, J. Senkungu, A. Kawuma, E. A. Frongillo, and S. D. Weiser. 2011. Food insecurity and sexual risk in an HIV endemic community in Uganda. *AIDS and Behavior* 15 (7):1512–9.

Mills, E. J., J. B. Nachega, I. Buchan, J. Orbinski, A. Attaran, S. Singh, and D. R. Bangsberg. 2006. Adherence to antiretroviral therapy in sub-Saharan Africa and North America: A meta-analysis. *JAMA* 296 (6):679–90.

Must, A., J. Spadano, E. H. Coakley, A. E. Field, G. Colditz, and W. H. Dietz. 1999. The disease burden associated with overweight and obesity. *JAMA* 282 (16):1523–29.

Neel, J. V. 1962. Diabetes mellitus: A "thrifty" genotype rendered detrimental by "progress"? *American Journal of Human Genetics* 14 (4):353.

Nelson, K., M. E. Brown, and N. Lurie. 1998. Hunger in an adult patient population. *JAMA* 279 (15):1211–4.

Nixon, D. E. and A. L. Landay. 2010. Biomarkers of immune dysfunction in HIV. *Current Opinion in HIV and AIDS* 5 (6):498–503.

Nord, M., A. Coleman-Jensen, M. Andrews, and S. Carlson. 2010. Household food security in the United States, 2009. Washington, DC: United States Department of Agriculture (USDA).

Oyefara, J. L. 2007. Food insecurity, HIV/AIDS pandemic and sexual behaviour of female commercial sex workers in Lagos metropolis, Nigeria. *SAHARA Journal* 4 (2):626–35.

Paes-Sousa, R., L. M. Santos, and E. S. Miazaki. 2011. Effects of a conditional cash transfer programme on child nutrition in Brazil. *Bulletin of the World Health Organization* 89 (7):496–503. doi: 10.2471/BLT.10.084202.

Palar, K., G. Wagner, B. Ghosh-Dastidar, and P. Mugyenyi. 2012. Role of antiretroviral therapy in improving food security among patients initiating HIV treatment and care. *AIDS* 26 (18):2375–81.

Peretti-Watel, P., B. Spire, M. A. Schiltz, A. D. Bouhnik, I. Heard, F. Lert, and Y. Obadia. 2006. Vulnerability, unsafe sex and non-adherence to HAART: Evidence from a large sample of French HIV/AIDS outpatients. *Social Science & Medicine* 62 (10):2420–33. doi: 10.1016/j.socscimed.2005.10.020.

Physicians for Human Rights. 2007. *Epidemic of Inequality: Women's Rights and HIV/AIDS in Botswana & Swaziland: An Evidence-Based Report on the Effects of Gender Inequity, Stigma and Discrimination.* Cambridge, MA.

Radimer, K. L., C. M. Olson, J. C. Greene, C. C. Campbell, and J. P. Habicht. 1992. Understanding hunger and developing indicators to assess it in women and children. *Journal of Nutrition Education* 24 (1 suppl.):36S–44S.

Rose, D. 1999. Economic determinants and dietary consequences of food insecurity in the United States. *Journal of Nutrition* 129 (2S Suppl):517S–20S.

Rose-Jacobs, R., M. M. Black, P. H. Casey, J. T. Cook, D. B. Cutts, M. Chilton, and D. A. Frank. 2008. Household food insecurity: Associations with at-risk infant and toddler development. *Pediatrics* 121 (1):65–72. doi: 10.1542/peds.2006-3717.

Rosmond, R., M. F. Dallman, and P. Bjorntorp. 1998. Stress-related cortisol secretion in men: Relationships with abdominal obesity and endocrine, metabolic and hemodynamic abnormalities. *The Journal of Clinical Endocrinology and Metabolism* 83 (6):1853–9.

Royce, R. A., A. Sena, W. Cates, Jr., and M. S. Cohen. 1997. Sexual transmission of HIV. *New England Journal of Medicine* 336 (15):1072–8. doi: 10.1056/NEJM199704103361507.

Schaible, U. E. and H. E. Stefan. 2007. Malnutrition and infection: Complex mechanisms and global impacts. *PLOS Medicine* 4 (5):e115.

Schectman, J. M., M. M. Nadkarni, and J. D. Voss. 2002. The association between diabetes metabolic control and drug adherence in an indigent population. *Diabetes Care* 25 (6):1015–21.

Schreck, R., P. Rieber, and P. A. Baeuerle. 1991. Reactive oxygen intermediates as apparently widely used messengers in the activation of the NF-kappa B transcription factor and HIV-1. *EMBO Journal* 10 (8):2247–58.

Seligman, H. K., A. B. Bindman, E. Vittinghoff, A. M. Kanaya, and M. B. Kushel. 2007. Food insecurity is associated with diabetes mellitus: Results from the National Health Examination and Nutrition Examination Survey (NHANES) 1999–2002. *Journal of General Internal Medicine* 22 (7):1018–23.

Seligman, H. K., B. A. Laraia, and M. B. Kushel. 2010. Food insecurity is associated with chronic disease among low-income NHANES participants. *Journal of Nutrition* 140 (2): 304–10. doi: 10.3945/jn.109.112573.

Seligman, H. K., E. A. Jacobs, A. López, J. Tschann, and A. Fernandez. 2012. Food insecurity and glycemic control among low-income patients with type 2 diabetes. *Diabetes Care* 35 (2):233–8.

Seligman, H. K., T. C. Davis, D. Schillinger, and M. S. Wolf. 2010. Food insecurity is associated with hypoglycemia and poor diabetes self-management in a low-income sample with diabetes. *Journal of Health Care for the Poor and Underserved* 21 (4):1227. doi: 10.1353/hpu.2010.0921.

Shannon, K., T. Kerr, M.-J. Milloy, A. Anema, R. Zhang, J. S. G. Montaner, and E. Wood. 2011. Severe food insecurity is associated with elevated unprotected sex among HIV-seropositive injection drug users independent of HAART use. *AIDS* 25 (16):2037–42.

Singh, S. 2003. Food crisis and AIDS: The Indian perspective. *Lancet* 362 (9399):1938–9. doi: 10.1016/S0140-6736(03)14980-X.

Sopheab, H., K. Fylkesnes, M. C. Vun, and N. O'Farrell. 2006. HIV-related risk behaviors in Cambodia and effects of mobility. *JAIDS Journal of Acquired Immune Deficiency Syndromes* 41 (1):81–6.

Steptoe, A., L. Perkins-Porras, C. McKay, E. Rink, S. Hilton, and F. P. Cappuccio. 2003. Behavioural counselling to increase consumption of fruit and vegetables in low income adults: Randomised trial. *BMJ* 326 (7394):855.

Stuff, J. E., P. H. Casey, C. L. Connell, C. M. Champagne, J. M. Gossett, D. Harsha, and K. L. Szeto. 2007. Household food insecurity and obesity, chronic disease, and chronic disease risk factors. *Journal of Hunger & Environmental Nutrition* 1 (2):43–62.

Stuff, J. E., P. H. Casey, K. L. Szeto, J. M. Gossett, J. M. Robbins, P. M. Simpson, and M. L. Bogle. 2004. Household food insecurity is associated with adult health status. *Journal of Nutrition* 134 (9):2330–35.

Sztam, K. A., W. W. Fawzi, and C. Duggan. 2010. Macronutrient supplementation and food prices in HIV treatment. *Journal of Nutrition* 140 (1):213S–23S. doi: 10.3945/jn.109.110569.

Tarasuk, V., A. Mitchell, L. McLaren, and L. McIntyre. 2013. Chronic physical and mental health conditions among adults may increase vulnerability to household food insecurity. *Journal of Nutrition*. 113.178483.

Taylor, L., J. Seeley, and E. Kajura. 1996. Informal care for illness in rural southwest Uganda: The central role that women play. *Health Transition Review* 6 (1):49–56.

Tegger, M. K., H. M. Crane, K. A. Tapia, K. K. Uldall, S. E. Holte, and M. M. Kitahata. 2008. The effect of mental illness, substance use, and treatment for depression on the initiation of highly active antiretroviral therapy among HIV-infected individuals. *AIDS Patient Care STDS* 22 (3):233–43. doi: 10.1089/apc.2007.0092.

Tsai, A. C., D. R. Bangsberg, E. A. Frongillo, P. W. Hunt, C. Muzoora, J. N. Martin, and S. D. Weiser. 2012. Food insecurity, depression and the modifying role of social support among people living with HIV/AIDS in rural Uganda. *Social Science & Medicine* 74 (12):2012–19.

Tsai, A. C., D. R. Bangsberg, N. Emenyonu, J. K. Senkungu, J. N. Martin, and S. D. Weiser. 2011. The social context of food insecurity among persons living with HIV/AIDS in rural Uganda. *Social Science & Medicine* 73 (12):1717–24.

Tsai, A. C., K. J. Hung, and S. D. Weiser. 2012. Is food insecurity associated with HIV risk? Cross-sectional evidence from sexually active women in Brazil. *PLOS Medicine* 9 (4):e1001203. doi: 10.1371/journal.pmed.1001203.

Tsai, A. C., K. Leiter, M. Heisler, V. Iacopino, W. Wolfe, K. Shannon, and S. Weiser. 2011. Prevalence and correlates of forced sex perpetration and victimization in Botswana and Swaziland. *American Journal of Public Health* 101 (6):1068.

Tsai, A. C., S. D. Weiser, M. L. Petersen, K. Ragland, M. B. Kushel, and D. R. Bangsberg. 2010. A marginal structural model to estimate the causal effect of antidepressant medication treatment on viral suppression among homeless and marginally housed persons with HIV. *Archives of General Psychiatry* 67 (12):1282.

Tucker, J. S., M. A. Burnam, C. D. Sherbourne, F. Y. Kung, and A. L. Gifford. 2003. Substance use and mental health correlates of nonadherence to antiretroviral medications in a sample of patients with human immunodeficiency virus infection. *American Journal of Medicine* 114 (7):573–80. doi: S0002934303000937 [pii].

van der Sande, M. A., M. F. Schim van der Loeff, A. A. Aveika, S. Sabally, T. Togun, R. Sarge-Njie, and H. C. Whittle. 2004. Body mass index at time of HIV diagnosis: A strong and independent predictor of survival. *JAIDS Journal of Acquired Immune Deficiency Syndromes* 37 (2):1288–94.

Vogenthaler, N. S., C. Hadley, A. E. Rodriguez, E. E. Valverde, C. del Rio, and L. R. Metsch. 2011. Depressive symptoms and food insufficiency among HIV-infected crack users in Atlanta and Miami. *AIDS and Behavior* 15 (7):1520–26.

Vogenthaler, N. S., M. B. Kushel, C. Hadley, E. A. Frongillo, E. D. Riley, D. R. Bangsberg, and S. D. Weiser. 2013. Food insecurity and risky sexual behaviors among homeless and marginally housed HIV-infected individuals in San Francisco. *AIDS and Behavior* 17 (5):1688–93. doi: 10.1007/s10461-012-0355-2.

Walsemann, K. M., J. A. Ailshire, B. A. Bell, and E. A. Frongillo. 2012. Body mass index trajectories from adolescence to midlife: Differential effects of parental and respondent education by race/ethnicity and gender. *Ethnicity & Health* 17 (4):337–62.

Webb-Girard, A., A. Cherobon, S. Mbugua, E. Kamau-Mbuthia, A. Amin, and D. W. Sellen. 2012. Food insecurity is associated with attitudes towards exclusive breastfeeding among women in urban Kenya. *Maternal & Child Nutrition* 8 (2):199–214.

Weiser, S. D., A. C. Tsai, R. Gupta, E. A. Frongillo, A. Kawuma, J. Senkungu, and D. R. Bangsberg. 2012. Food insecurity is associated with morbidity and patterns of health-care utilization among HIV-infected individuals in a resource-poor setting. *AIDS* 26 (1):67–75. doi: 10.1097/QAD.0b013e32834cad37.

Weiser, S. D., C. Yuan, D. Guzman, E. A. Frongillo, E. D. Riley, D. R. Bangsberg, and M. B. Kushel. 2013. Food insecurity and HIV clinical outcomes in a longitudinal study of homeless and marginally housed HIV-infected individuals in San Francisco. *AIDS* 27 (18):2953–8. doi: 10.1097/01.aids.0000432538.70088.a3.

Weiser, S. D., D. M. Tuller, E. A. Frongillo, J. Senkungu, N. Mukiibi, and D. R. Bangsberg. 2010. Food insecurity as a barrier to sustained antiretroviral therapy adherence in Uganda. *PLOS ONE* 5 (4):e10340. doi: 10.1371/journal.pone.0010340.

Weiser, S. D., D. R. Bangsberg, S. Kegeles, K. Ragland, M. B. Kushel, and E. A. Frongillo. 2009. Food insecurity among homeless and marginally housed individuals living with HIV/AIDS in San Francisco. *AIDS and Behavior* 13 (5):841–8. doi: 10.1007/s10461-009-9597-z.

Weiser, S. D., E. A. Frongillo, K. Ragland, R. S. Hogg, E. D. Riley, and D. R. Bangsberg. 2009. Food insecurity is associated with incomplete HIV RNA suppression among homeless and marginally housed HIV-infected individuals in San Francisco. *Journal of General Internal Medicine* 24 (1):14–20.

Weiser, S. D., K. Leiter, D. R. Bangsberg, L. M. Butler, F. Percy-de Korte, Z. Hlanze, and M. Heisler. 2007. Food insufficiency is associated with high-risk sexual behavior among women in Botswana and Swaziland. *PLOS Medicine* 4 (10):1589–97; discussion 1598. doi: 10.1371/journal.pmed.0040260.

Weiser, S. D., K. Palar, E. A. Frongillo, A. C. Tsai, E. Kumbakumba, S. Depee, and D. R. Bangsberg. 2014. Longitudinal assessment of associations between food insecurity, antiretroviral adherence and HIV treatment outcomes in rural Uganda. *AIDS* 28 (1):115–20. doi: 10.1097/01.aids.0000433238.93986.35.

Weiser, S. D., K. A. Fernandes, E. K. Brandson, V. D. Lima, A. Anema, D. R. Bangsberg, and R. S. Hogg. 2009. The association between food insecurity and mortality among HIV-infected individuals on HAART. *JAIDS Journal of Acquired Immune Deficiency Syndromes* 52 (3):342–9.

Weiser, S. D., R. Gupta, A. C. Tsai, E. A. Frongillo, N. Grede, E. Kumbakumba, and D. R. Bangsberg. 2012. Changes in food insecurity, nutritional status, and physical health status after antiretroviral therapy initiation in rural Uganda. *JAIDS Journal of Acquired Immune Deficiency Syndromes* 61 (2):179–86.

Weiser, S. D., S. L. Young, C. R. Cohen, M. B. Kushel, A. C. Tsai, P. C. Tien, and D. R. Bangsberg. 2011. Conceptual framework for understanding the bidirectional links between food insecurity and HIV/AIDS. *American Journal of Clinical Nutrition* 94 (6):1729S–39S.

Whitaker, R. C. 2004. Predicting preschooler obesity at birth: The role of maternal obesity in early pregnancy. *Pediatrics* 114 (1):e29–e36.

Whitaker, R. C., S. M. Phillips, and S. M. Orzol. 2006. Food insecurity and the risks of depression and anxiety in mothers and behavior problems in their preschool-aged children. *Pediatrics* 118 (3):e859–68. doi: 10.1542/peds.2006-0239.

WHO. 2003. *Joint WHO/FAO Expert Consultation on Diet, Nutrition and the Prevention of Chronic Diseases*. Geneva: World Health Organization,.

Wilde, P. E. and C. K. Ranney. 2000. The monthly food stamp cycle: Shopping frequency and food intake decisions in an endogenous switching regression framework. *American Journal of Agricultural Economics* 82 (1):200–213.

Wilde, P. E. and J. N. Peterman. 2006. Individual weight change is associated with household food security status. *Journal of Nutrition* 136 (5):1395–1400.

Wolongevicz, D. M., L. Zhu, M. J. Pencina, R. W. Kimokoti, P. K. Newby, R. B. D'Agostino, and B. E. Millen. 2010. Diet quality and obesity in women: The Framingham Nutrition Studies. *British Journal of Nutrition* 103 (08):1223–29.

Womack, J., P. C. Tien, J. Feldman, J. H. Shin, K. Fennie, K. Anastos, and H. Minkoff. 2007. Obesity and immune cell counts in women. *Metabolism* 56 (7):998–1004. doi: 10.1016/j.metabol.2007.03.008.

World Health Organization. 2013. *Noncommunicable Diseases: Fact Sheet*. WHO Accessed August 29. http://www.who.int/mediacentre/factsheets/fs355/en/.

Yamano, T. and T. S. Jayne. 2004. Measuring the impact of working-age adult mortality on small-scale farm households in Kenya. *World Development* 32 (1):91–119.

Yamano, T. and T. S. Jayne. 2005. Working-age adult mortality and primary school attendance in rural Kenya. *Economic Development and Cultural Change Change* 53 (3):619–54.

Young, S., A. C. Wheeler, S. I. McCoy, and S. D. Weiser. 2014. A review of the role of food insecurity in adherence to care and treatment among adult and pediatric populations living with HIV and AIDS. *AIDS and Behavior* 18 (Suppl 5):S505–15. doi: 10.1007/s10461-013-0547-4.

Young, S. L., M. N. N. Mbuya, C. J. Chantry, E. P. Geubbels, K. Israel-Ballard, D. Cohan, and M. C. Latham. 2011. Current knowledge and future research on infant feeding in the context of HIV: Basic, clinical, behavioral, and programmatic perspectives. *Advances in Nutrition: An International Review Journal* 2 (3):225–43.

Zachariah, R., M. Fitzgerald, M. Massaquoi, O. Pasulani, L. Arnould, S. Makombe, and A. D. Harries. 2006. Risk factors for high early mortality in patients on antiretroviral treatment in a rural district of Malawi. *AIDS* 20 (18):2355–60. doi: 10.1097/QAD.0b013e32801086b0.

3 Food Insecurity Measurement

Jennifer Coates

CONTENTS

EVOLUTION OF FOOD SECURITY DEFINITIONS

The most widely accepted definition of food security is "a state in which all people, at all times, have physical and economic access to sufficient, safe, and nutritious food to meet their dietary needs and food preferences for an active and healthy life" (Food and Agriculture Organization 1996). But it was not always conceived this way, nor was there always such agreement. In the 1990s, Maxwell and Frankenberger identified over 200 variations of the definition, many of them similar but emphasizing different elements of the complex construct (1992). In fact, the food insecurity definition, and the policy focus that emerged from it, has evolved tremendously since the 1970s when the term was first used to describe a problem of national and global food availability. By the 1980s, the focus of definition (and the emphasis of the policy response) shifted to describe problems of food access (World Bank 1986). The 1990s ushered in an increasingly holistic definition, both in the United States and internationally, that incorporated elements of preference, quality, safety, and an emphasis on the stability of food access. Food *insecurity* was increasingly viewed as a more dynamic concept in the context of risk and risk management, with distinctions made about its severity, duration, and periodicity.

Though food insecurity is often described as having three pillars (availability, access, and utilization), arguably the ultimate objective is to ensure that individuals can utilize food of sufficient (1) quantity, (2) quality, (3) acceptability, and (4) safety in (5) a secure and stable way. Disaggregating these dimensions and measuring them accordingly should be the objective of any food security measurement effort. At the same time, assessing food availability and household access issues can help to elucidate the *causes* of individual food insecurity, while malnutrition and other public health outcomes should be considered as potential consequences of the problem.

MEASUREMENT OF FOOD INSECURITY

CONSIDERATIONS IN CHOOSING FOOD SECURITY INDICATORS: VALIDITY AND RELIABILITY

Validity is defined as the extent to which a method captures the phenomenon it is trying to measure for a particular purpose (Messick 1995; Goodwin and Leech 2003). A method is "neither valid nor invalid in and of itself, but only in regard to how it is used and what interpretations are given to the scores for particular groups of people" (Streiner and Norman 2006). Unfortunately, measures are often used without proper validation. For example, Hinkin reviewed 277 measures from over 75 academic journals relating to the behavioral sciences and concluded that only 17% had demonstrated any evidence of content validity (Hinkin 1995). It is important to know something about standards of validity and reliability in order to evaluate the merits of various food security indicators. This section briefly reviews definitions of these two terms and describes criteria that are used to assess them.

There are three main types of validity: "content," "construct," and "criterion" (De Vellis 1991). "Content validity" is the degree to which the questions that comprise a measure are *representative* of the phenomenon of interest (in this case, food insecurity). Creating a measure with content validity requires a solid theoretical understanding of the dimensions and boundaries of the construct to be measured, as well as the ability to develop questions that capture these dimensions. To establish content validity, one can rely on the literature and on expert input. A complementary approach, called cognitive debriefing, considers qualitative feedback provided by respondents about whether a set of questions makes sense and fully captures what they believe to be the important aspects of the construct.

A measure exhibits "construct validity," when it is associated as expected with other theoretically related variables (De Vellis 1991). For instance, one might expect an indicator of food security to be significantly correlated with income, or with nutrient intake. If they are not correlated, then this may indicate a problem with the metric being tested. This criterion is a relatively low bar, however; there is no standard for how strong the statistical relationship must be in order to serve as acceptable evidence of construct validity.

"Criterion validity" is more challenging to establish. It requires evidence of a strong correlation between the phenomenon of interest and a definitive benchmark (De Vellis 1991). Criterion validity is not typically assessed in evaluating food security indicators, because there is no one widely accepted gold standard against which to make comparisons. Caloric adequacy used to be considered a good "gold standard," but fell out of favor after researchers recognized that it only indicates the "quantity" dimension of a multidimensional issue.

"Reliability" differs from validity, in that it describes the ability of an indicator to yield consistent results when the underlying condition is unchanging (De Vellis 1991). It is possible for an indicator to be reliable (yielding consistent measures) but not valid (i.e., consistently not measuring what it is intended to measure). The sensitivity of a measure to change is also important in food security measurement; while we want to ensure that an indicator does not give different results when the underlying food security situation is the same, we often do need to identify measures that are able to detect relatively small shifts in food insecurity when the situation is changing. This measurement characteristic is important for purposes such as early warning and situation monitoring, as well as for program impact evaluation.

OTHER CONSIDERATIONS FOR CHOOSING INDICATORS

There are other important factors that must be considered in selecting food insecurity indicators. As shown in Figure 3.1, food security is measured for many different purposes. Knowing the objective of the measurement effort helps to dictate which indicator(s) are most appropriate. For instance, some indicators are not comparable across different geographic contexts and would not enable valid comparisons of prevalence estimates for geographic targeting. Such indicators would be better suited for tracking changes over time in a narrower setting, as is done in localized program monitoring and evaluation or as part of an early warning system.

It is also useful to keep in mind that not all programmatic decisions require "gold standard" data. Program planners and managers must be able to select the most suitable food security metric for their objectives, while bearing in mind the degree of confidence needed in the results (Habicht and Pelletier 1990; Habicht et al. 1999). There is often an inverse relationship between the resources required to measure something and the degree of accuracy and precision obtained. Fortunately, this trade-off has been somewhat reduced in the realm of food security measurement with the rise of a small set of valid, simple, low-cost instruments.

Population level:

- Estimation of prevalence (How many people are affected?)
- Determination of causes (Why are people affected?)
- Targeting (Who is affected?)
- Monitoring and early warning (How is the situation changing?)
- Evaluation of programs (Who has benefited and how?)

Individual level:

- Screening (Is the person at risk?)
- Diagnosis (Does the person have the problem?)
- Monitoring (Is the person/population's situation improving?)

FIGURE 3.1 Purposes of food security measurement. (From Frongillo, E.A. 1999. Validation of measures of food insecurity and hunger. *Journal of Nutrition* 129 (2):506S–509S.)

A related consideration has to do with the notion of "proxy" indicators, or indicators that are used as substitutes for the real thing because they are more feasible to implement. While in certain contexts a proxy measure may be necessary, all else equal a direct measure is preferred, and a "proximate" (close) proxy is preferred to a "distal" (distantly related) proxy. The main reason for this is that proxies tend to be less accurate than direct measures. The more directly we can measure something, the better we can count it, and the more effectively we can distinguish how it interacts with other closely related phenomena. For instance, having direct measures of food insecurity allows us to understand more about the relationship between food security and malnutrition than if malnutrition was used as a proxy indicator of food security. A final consideration in selecting indicators has to do with the extent to which measurement results can be easily and convincingly communicated for the purpose of influencing decision making. The FAO undernourishment measure is also called a "hunger measure," in part because hunger is an emotive term that is useful for advocacy purposes.

COMMON FOOD SECURITY METRICS

Barrett (2002) describes a generational transition in approaches to measuring food insecurity that largely paralleled developments in the definitions and usage of the concept. The first generation focused largely on measures of food *availability* at the national level, while the second generation of indicators reflected a renewed attention to the *access* dimension of household insecurity. The third generation has seen a shift toward understanding the behavior of individuals faced with uncertainty and constraints on choice. A fourth generation, still emerging, has concentrated on identifying universal indicators that can be applied without regard for context.

Barrett's use of the word "generations" should not be interpreted to mean that entire cohorts of metrics have come and gone, replaced by better and newer methods; the three different classes of measurement approaches are still in widespread, concurrent use by different people and for varying objectives. Rather than championing one approach to over all others, leaders in the field recognize that the multi-dimensional concept cannot be sufficiently captured by one indicator (Food and Agriculture Organization of the United Nations 2002; Carletto et al. 2013; Coates 2013). Nonetheless, it is true that each new generation has evolved to improve upon perceived conceptual and methodological shortcomings of the previous generation of measures. The generational distinction serves as a useful organizing framework for this section, which examines these methodological developments and highlights some of the key strengths and weaknesses associated with each stage of food security measurement's evolution.

First Generation: Measures of Food Availability

The principal measure of food availability at the national level is derived through food balance sheets. Food balance sheets are national-level accounts that track food production, imports, exports, waste/animal feed/seed, and stock holdings. Subtracting all sources of food supply from all sources of utilization yields an estimate of the amount of food available for human consumption. Per capita dietary energy supply (called DES) is estimated by converting this quantity of available food into its calorie equivalent, transforming the result from an annual to a daily figure, and factoring in the population size to produce a per capita indicator.

Despite widespread recognition that food insecurity can occur in locations where food is plentiful, and that national-level data does not accurately detect subnational and intrahousehold inequalities in food access, this approach is used to generate high-profile indicators of food insecurity. Following the UN World Food Summit in 1996, the Food and Agricultural Organization (FAO) was charged with the task of monitoring global and national progress toward the objective of halving hunger by 2015 (Food and Agriculture Organization 2004). The FAO measure of undernourishment is its indicator of hunger for this purpose. The measure is constructed by calculating total dietary energy supply (derived from food balance sheets) and adjusting this figure for distribution effects by estimating a coefficient of variation parameter for the "usual food consumption" of different income strata (from a household income/expenditure survey or using a theoretical modeling approach when survey data are not available). This adjusted supply figure is then compared against age- and sex-specific energy requirements that have been weighted according to their distribution in the population and then aggregated (Naiken 2002; Food and Agriculture Organization 2012). The estimation of supply relative to need produces an indicator of the prevalence and number of people who are undernourished, which is reported annually by FAO for most countries and regions around the world.

This FAO undernourishment measure provides useful data for assessing trends over time and across countries for purposes of monitoring progress toward, and advocating for attention to, international targets. Despite these advantages, the FAO measure has been criticized on a number of fronts. For instance, the food balance data used to estimate dietary energy supply are often of dubious quality (Food and Agriculture Organization 2004). The adjustments for inequality typically relied heavily on theoretical distributions whose parameters were modeled, introducing un quantified errors. Furthermore, the inequality coefficients that were derived from the expenditure data were not routinely updated to account for shifts in income distribution over time (Smith 2002).

Recently, FAO has revised aspects of its method of generating undernourishment estimates to improve on the quality of its results. Changes include: revised estimates of population size and structure and estimated dietary requirements based on new data on average height; changes in estimated dietary energy supply, accounting for food losses during retail distribution; and improved statistical estimation techniques, including a greater reliance on household consumption and expenditure surveys to provide more accurate information on the distribution of available energy (Food and Agriculture Organization, World Food Programme, and International Fund for Agricultural Development 2012). Following the introduction of this new method, FAO statisticians recalculated undernourishment trends from 1990 to 2012. The revised estimates suggest that undernourishment has declined more steeply than previously thought and that it did not spike in 2007/2008 following the global food price crisis. However, this approach continues to be criticized on various fronts. For instance, estimates of energy requirements assume only "sedentary" levels of energy expenditure. Lappé et al. (2013) point out that a more realistic assumption of "moderate" levels of energy expenditure for much of the global population would yield a very significant increase in number of people in the world deemed to be undernourished. Furthermore, this indicator takes into account only chronic food insecurity of at least a year, and cannot detect effects of rapid, shorter-term shocks like food price inflation.

Second Generation: Measures of Food "Access"

The second generation of food insecurity metrics focuses on capturing economic access to sufficient food as well as the individual consequences of insufficient access. Measures belonging to this category include household and individual-level indicators of calorie and nutrient adequacy, income, food expenditure, assets, anthropometric status, and related proxies.

Dietary data collected through individual or household-level 24-hour dietary recalls can be used to construct *caloric adequacy* indicators, which were considered for a long time to be a food security "gold standard" (Chung et al. 1997; Maxwell et al. 1999; Swindale and Ohri-Vachaspati 2000). But while caloric adequacy contributes information about whether the quantity of food consumed is sufficient at one time point (typically the previous 24-hours), it does not yield information about the nutritional quality of the diet or the stability of consumption over time. Equally important to note is that collecting and analyzing quantifiable information on dietary intake is very time consuming and requires highly trained staff. For this reason, it is not often done outside of research contexts.

A recent set of initiatives has aimed to highlight the potential for harnessing national-level household consumption and expenditure survey (HCES) data for estimating household-level caloric adequacy. This type of survey is undertaken every 4–5 years by many governments in order to track the consumer price index and national poverty levels. These surveys are not designed specifically for the purpose of estimating caloric or nutrient adequacy and, as such, are not always constructed to facilitate highly accurate estimates. However, there is ongoing advocacy by FAO, the World Bank, and others to support governments in instituting relatively minor survey design tweaks that would greatly increase the surveys' usefulness for food security and nutrition purposes (Fiedler et al. 2012). Additionally, the food security and nutrition communities have published guidance for harnessing existing HCES data into useful food security measures (Smith and Subandoro 2007; Fiedler et al. 2012). While using a secondary data source dramatically reduces the overall cost, the analytical burden can still be fairly substantial. Calculating caloric adequacy from HCES data as one of a dashboard of food security indicators can be useful for national-level policy design or global monitoring. It is less useful for programmatic purposes where simpler, more frequent feedback on progress is required.

A *Dietary Diversity Index* is a simple method, calculated from a short questionnaire, that asks which food groups the household (or an individual in the household) has consumed over some time period, typically either 24 hours or 7 days (Coates et al. 2007). This type of indicator can also be constructed from more in-depth 24-hour recall data or household food consumption and expenditure surveys. When measured at the household level, dietary diversity is considered to be an indicator of household food access. One reason for this is that resource-constrained households tend to first focus on ensuring they have "enough" food to eat by consuming calorie-rich staple foods. Only once energy needs are relatively adequate do they typically diversify their consumption to more micronutrient-rich fruits, vegetables, and animal products that are considered "luxury goods" in many settings (Hoddinott and Yohannes 2002). A higher dietary diversity score is typically associated with greater economic access, higher calorie consumption, as well as the consumption of a more nutritionally well-rounded diet (Hoddinott and Yohannes 2002; Ruel 2003; Coates et al. 2007). This type of measure has been widely promoted by FANTA and FAO (Swindale and Bilinsky 2006b; Kennedy et al. 2013). Such measures are quick and easy to implement and tabulate and are sensitive to fluctuations in dietary patterns across seasons and following shocks. For these reasons, dietary diversity indices are now in widespread use.

However, measures of dietary diversity do not show a consistent association with caloric adequacy across different cultures. For instance, in Bangladesh, a high average dietary diversity score was found to be associated with caloric insufficiency, whereas in other countries, caloric sufficiency was associated with a much lower dietary diversity score (Coates et al. 2007). One of the reasons for this phenomenon is that the dietary diversity questionnaire does not consider minimum portion sizes, so cultures that consume small amounts of many different types of foods and condiments, as in Bangladesh, can appear to have good dietary diversity when their caloric and overall nutrient intake is still relatively low. This issue is not so critical when the measure will be used in just one culture, but it does become important when seeking to compare the scores of households from different contexts. It is difficult to say whether households with the same index score are equally "food-insecure," and it is not possible to draw one universal cut off on the index in order to distinguish food-secure from food-insecure households across different settings.

A second important factor is that this type of measure, implemented at the household level, does not reflect intra household food distribution. For this reason, individual dietary diversity scores *(IDDS)* have been developed for target individuals in the household (e.g., women, children) as a complement to, or substitute for, household-level information. Studies have shown that these scores do a good job at predicting maternal micronutrient adequacy and child malnutrition (Arimond and Ruel 2004; Arimond et al. 2010; Kennedy et al. 2010).

The *Food Consumption Score*, promoted by the UN World Food Program, is similar to the household dietary diversity index except that it weights the consumption of different food groups differently—those that are considered more nutritionally desirable, such as pulses or vegetables, receive a higher weight. The FCS also prescribes cutoffs on this index score that categorize households as having "poor," "borderline," or "acceptable" food consumption (World Food Programme VAM Unit 2008). Validation studies of the FCS have demonstrated its association with caloric adequacy. However, the authors found that an unweighted version of the index performed just as well as the weighted one (Coates et al. 2007; Wiesmann et al. 2008). As mentioned above, thresholds for a categorical indicator such as these are arbitrary—they do not consistently correspond to "acceptable" caloric or nutrient intake in all cultures and would need to be adjusted to be contextually appropriate.

Measures of *total household income, expenditure, and assets* offer a well-rounded picture of a household's entitlement bundle—its economic potential to command food. Expenditure data are typically considered more reliable than income data for this purpose, but measures of asset holdings are seen as a better way of assessing household stochastic poverty, as asset holdings capture a household's situation net of regular fluctuations that occur in income and expenditures over time (Carter and Barrett 2006). People studying food security dynamics, therefore, appreciate measures of assets.

A more direct indicator is total per capita *food expenditure*, which assesses the amount of money a household spends in a given time period on food. As a way of standardizing comparisons across households, this indicator is often transformed into "the *proportion of total expenditures (or total income) devoted to food*" (Smith and Subandoro 2007). Most poor, food-insecure households spend a relatively large portion of their overall budget on food. The higher the proportion, the more challenged a household is likely to be in meeting its food needs. Like many other indicators, this relationship does not hold in all contexts. For instance, the *Economist* reported that the average household in Russia spends a greater share of income on food than its counterpart in India (Economist.com 2013).

A major challenge with relying on indicators of income and expenditure for programmatic purposes is that the data, supplied through household surveys, are labor intensive and costly to collect accurately. While the aforementioned initiatives to harness national-level HCES data for assessing food security are very useful for national policy making, they are less helpful for measuring program impact or for monitoring shorter-term fluctuations in food security. Another problem is that such indicators are suggestive of overall household economic access, but do not reveal anything about other key food security dimensions, such as stability, safety, or food preferences.

Anthropometric indicators, also a member of "second generation" of measures, are often championed as an expedient way of capturing what many perceive to be not only a conceptually close correlate of food security, but also the outcome of greatest interest. Yet, like other indicators of this generation, they are not very specific measures of food insecurity. Poor nutrition outcomes can be caused by many other factors in addition to food insecurity, including poor health, insufficient hygiene and sanitation, and poor caring practices. As discussed later in this chapter, food insecurity can also result in other important outcomes aside from those manifesting in malnutrition.

With the exception of dietary diversity indices, these second-generation measures are not ideal for programmatic contexts due to a combination of factors: (1) they are unidimensional, capturing but one aspect of food insecurity; (2) they are resource intensive to estimate (particularly caloric adequacy, income, expenditure, and assets); (3) they are distal and nonspecific measures: that is, they do not measure food security directly. Hence, over the past decade, there has been a convergence of interest on the part of academics and practitioners to produce simple, scientifically developed, and validated approaches to capturing the multiple dimensions of food insecurity that are largely missing from second-generation measures. Progress on this front has been made via this class of "third-generation" indicators, described below.

Third Generation: Experiential Measures

The third-generation measures of food insecurity are characterized by an increased focus on the "vulnerability" dimension inherent in food insecurity, an emphasis on individual subjective perceptions of insecurity, and attempts to capture these elements of the food insecurity experience through more direct, "fundamental" measures. Two notable members of the third generation, the Coping Strategies Index (CSI) and several experiential food insecurity scales, are described here.

The Coping Strategies Index

The CSI was developed by Daniel Maxwell and colleagues in the latter half of the 1990s (Maxwell 1996; Maxwell et al. 1999, 2003). In recent years, it has become a popular third-generation food insecurity measurement tool, having been adopted by WFP/VAM (World Food Programme/Vulnerability Analysis Mapping Unit), FAO/FSNAU (UN Food and Agriculture Organization/Food Security and Nutrition Analysis Unit for Somalia), and the Global IPC (Integrated Phase Classification) team, among others (Maxwell et al. 2013).

The CSI method grew out of a body of work from the 1980s on the behavioral responses to famine which contended that, in contrast to widely held perceptions, people subjected to daily risks were not passive victims of sudden events, or exhibitors of bizarre and inexplicable behaviors, but were active participants in managing the risks that they faced in their daily lives (see Watts 1983; Longhurst 1986; Corbett 1988; De Waal 1989). Their work, along with even earlier work by Currey on the geographic distribution of these responses (Currey 1979; Currey and Hugo 1984), was influential in shaping the modern form of famine early warning systems, which previously had been largely dependent on aggregate indicators of food availability. Monitoring self-reported behavioral responses to food stress along with other proxies of entitlement decline showed promise as an alternative and more leading indicator of impending food crisis. During the late 1980s and early 1990s, the measurement of coping strategies began to be codified into vulnerability assessments, as well as food security and nutrition monitoring and early warning systems (Babu and Pinstrup-Andersen 1994; Eele 1994; Haddad et al. 1994; Quinn and Kennedy 1994; Davies 1996; Webb and Harinarayan 1999). Maxwell and colleagues advanced this work through a methodologically more sophisticated approach that could quantify what had previously produced largely qualitative results. The resulting tool is grounded in local food insecurity experience and can be used in a variety of settings for purposes ranging from food aid monitoring to early warning (Maxwell et al. 2003).

The CSI method typically begins with key informant interviews to develop a list of coping strategies that are commonly used in response to food insecurity. Following this step, participatory ranking exercises are conducted to achieve a consensus around the relative severity indicated by each coping strategy on the list. This list of coping strategies questions is later administered to a sample of households, and an index is calculated by weighting each of the responses by the severity weights determined from the focus groups, by multiplying the weighted responses by the frequency of each strategy's occurrence, and by summing the results.

The CSI is quick and easy to implement, once it has been contextually adapted. It is useful for tracking changes in food security over time, though not as useful for cross-cultural comparisons of food security prevalence due to its context specificity (see discussion in the following section about a "reduced" CSI composed of contextually invariant items that can be used for spatial comparisons).

One caution in using the CSI is that certain types of responses are difficult to interpret. In any given context, there are supply and access constraints to adopting coping strategies that may affect the meaning of reported responses in unpredictable ways. To take a common example, highly food-insecure households might be desperate enough to dispose of productive assets but might have nothing left to sell. Very food-secure households may have no need to sell assets in the first place. Yet, both groups would respond in the negative to a question about asset disposal, rendering it difficult to discriminate between two very different types of households. For this reason, the developers of the CSI advise a focus on consumption strategies, rather than on a broader category of "resource augmentation strategies" that can yield these ambiguous results.

An additional challenge with the CSI is its approach to scoring. Because the severity of coping strategies and their frequency were considered to be two important dimensions of food insecurity, the CSI attempts to capture both in the same measure. One problem with this additive approach is that potentially important information is lost or disguised. It is impossible to tell from the overall total whether the score represents the frequent occurrence of low-severity strategies or the infrequent occurrence of highly severe strategies. These two scenarios might describe very different types of households on different trajectories with different implications. Additionally, because the score is a continuous indicator with no cut-points or categories to distinguish the food-secure from the food-insecure, it is most useful for reporting the degree of change in the score over time.

Experiential Food Insecurity Scales

The U.S. Household Food Insecurity Survey Measure, the first and most well-known experiential food insecurity scale, was developed by a government–university partnership in the United States after the country had spent nearly three decades grappling with food security measurement issues. Only within the last 15 years has this scaled approach to U.S. national food security measurement achieved broad consensus.

The tool of choice used by the USDA to monitor national food security, inserted since 1995 into the annual Current Population Survey, is a validated scale of 18 items about behaviors and attitudes that collectively distinguish households experiencing different degrees of food insecurity. Building on the theoretical groundwork of Kathy Radimer and colleagues at Cornell University (Radimer et al. 1990, 1992) and the advocacy-oriented Community Childhood Hunger Identification Project (CCHIP) (Wehler et al. 1992), the USDA Household Food Security Survey Module is underpinned by the notion that the experience of insecurity prompts predictable responses (relating to four dimensions: insufficient quantity and quality of food, having to procure food through personally and socially unacceptable means, and feeling worried over uncertain access) that are quantifiable in a way that "food security" itself is not. Each of these behavioral or attitudinal responses is assumed to represent a particular, predictable point on a continuum of severity. The self-reported responses of a household representative about the household members' experience with the set of presumably common food insecurity manifestations are summarized in a scale of severity, and cut-points on the scale categorize households as food-secure, food-insecure, or very low food-insecure (Coleman-Jenson et al. 2013). In the United States, these data are used to report on national food insecurity prevalence and to monitor the household effects of food assistance programs.

Household Food Insecurity Access Scale (HFIAS). Stymied by the lack of simple, valid, direct measures of food insecurity and inspired by the US HFSSM, in the early 2000s, international development organizations began to seize upon the US 18-question scale as an apparent solution, implementing it in myriad countries without any assessment first of its suitability for chronically and acutely food-insecure settings. Cognizant of the need for a more scientific approach, the FANTA Project sponsored a decade-long initiative of scale development and validation testing (Swindale and Bilinsky 2006a; Deitchler et al. 2010). The first phase involved multi year validation studies in Bangladesh and Burkina Faso. The results of these studies and others were harmonized to produce a nine-item scale, the Household Food Insecurity Access Scale, which has since been widely adopted for assessing the impacts of programs seeking to affect food security. It is conceptually similar to the CSI, except that it was intentionally developed to reflect the four key underlying dimensions of food insecurity that appeared to be universal from a review of ethnographic work on the subject: quantity, quality, preferences, and worry/uncertainty (Coates et al. 2006). As such, it includes a question about the psychological aspects of the food insecurity experience in addition to questions about behavioral responses. The guidance for use of the HFIAS also contains instructions for calculating a categorical indicator that can be used to assess the prevalence of food insecurity based on the pattern of responses to these nine questions (Coates et al. 2007).

In seeking to capture multiple dimensions of food insecurity, the HFIAS represents a big improvement over uni dimensional and less direct food insecurity metrics. It is simple and quick to administer, and can be used for population-based targeting, monitoring, and evaluation. Though individual questions that form the HFIAS nine-item scale were tested across a range of contexts, the HFIAS was not validated as a whole before being promoted widely by FANTA, thus there remained uncertainty about its cross-cultural validity, which FANTA expected to further assess once data sets became available. As such, the guidance for the HFIAS recommends an adaptation process that, for the first time using it in a new setting, can add an additional time burden. One of the potential weaknesses of the HFIAS is that it contains a few subjective questions (e.g., did you ever worry about not having food) that could be easy for respondents to manipulate in the expectation of a benefit, thus introducing respondent bias. For this reason, it is not generally recommended for screening households for program eligibility. Another issue to be aware of is that the HFIAS approach to categorizing households as "food-insecure," like all such indices or scales, relies on a set of thresholds that were set by a group of experts based on their judgment of what should constitute a classification of food-insecure vs. food-secure. Like other food security measures, this classification scheme is not calibrated to a functional outcome, or to a strict definition of food insecurity, and thus remains rather arbitrary. One perception shared by users of the HFIAS is that it tends to overestimate estimates of food insecurity. This argument is not well supported, however. The HFIAS categories have stricter criteria than the official food security definition (i.e., the HFIAS only classifies households as food-insecure that exhibit various manifestations of food insecurity, whereas the definition considers any individual experiencing any of the defined conditions at any time to be insecure). That said, the sensitivity of the categorization approach to relatively mild food insecurity means that it is less discriminating for targeting purposes in contexts where the majority of the population exhibits at least some food insecurity conditions on a regular basis.

Fourth Generation: Culturally Invariant Measures

Though the fourth generation of food insecurity measures is still emerging, over the last few years, there has been progress in the search for the "holy grail" of food security measurement—simple, direct, valid, multidimensional measures that are also cross-culturally comparable. These fourth-generation measures are all direct descendants of the third generation. Indicators grouped in this category include the *Household Hunger Scale*, a subset of three items from the HFIAS that were shown to be culturally invariant after a comparative validation study of HFIAS results from seven countries (Deitchler et al. 2010, 2011). The *Reduced CSI*, also in this category, emerged from the pooling of CSI data across 15 countries to identify those items that appeared to be common to most cultures and to represent similar levels of severity in different contexts (Maxwell et al. 2008).

The Latin American and Caribbean Food Security Scale (ELCSA) has been validated for use in assessing national-level food insecurity across several countries (Perez-Escamilla et al. 2004, 2007; Segall-Correa and Marin 2009; Food and Agriculture Organization 2010). And, more recently, the Food and Agriculture Organization (FAO) has launched an initiative to insert an 8-question experiential food insecurity scale into the Gallup World Poll as a complement to FAO's existing undernourishment measure (Food and Agriculture Organisation 2013). To be piloted initially in four countries, the FAO hopes to scale-up the use of this measure to 150 countries, annually.

Though this generation of indicators has expanded the usefulness of food security measures by enabling comparisons across space as well as over time, there are aspects that have been sacrificed in the search for "universal" measures. In the case of the HFIAS, for example, the impetus to create a scale with cross-cultural properties meant that items that were not cross-culturally invariant were omitted. The resultant "Household Hunger Scale" (Deitchler et al. 2010) contains only items pertaining to reduced quantity of food consumed, with no items capturing quality, safety, stability, or preferences. As a result, the HHS measures only the most severe end of the food insecurity spectrum, which may be useful in severe acute contexts but not in contexts suffering from milder, chronic food insecurity. Interestingly, the reduced CSI captures food insecurity only on the less severe end of the spectrum, implying that the two metrics may be complementary but are not perfect substitutes (Maxwell et al. 2013). On the other hand, the use of measures such as the ELCSA and the forthcoming FAO Food Insecurity Experience Scale at national and global levels promises to introduce a much-needed complement to global food security tracking currently done through national-level caloric availability data.

CONTINUED MEASUREMENT CHALLENGES AND RECENT ADVANCES

As the previous sections have discussed, there have been a great deal of promising advances made in food security measurement, particularly over the past decade. There is increasing convergence around a smaller set of indicators, and more conceptual clarity around the ways in which current measures do, and do not, capture the breadth and depth of the holistic food security construct. A set of measures has emerged that can be used not just for tracking changes over time, but also for making spatial comparisons. These fourth-generation measures have been scientifically validated, are simple to use, and have gained widespread backing of key institutions. However, important challenges remain. This section will briefly touch on some of these issues and will describe some steps being taken to address them.

- *Continued incongruence between metrics and definition:* While it is widely recognized that no single indicator captures all food security dimensions, in practice, indicators are used without understanding or recognition of what exactly they are measuring and what they are not. Such indiscriminate use of indicators has the following implications (Coates 2013): first, estimates of the food-insecure for policy and programmatic purposes are underestimated when only certain dimensions are measured. Second, using single indicators interchangeably or lumping them together indiscriminately makes diagnostics difficult; this approach obscures potentially significant relationships between functionally important causes and consequences of individual elements of food security; third, errors in diagnostics risk leading to the design of "one-size-fits-all" interventions for households or individuals facing different types of food insecurity, and finally, a misalignment of impact metric for a given policy or program design can bias the impact estimate and obfuscate which elements of food security have been most improved, or not, by a given intervention.
- *Which one to choose?* There is recent convincing evidence to suggest these measures are not capturing the same thing. A recent paper by Maxwell et al. demonstrates that households are classified very differently by different measures (Maxwell et al. 2013). Different indicators also use different approaches to categorizing households as food-insecure. One of the reasons for the cherry picking of indicators is that there is a lack of clear guidance around which indicators to use for which purposes. The aggregation of items into a multidimensional index like the HFIAS or CSI is useful for communicating a summary result, but aggregation also reduces clarity about which dimensions are being captured. One way of moving forward is to deconstruct food insecurity to measure its component parts separately and well through a dashboard of indicators. This idea has been put forward for some time within the food security community (Kennedy 2002) but has

regained traction recently (Carletto et al. 2013; Coates 2013). The recognition that multidimensional constructs should perhaps not be measured with multidimensional indices has also been echoed among those working in poverty measurement (Ravallion 2011).

- *Household vs. individual:* Despite ample evidence to suggest that food insecurity is experienced differently by different household members (Hadley et al. 2008; Wutich 2009; Coates et al. 2010; Kuku et al. 2011; Bernal et al. 2012; Quisumbing 2013), food insecurity continued to be measured primarily at the household level and above. The main reason for this is that the household has long been the economic unit of interest to economists, and the feasibility of generating individual-level information on various household members through surveys is more challenging. That being said, measures like the IDDS are already tailored for individual use, and in theory there is no reason why other measures could not be used on individuals.

- *Attention needed to public health (nonnutrition) outcomes:* According to Dery, "definition implies a choice, a particular way of seeing a problem among a range of alternatives. Policy is determined in part by that choice." (1984, p. xii). The way in which food security is measured also informs what we know about its functional consequences. For instance, developing country research into food security outcomes has been almost entirely focused on its nutrition effects, in part because food security is often operationalized in terms of dietary indicators or anthropometrics (Weaver and Hadley 2009). Measures that take into account the psychological dimensions of food insecurity are more likely to detect its effects on important functional outcomes such as mental health, as demonstrated by a growing body of developed and developing country literature (Weaver and Hadley 2009; Cole and Tembo 2011; Nanama and Frongillo 2012; Tsai et al. 2012). There is a growing body of evidence between food insecurity and other public health impacts, mostly from developed country studies. These include (to name just a few) associations between food insecurity and antiretroviral adherence, HIV status, obesity chronic disease, homelessness, and intimate partner violence. In order to be able to continue to understand the mechanisms of these and other relationships in developing country contexts, it will be necessary to choose the metrics discerningly.

REFERENCES

Arimond, M., D. Wiesmann, E. Becquey, A. Carriquiry, M. C. Daniels, M. Deitchler, and L. E. Torheim. 2010. Simple food group diversity indicators predict micronutrient adequacy of women's diets in 5 diverse, resource-poor settings. *Journal of Nutrition* 140 (11):2059S–2069S. doi: 10.3945/jn.110.123414.

Arimond, M. and M. T. Ruel. 2004. Dietary diversity is associated with child nutritional status: Evidence from 11 demographic and health surveys. *Journal of Nutrition* 134 (10):2579–2585.

Babu, S. C. and P. Pinstrup-Andersen. 1994. Food security and nutrition monitoring: A conceptual framework, issues and challenges. *Food Policy* 19 (3):218–233.

Barrett, C. B. 2002. Food security and food assistance programs. In *Handbook of Agricultural Economics*. B. L. Gardner and G. C. Rausser, eds. Amsterdam, Netherlands: Elsevier.

Bernal, J., E. A. Frongillo, H. Herrera, and J. Rivera. 2012. Children live, feel, and respond to experiences of food insecurity that compromise their development and weight status in Peri-Urban Venezuela. *Journal of Nutrition* 142 (7):1343–1349.

Carletto, C., A. Zezza, and R. Banerjee. 2013. Towards better measurement of household food security: Harmonizing indicators and the role of household surveys. *Global Food Security* 2:30–40.

Carter, M. R. and C. B. Barrett. 2006. The economics of poverty traps and persistent poverty: An asset-based approach. *Journal of Development Studies* 42 (2):178–199.

Chung, K., L. Haddad, J. Ramakrishna, and F. Reily. 1997. *Identifying the Food Insecure: the Application of Mixed-Method Approaches in India*. Washington, DC: International Food Policy Research Institute.

Coates, J. 2013. Build it back better: Deconstructing food security for improved measurement and action. *Global Food Security* 2 (3):188–194. doi: 10.1016/j.gfs.2013.05.002.

Coates, J., A. Swindale, and P. Bilinsky. 2007. Household Food Insecurity Access Scale (HFIAS) for Measurement of Household Food Access: Indicator Guide (v. 3). Food and Nutrition Technical Assistance Project (FANTA)/AED.

Coates, J., B. L. Rogers, P. Webb, D. Maxwell, R. Houser, and C. McDonald. 2007. Diet Diversity Study. World Food Programme, Emergency Needs Assessment Service (ODAN).

Coates, J., E. A. Frongillo, B. L. Rogers, P. Webb, P. E. Wilde, and R. Houser. 2006. Commonalities in the experience of household food insecurity across cultures: What are measures missing? *Journal of Nutrition* 136:1428S–1448S.

Coates, J., P. Webb, R. Houser, B. L. Rogers, and P. Wilde. 2010. He said she said: Who should speak for households about experiences of food insecurity in Bangladesh? *Food Security Journal* 2:81–95.

Cole, S. M. and G. Tembo. 2011. The effect of food insecurity on mental health: Panel evidence from rural Zambia. *Social Science & Medicine* 73 (7):1071–1079.

Coleman-Jenson, A., M. Nord, and A. Singh. 2013. Household Food Security in the United States in 2012. In *Economic Research Report No. (ERR-155) 41*.

Corbett, J. 1988. Famine and household coping strategies. *World Development* 16 (9):1099–1112.

Currey, B. 1979. Mapping areas liable to famine in Bangladesh. PhD dissertation, University of Honolulu, Honolulu, Hawaii.

Currey, B. and G. Hugo. 1984. *Famine as a Geographical Phenomenon*. Dordrecht: Reidel.

Davies, S. 1996. *Adaptable Livelihoods: Coping with Food Insecurity in the Malian Sahel*. New York: St. Martin's Press.

De Vellis, R. F. 1991. Scale development: Theory and applications. L. Bickman and D. J. Rog, eds. *Applied Social Research Methods Series*. Vol. 26. London: Sage Publications.

De Waal, A. 1989. *Famine That Kills: Darfur, Sudan, 1984–1985*. Oxford: Clarendon Press.

Deitchler, M., T. Ballard, A. Swindale, and J. Coates. 2010. Validation of a measure of household hunger for cross-cultural use. Food and Nutrition Technical Assistance II Project (FANTA-2)/Academy for Educational Development. Accessed September 10, 2014. http://www.state.gov/documents/organization/148436.pdf.

Deitchler, M., T. Ballard, A. Swindale, and J. Coates. 2011. Introducing a Simple Measure of Household Hunger for Cross-Cultural Use. [Technical Note No. 12]. Food and Nutrition Technical Assistance II Project (FANTA-2)/Academy for Educational Development.

Dery, D. 1984. *Problem Definition in Policy Analysis*. Lawrence: University Press of Kansas.

Economist.com. 2013. Thought for food: How much people in different countries spend on food. [Graphic]. Accessed September 10, 2014. http://www.economist.com/blogs/graphicdetail/2013/03/daily-chart-5.

Eele, G. 1994. Indicators for food security and nutrition monitoring: A review of experience from Southern Africa. *Food Policy* 19 (3):314–328.

Fiedler, J., C. Carletto, and O. Dupriez. 2012. Still waiting for Godot? Improving household consumption and expenditures surveys (HCES) to enable more evidence-based nutrition policies, *Food and Nutrition Bulletin* 33 (S2):242S–251S.

Fiedler, J., K. Lividini, O. Bermudez, and M.-F. Smitz. 2012. Household consumption and expenditures surveys (HCES): A primer for food and nutrition analysts in low- and middle-income countries. *Food and Nutrition Bulletin* 33 (S2):170S–184S(15).

Food and Agriculture Organization. 1996. Rome declaration on world food security, World Food Summit. Rome.

Food and Agriculture Organization. 2004. The State of Food Insecurity in the World 2004. Accessed September 10, 2014. ftp://ftp.fao.org/docrep/fao/007/y5650e/y5650e00.pdf.

Food and Agriculture Organization. 2010. Informe sobre el taller regional: Armonización de la Escala Latinoamericana y Caribeña de Seguridad Alimentaria—ELCSA. Report of workshop, National Institute of Public Health, Cuernavaca, Mexico.

Food and Agriculture Organization. 2012. The State of Food Insecurity in the World 2012 Technical note: FAO methodology to estimate the prevalence of undernourishment. Food and Agriculture Organization. Accessed September 10, 2014. http://www.fao.org/fileadmin/templates/es/SOFI_2012/sofi_technical_note.pdf.

Food and Agriculture Organisation. 2013. New metric to be launched on hunger and food insecurity: FAO's Voices of the Hungry project to be tested on a pilot basis. [News article]. Accessed September 10, 2014. http://www.fao.org/news/story/en/item/171728/icode/.

Food and Agriculture Organization of the United Nations. 2002. *Proceedings of the International Scientific Symposium on Measurement and Assessment of Food Deprivation and Undernutrition*, Rome, Italy, June 26–28.

Food and Agriculture Organization, World Food Programme, and International Fund for Agricultural Development. 2012. The State of Food Insecurity in the World 2012: Economic growth is necessary but not sufficient to accelerate reduction of hunger and malnutrition. Food and Agriculture Organization. Accessed September 10, 2014. http://www.fao.org/docrep/016/i3027e/i3027e.pdf.

Frongillo, E. A. 1999. Validation of measures of food insecurity and hunger. *Journal of Nutrition* 129 (2):506S–509S.

Goodwin, L. D. and N. L. Leech. 2003. The meaning of validity in the new standards for educational and psychological testing: Implications for measurement courses. *Measurement and Evaluation in Counseling and Development* 36:181–191.

Habicht, J. P., C. G. Victora, and J. P. Vaughan. 1999. Evaluation designs for adequacy, plausibility and probability of public health programme performance and impact. *International Journal of Epidemiology* 28 (10–8):10–18.

Habicht, J. P. and D. L. Pelletier. 1990. The importance of context in choosing nutritional indicators. *Journal of Nutrition* 120 (11):1519–1524.

Haddad, L., E. Kennedy, and J. Sullivan. 1994. Choice of indicators for food security and nutrition monitoring. *Food Policy* 19 (3):329–343.

Hadley, C., D. Lindstrom, F. Tessema, and T. Belachew. 2008. Gender bias in the food insecurity experience of Ethiopian adolescents. *Social Science & Medicine* 66 (2):427–438.

Hinkin, T. R. 1995. A review of scale development practices in the study of organizations. *Journal of Management* 21 (5):967–989.

Hoddinott, J. and Y. Yohannes. 2002. Dietary diversity as a food security indicator. In *IFPRI Discussion Paper*. Washington, DC: International Food Policy Research Institute.

Kennedy, E. 2002. Qualitative measures of food insecurity and hunger. *Proceedings of the International Scientific Symposium on Measurement and Assessment of Food Deprivation and Undernutrition*, Rome, June 26–28, 2002.

Kennedy, G., N. Fanou-Fogny, C. Seghieri, M. Arimond, Y. Koreissi, R. Dossa, and I. D. Brouwer. 2010. Food groups associated with a composite measure of probability of adequate intake of 11 micronutrients in the diets of women in Urban Mali. *Journal of Nutrition* 140 (11):2070S–2078S.

Kennedy, G., T. Ballard, and M. C. Dop. 2013. *Guidelines for Measuring Household and Individual Dietary Diversity*. Rome: Food and Agriculture Organization.

Kuku, O., C. Gundersen, and S. Garasky. 2011. Differences in food insecurity between adults and children in Zimbabwe. *Food Policy* 36 (2):311–317. doi: 10.1016/j.foodpol.2010.11.029.

Lappé, F. M., J. Clapp, M. Anderson, R. Lockwood, R. Forster, D. Nierenberg, and T. Nuova. 2013. Framing Hunger: A Response to The State of Food Insecurity in the World 2012. Accessed September 10, 2014. http://www.ase.tufts.edu/gdae/Pubs/rp/FramingHunger.pdf.

Longhurst, R. 1986. Household food strategies in response to seasonality and famine. *IDS Bulletin* 17 (3):67–71.

Maxwell, D. 1996. Measuring food insecurity: The frequency and severity of coping strategies. *Food Policy* 21 (3):291–303.

Maxwell, D., B. Watkins, R. Wheeler, and G. Collins. 2003. The Coping Strategies Index: A Tool for Rapidly Measuring Food Security and the Impact of Food aid Programs in Emergencies. Nairobi: CARE Eastern and Central Africa Regional Management Unit and the World Food Programme Vulnerability Assessment and Mapping Unit.

Maxwell, D., C. Ahiadeke, C. Levin, M. Armar-Klemesu, S. Zakariah, and G. M. Lamptey. 1999. Alternative food-security indicators: Revisiting the frequency and severity of "coping strategies". *Food Policy* 24 (4):411–429.

Maxwell, D., J. Coates, and B. Vaitla. 2013. How do different indicators of household food security compare? Empirical evidence from Tigray. In *Feinstein International Center Working Paper 13*. Medford: Tufts University Friedman School of Nutrition Science and Policy.

Maxwell, D., R. Caldwell, and M. Langworth. 2008. Measuring food insecurity: Can an indicator based on localized coping behaviors be used to compare across contexts? *Food Policy* 33 (6):533–540.

Maxwell, S., and T. Frankenberger. 1992. *Household Food Security: Concepts, Indicators, Measurements; A Technical Review*. New York and Rome: UNICEF Programme Publications and IFAD.

Messick S. 1995. Validity of psychological assessment: Validation of inferences from persons' responses and performance as scientific inquiry into score meaning. *American Psychology* 50:741–9.

Naiken, L. 2002. FAO methodology for estimating the prevalence of undernourishment. *Proceedings of the International Scientific Symposium on Measurement and Assessment of Food Deprivation and Undernutrition*, Rome, 26–28 June.

Nanama, S. and E. A. Frongillo. 2012. Altered social cohesion and adverse psychological experiences with chronic food insecurity in the non-market economy and complex households of Burkina Faso. *Social Science & Medicine* 74 (3):444–451. doi: 10.1016/j.socscimed.2011.11.009.

Perez-Escamilla, R., A. M. Segall-Correa, L. K. Maranha, M. de Fatima Archanjo Sampaio, L. Marin-Leon, and G. Panigassi. 2004. An adapted version of the U.S. Department of Agriculture Food Insecurity Module is a valid tool for assessing household food insecurity in Campinas, Brazil. *Journal of Nutrition* 134 (8):1923–1928.

Perez-Escamilla, R., H. Melgar-Quinonez, M. Nord, M. C. Uribe Alvarez, and A. M. Segall-Corrêa. 2007. Escala Latinoamericana y Caribena de Seguridad Alimentaria (ELCSA) [Latinamerican and Caribbean Food Security Scale]. *Perspectives en Nutricion Humana (Colombia)*:S117–S134.

Quinn, V. J. and E. Kennedy. 1994. Food security and nutrition monitoring systems in Africa: A review of country experiences and lessons learned. *Food Policy* 19 (3):234–254.

Quisumbing, A. R. 2013. Generating evidence on individuals' experience of food insecurity and vulnerability. *Global Food Security* 2 (1):50–55.

Radimer, K. L., C. M. Olson, and C. C. Campbell. 1990. Development of indicators to assess hunger. *Journal of Nutrition* 120 (11):1544–1548.

Radimer, K. L., C. M. Olson, J. C. Greene, C. C. Campbell, and J. P. Habicht. 1992. Understanding hunger and developing indicators to assess it in women and children. *Journal of Nutrition Education* 24 (1 suppl):36S–44S.

Ravallion, M. 2011. On multidimensional indices of poverty. In *Policy Research Working Paper 5580*. Washington, DC: World Bank.

Ruel, MT. 2003. Is dietary diversity an indicator of food security or dietary quality? A review of measurement issues and research needs. *Food and Nutrition Bulletin* 24 (2):231–2.

Segall-Correa, A. M. and L. Marin. 2009. Household food security measurement in Brazil: Informing policy makers. *Annals of Nutrition and Metabolism* 55:70–70.

Smith, L. C. 2002. The use of household expenditure surveys for the assessment of food insecurity. *Proceedings of the International Scientific Symposium on Measurement and Assessment of Food Deprivation and Undernutrition*, Rome, June 26–28.

Smith, L. C. and A. Subandoro. 2007. *Measuring Food Security Using Household Expenditure Surveys, Food Security in Practice Technical Guide Series*. Washington, DC: International Food Policy Research Institute.

Streiner, D. L., and G. R. Norman. 2006. "Precision" and "accuracy": Two terms that are neither. *Journal of Clinical Epidemiology* 59:327–330.

Swindale, A. and P. Ohri-Vachaspati. 2000. *Measuring Household Food Consumption: A Technical Guide*. Washington, DC: Food and Nutrition Technical Assistance (FANTA) Project.

Swindale, A. and P. Bilinsky. 2006a. Development of a universally applicable household food insecurity measurement tool: Process, current status, and outstanding issues *Journal of Nutrition* 136 (5):1449S–1452S.

Swindale, A. and P. Bilinsky. 2006b. *Household Dietary Diversity Score (HDDS) for Measurement of Household Food Access: Indicator Guide (v.2)*. Washington, D.C.: FHI 360/FANTA.

Tsai, A. C., D. R. Bangsberg, E. A. Frongillo, P. W. Hunt, C. Muzoora, J. N. Martin, and S. D. Weiser. 2012. Food insecurity, depression and the modifying role of social support among people living with HIV/AIDS in rural Uganda. *Social Science & Medicine* 74 (12):2012–2019.

Watts, M. 1983. *Silent Violence: Food, Famine, and Peasantry in Northern Nigeria*. Berkeley: University of California Press.

Weaver, L. J. and C. Hadley. 2009. Moving beyond hunger and nutrition: A systematic review of the evidence linking food insecurity and mental health in developing countries. *Ecology of Food and Nutrition* 48 (4):263–284. doi: 10.1080/03670240903001167.

Webb, P. and A. Harinarayan. 1999. A measure of uncertainty: The nature of vulnerability and its relationship to malnutrition. *Disasters* 23 (4):292–305.

Wehler, C., R. Scott, and J. Anderson. 1992. The community childhood hunger identification project: A model of domestic hunger—Demonstration project in Seattle, Washington. *Journal of Nutrition Education* 24:29S–35S.

Wiesmann, D., L. Bassett, Lucy, T. Benson, and J. Hoddinott. 2009. Validation of the World Food Programme's Food Consumption Score and Alternative Indicators of Household Food Security. *IFPRI Discussion Paper No. 870*, Washington, D.C.: International Food Policy Research Institute.

World Bank. 1986. Poverty and hunger: Issues and options for food security in developing countries. In *World Bank Policy Study*. Washington, DC.

World Food Programme VAM Unit. 2008. *Food Consumption Analysis: Calculation and Use of the Food Consumption Score*. Rome: United Nations World Food Programme.

Wutich, A. 2009. Intrahousehold disparities in women and men's experiences of water insecurity and emotional distress in Urban Bolivia. *Medical Anthropology* 23 (4):357–516.

4 Nutrition, Food Security, Social Protection, and Health Systems Strengthening for Ending AIDS

Divya Mehra, Saskia de Pee, and Martin W. Bloem

CONTENTS

INTRODUCTION

The HIV/AIDS response has been one of the most significant social movements in recent times. It has provided a benchmark for global leadership on what can be accomplished through a unique model of partnership. Remarkable success has been achieved in the past decade; in 2013, almost 10 million of the approximately 35 million people living with HIV (PLHIV) were receiving treatment. New infections and mortality due to AIDS-related causes have declined by 33% since 2001 and by 30% since 2005, respectively (UNAIDS 2013). As a result of recent advances in access to antiretroviral treatment (ART), HIV-positive people now live longer and healthier lives. ART, in turn, prevents onward transmission of HIV. Since 1996, ART has averted 6.3 million deaths related to AIDS. Policy frameworks accompanying the programs have also accelerated the progress in combatting the epidemic.

It is now possible to envision a world with "zero new infections" and "zero AIDS-related deaths" given the progress made on improved treatment. The rhetoric around "the end of AIDS" is gaining significant momentum. The implementation of the WHO 2010 guidelines for the prevention of mother-to-child transmission (PMTCT) can reduce the risk of transmission from 35% to less than 5% when breastfeeding, and from 25% to less than 2% in non breastfeeding infants. The most recent UNAIDS report estimates ART coverage among pregnant women living with HIV in 2012 at 62%. It is projected that this could reach up to 90% by 2015 (UNAIDS 2013).

Despite significant progress, HIV and access to ARV treatment remains one of the great challenges of our times. HIV/AIDS has claimed 36 million lives so far; it is the leading cause of death among women aged 15–49 years worldwide. Sub-Saharan Africa is the most affected region, with a small population (12% of the world's population) but high proportion of people living with HIV (71% of all PLHIV in 2012) (UNAIDS 2013). The 2013 WHO guidelines have recommended earlier initiation of ART at CD4 count of 500 cells/μL or less for all adults and children above 5 years based on the recent findings that treatment is an important prevention strategy. Under these guidelines, over 16 million PLHIV who are in need of ART do not have access yet. In fact, under the 2013 guidelines, treatment coverage in low- and middle-income countries represented only 34% of their 28.3 million eligible people. A large number of eligible people in need of ART do not start treatment because of low rates of testing and losses that occur between the diagnosis of HIV and initiation of treatment. Issues of retention in ART programs and long-term adherence to treatment care regimens have often been ignored. To date, only 65% of people living with HIV in Africa who enrolled on ART remain on treatment, as assessed after 3 years (Kranzer et al. 2012). Therefore, programs that achieve high retention rates and good long-term adherence are needed and can serve as models for other programs.

Treatment is rightly the cornerstone of an effective response. As mentioned previously, adequate treatment not only allows people to live longer and healthier lives, but also curbs the transmission of HIV (Karim and Karim 2011). UNAIDS' Treatment 2015 provides a framework for scaling up treatment with three pillars: demand (enhance the demand for HIV testing and treatment services), invest (mobilize sufficient resources for expediting the scaling up of treatment and to enhance the effectiveness and efficiency of spending), and deliver (close gaps in the HIV treatment continuum within health and community systems) (UNAIDS 2012). Underpinning these pillars is an emphasis on a rights-based approach that ensures equity, critical in ensuring universal access. UNAIDS' expanded understanding of treatment is also meant to incorporate nonclinical issues, which may often act as barriers in achieving HIV treatment goals. Here, communities, and not necessarily health systems, are important in providing leadership, for example, for key populations, such as sex workers, men who have sex with men (MSM), or injecting drug users (IDU). A better understanding of barriers to testing and treatment will reduce patient loss through the continuum of care. Global efforts are channeled toward biomedical treatment interventions, while significant work remains to be done for getting people on treatment and retaining them on care.

CURRENT CONTEXT FOR HIV AND NUTRITION

HUMAN IMMUNODEFICIENCY VIRUS

While much remains to be done for the HIV/AIDS response, strategic shifts are occurring in the field of HIV/AIDS, as well as to global health and development in general.

First, we know that strengthening the disease-specific vertical approach for AIDS will not be enough to successfully combat the epidemic; health systems will need to be strengthened too. In 2011, a new investment framework was proposed for the HIV response outlining cost-effective interventions for HIV prevention, treatment, care, and support. Based on evidence from the last 30 years, the framework models the total investment required for a basic set of program activities, along with the "critical enablers" and "synergies with development sectors" (Schwartlander et al. 2011). While the evidence on program activities is abundant, operationalization of "critical enablers" and "development synergies" is a limitation of the investment framework. Nonetheless, the importance of integrating HIV in other sectors has been recognized.

Second, under the new WHO guidelines, more people are on treatment than ever before. People are starting treatment earlier and live longer. HIV is emerging as a chronic disease with a set of new complications and comorbidities that require sophisticated and integrated systems and expertise for disease management (Deeks et al. 2013). Deeks et al. argue for the need to rethink and develop chronic-care models for HIV and to link HIV treatment facilities with services for chronic diseases. This will pose to be a significant challenge in low-resource settings where the health care systems are already overburdened and usually equipped to only handle acute or disease-specific care. While it is imperative to appreciate the "HIV as a chronic disease" paradigm, it also assumes that people are already accessing and adhering to treatment optimally, which is often not the case among the most vulnerable populations.

Third, as a consequence of the difficult global economic situation in recent years, HIV programming is under increasing financial strain. It can be expected that future funding levels from traditional donors will stagnate or decline. Global health funding is shifting away from large-scale investment in vertical approaches that target single disease, to horizontal approaches that reinforce the integration of services, maternal and child health programs, primary care, and efforts to strengthen health systems overall. The largest funder of the HIV/AIDS response, the U.S. President's Emergency Plan for AIDS Relief (PEPFAR), has scaled back its support in some countries. While 2011 saw global financial assistance for HIV/AIDS decline for the first time, it was also the first time that a larger share of the resources came from domestic rather than international sources as domestic funding increased. This trend will likely continue, where low- and middle-income country governments will pick up a larger share of the total cost of the response.

Finally, the post-2015 development agenda, which builds on the original eight Millennium Development Goals (MDGs) agreed upon in 2000 by member states, of which MDG 6 is on the HIV/AIDS response,* will now be concentrated on social, economic, and environmental issues, and peace and security. To formulate the post-2015 development agenda, an inclusive and participatory consultation process was initiated by the UN Development Group (UNDG) in 2012. Stakeholders were invited to participate in web-based consultations, which ultimately contributed to the content of the High-Level Panel (HLP) report on the post-2015 development agenda (United Nations 2013). The report, "A New Global Partnership: Eradicate Poverty and Transform Economies through Sustainable Development," outlines recommendations for the next global development agenda, sets out proposed strategic shifts in development planning for the accelerated reduction of poverty, and proposes illustrative goals to follow on the Millennium Development Goals from 2015. HIV/AIDS has received limited visibility in this report; instead, HIV is mentioned as a target in a health-related goal, "Ensure Healthy Lives," which focuses on universal access to health, reducing maternal and child mortality, and improving reproductive and sexual health and rights. The target calls for a reduction in the burden of disease from HIV/AIDS, tuberculosis, malaria, neglected tropical diseases, and priority noncommunicable diseases, with indicators still to be proposed.

NUTRITION

While HIV/AIDS is moving toward health systems integration, food security and nutrition have been gaining momentum. The HLP report on the post-2015 sustainable development goals has a specific goal focused on "Ensuring Food Security and Good Nutrition." The United Nations Secretary General's Zero Hunger Challenge is aiming to achieve the vision of a Zero Hunger world by uniting around clear, measureable, zero-based targets that would reject inequities and aim to eliminate childhood stunting; ensure that food is accessible to all; and that food systems are sustainable. Concurrently, the Scaling up Nutrition (SUN) Movement is galvanizing unprecedented political momentum, with national governments taking the lead to comprehensively address undernutrition among their populations. All of this has been bolstered by updated evidence in the 2013 Lancet Series on Maternal and Child

---

* MDG 6: combat HIV/AIDS, malaria, and other diseases. Target 6A: Have halted by 2015 and begun to reverse the spread of HIV/AIDS. Target 6B: Achieve, by 2010, universal access to treatment for HIV/AIDS for all those who need it.

Nutrition, now emphasizing the importance of intervening during pregnancy and prepregnancy (adolescence) for improved nutrition outcomes among children. With nutrition high on the global agenda, funding is following suit. At the Nutrition for Growth Summit in London, a commitment of USD 4.15 billion for directly tackling undernutrition, and an additional estimated $19 billion for improved nutrition outcomes through nutrition-sensitive investments by 2020, were pledged.

OPPORTUNITIES AHEAD

Given the global strategic shifts in HIV/AIDS, there seems to be a gap between what the investment framework proposes and the current global financial and political climate. As described in the UNAIDS investment framework, biomedical interventions and programs, such as voluntary medical male circumcision and emphasis on HIV treatment, seem to have the strongest evidence of reducing the transmission of HIV (UNAIDS 2013). But important facts are that 16 million people in need are not on treatment; retention on treatment among PLHIV after 3 years in sub-Saharan Africa has been reported to be 65%; and only 39% of PLHIV know their HIV status (Kranzer et al. 2012). One of the reasons for these staggering statistics is that public health resources are scarce, and as described by Magnani et al., surveillance has traditionally targeted the easily accessed populations for HIV. In resource-limited settings, surveillance for HIV has been limited to pregnant women seeking antenatal care, those seeking medical care for sexually transmitted diseases, and potential military recruits (Magnani et al. 2005). A new strategy based on context and "knowing the epidemic" is required for the hard-to-reach populations.

For such an approach, organizations and programs that are well equipped to access vulnerable populations need to be leveraged better. An HIV lens needs to be applied to existing initiatives, and beyond those that are focused on HIV as the primary interest. Looking ahead, there is a need to integrate HIV in poverty reduction, social protection and health systems, and other development sectors. One example, related to food and nutrition, is that while in the past, nutrition and food assistance programs were meant to be integrated within the HIV/AIDS response (as per the UNAIDS strategy), today's environment presents a unique opportunity for new approaches that focus on making the fields of nutrition and health more HIV-sensitive (a detailed description is provided in the following sections). Programs with goals beyond HIV can play a pivotal role in targeting hard-to-reach populations.

Another example is PMTCT: one of the basic program activities under the investment framework is eliminating new infections among children. However, investment allocation for PMTCT by Schwartländer and colleagues estimated the costs for the investment framework interventions as very small; $1.5 billion out of $22 billion in 2015 (England 2011; Schwartlander et al. 2011). It has been acknowledged that the elimination of pediatric AIDS in the coming years is possible, but this would require an integrated and comprehensive approach. This means that the HIV/AIDS treatment and care packages would have to be integrated with maternal, new-born, and child health care, and family planning services would have to be scaled up substantially.

COMPREHENSIVELY ADDRESSING HIV/AIDS: TREATMENT AND BEYOND

The HIV/AIDS movement has experienced enormous success and it is well positioned to be integrated with other sectors. The 2013 report from UNAIDS acknowledges a clear trend toward integration of HIV with different systems and sectors and it highlights that greater efforts are needed to ensure the integration of HIV in broad health and development efforts, including the removal of parallel mechanisms.

Kim et al. propose a framework to address the shortcomings in global health care delivery by applying a systems-level analysis to care delivery value chains (Kim et al. 2013). Their comprehensive approach proposes to not only integrate stand-alone approaches in the shared delivery infrastructure, but also to align these with the local context, including social and economic factors. They emphasize the need for diagonal approaches, which incorporate effective disease management with improved health systems over horizontal or vertical approaches. Their framework includes four components: continuum of care (from prevention and screening to disease management); shared delivery infrastructure to capture synergies in required resources and address multiple health problems; understanding barriers at the community level; and leveraging health care delivery systems for economic and social development. They use HIV/AIDS in resource-poor settings as an example to illustrate this framework.

The "cascade of care" and "test and treat" concepts provide a useful framework when considering integration of HIV in other sectors (Gardner et al. 2011; Mugavero et al. 2011). Before undertaking this, however, current gaps and the scope of the problem need to be defined. Kranzer et al. have systematically quantified the losses along the continuum of HIV care, that is, testing, eligibility for initiating ART, pre-ART care, ART, and long-term retention (Kranzer et al. 2012), recognizing that the pathway may not be a linear process since the patients may cycle in and out of care, as shown in Figure 4.1.

Applying the factors proposed by Kim et al. to the continuum of care described above, we propose a framework (Figure 4.2) that defines individual, household, community, and health systems-level considerations in all steps of the HIV cycle of care for a comprehensive response. At each step of the HIV cascade, from transmission to testing and from initiation of ART to on going disease management, it is instructive to analyze individual, household, community, and health systems-level factors in order to better prevent losses along the HIV care continuum.

Mugavero et al. have presented a comparable but distinct framework that shows the complex interplay between individual, community, relationship, health systems, and policy factors as part of a social–ecological perspective that impacts the process of engagement through the HIV care continuum (Mugavero et al. 2011). The authors use the framework to make a case for reforming the fragmented health care delivery system for HIV in the United States, which is wrought with gaps and problems such as: limited patient surveillance; lack of linkages between testing and medical services or support services that could enable individuals to remain in care facilities such as substance abuse treatment centers and housing assistance; funding challenges (e.g., insurance, government programs); and provider reimbursement issues. The case management for PLHIV is multifaceted and multidisciplinary. If there are

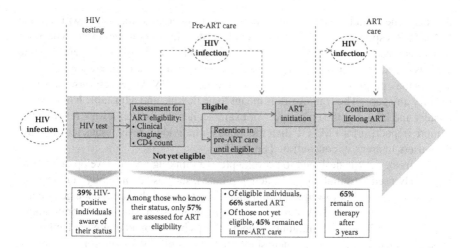

FIGURE 4.1 Losses along the HIV continuum of care. (From Kranzer, K. et al., 2012. *Journal of the International AIDS Society* 15 (2):17383.)

existing gaps in resource-rich settings, then these issues are only exacerbated in resource-limited settings.

The framework introduced here (Figure 4.2) draws on the considerations presented by Mugavero and colleagues, but presents a simple matrix so that each level can be parsed out throughout the care continuum to serve as a model for assessing current initiatives and identifying gaps for future programming in any given context.

	HIV Transmission	HIV Testing	Pre-ART Care	ART Initiation and Adherence

Individual level	• Socioeconomic status
	• Coping behavior
	• Position of women
	• Attitude/knowledge toward medical care
	• Medical history, STIs
	• Use of condoms
		• Socioeconomic status Knowledge
		• Stigma
		• Household support
		• Cultural beliefs
		• Identification of risk factors
			• Socioeconomic status Awareness /
			  knowledge of disease progression
			• Monitoring of indicators
			• Mental wellness
				• Socioeconomic status
				  Psychological preparedness
				• Substance abuse
				• Stigma
				• Cultural beliefs
				• Side effects

Household level	• Socioeconomic status • Support, relationships • Cultural beliefs • Education	• Socioeconomic status • Support • Attitude toward accessing health care	• Socioeconomic status • Food and nutrition security • HH/family support	• Socioeconomic status • Food and nutrition • HH/family support • Pressure to share • Cultural beliefs
Community level	• Social norms • Laws, policies • Support • Poverty, employment • Education	• Social norms toward health care • Poverty, employment • Laws, policies • Support	• Support groups • Community programs • Food assistance • Counseling	• Support groups • Community programs • Food assistance • Counseling
Health systems level	• Preventative facilities • Primary care clinics • PMTCT, prenatal care • Counseling • Availability/affordability of health care • Identification of high-risk individuals	• Availability of health care • Appropriate testing, sharing results • Treatment plan • Comorbidities, STIs • PMTCT, prenatal care • Identification of others at risk	• Availability of health care • Therapies for delaying progression • Treatment of comorbidities • Patient support • Ongoing disease management	• Medication, including second/third line • Disease management • Psychological support • Managing comorbidities • Nutrition support

FIGURE 4.2 Framework for HIV programming through the cascade of care: considerations at individual, household, community, and health systems levels.

Although the model presents a holistic framework to address the complexities of the HIV/AIDS response, it is by no means an exhaustive list of considerations. The 4 × 4 matrix is meant to serve as a conceptual model that can be used to operationalize various aspects within a program, as well as serve as a point of reference for where a particular program may/may not fit in the larger HIV/AIDS response and thus identify any gaps. The framework is meant to be flexible and adjustable based on the context and knowing the epidemic. For example, health systems-level strengthening is more impactful for PMTCT than the focus on individual-level issues for injecting drug users in areas of concentrated epidemics.

The framework is designed to provoke precise thinking and to develop definitions for loosely used terminology and catchall phrases, such as "community" or "stigma" or "social norms." For example, "community" may refer to the immediate geographical vicinity of where PLHIV may reside, but it could also mean virtual communities (Horvath et al. 2013), or community support groups built around treatment facilities if these happen to be away from where someone lives. Similarly, stigma could be present at the individual or community levels (shown only at individual level in the framework, Figure 4.2) and could impact the testing, pre-ART care, and ART adherence stages in the HIV cascade. The reason for being precise in understanding and defining these concepts is so that enabling (or disabling) factors that ultimately impact good HIV outcomes and support disease management can be identified. For example, understanding how communities can be effectively leveraged to support health systems and services can prove to be extremely powerful in not only reducing some of the burden on the health systems but also for making linkages with hard-to-reach vulnerable populations.

Finally, this framework encourages simultaneous thinking on supply and demand side enablers and barriers. To date, supply side- or biomedical treatment-focused interventions have been the emphasis of HIV programming. However, going forward, given that there is still much to be done, including retaining people on treatment and reaching the most vulnerable, providing treatment alone will not be enough; addressing the demand side factors will be equally important. The lack of focus on the demand side factors is reflected in UNAIDS' investment framework, where the critical enablers and synergies with the development sectors have not been fully operationalized, at least in terms of guidance for programming. This has led to a vicious circle: the enablers and barriers in the investment framework were not precisely defined (likely due to the lack of robust evidence); and now programming, which is based on the investment framework that has a biomedical/treatment focus, further precludes gaining expertise and generating evidence in this area.

APPLICATION OF THE MATRIX FRAMEWORK

HIV TRANSMISSION

At the individual and household levels, several factors may be responsible for HIV transmission. Given that transmission is inextricably linked to poverty and inequality, low socioeconomic status and food insecurity could easily result in resorting to risky coping behavior, such as unprotected transactional sex (Weiser et al. 2007). Women are particularly vulnerable in this situation due to systemic gender inequality, which may also hamper their negotiating power to use condoms. Education has been associated with a lower risk of acquiring HIV infection as it can impact an individual's knowledge of HIV/AIDS, as well as attitude toward medical care, importance of preventative care, and general well-being.

Community-level factors are equally important. These include the external political environment and local policies and laws, in addition to cultural beliefs and attitudes within a community. Cultural norms can determine local laws and, in turn, may perpetuate disabling environments that fail to address HIV. For example, stigma against MSM or IDU may result in punitive laws that would likely fail to curb transmission and lead to concentrated epidemics. Community-level considerations may also extend to the local attitude toward preventative behaviors; the use of health systems/medical care; as well as the availability of risk-reduction facilities within communities, for example, the availability of condoms, syringe exchange programs, planned parenthood, and resilience-building safety nets that link with health facilities to reduce risky copying behavior within communities.

Health systems can play an important preventative role. PMTCT, identification of high-risk individuals, and counseling would heavily rely on health care facilities as the point of contact.

HIV Testing

Only 39% of people infected with HIV are aware of their status (Kranzer et al. 2012). It is therefore important to understand the existing barriers that prevent people from getting tested. This can be examined both from the supply side as well as the demand side. On the supply side, the provision of quality health systems and facilities are at the core. But the availability of appropriate health systems, facilities, and community health workers depends on resources within a society. Furthermore, the types of available health services also depend on the level of awareness, attitudes, and cultural beliefs within a community.

If the availability of health systems is addressed alone, it provides no guarantee that it would be adequate to alleviate the problem of low testing. Analysis of the demand side is equally important. Individual-level factors such as socioeconomic status (including food security), physical health, mental well-being, knowledge, and perception of stigma based on cultural beliefs, can all act as barriers to HIV testing. The most important community-level barriers may be the cultural beliefs, attitudes, and stigma associated with HIV. They would determine the level of support that can be provided in a community, such as support groups and counseling centers. In addition, the cultural beliefs can also be reflected in enabling or punitive local laws and policies.

Pre-ART Care

In the continuum of the HIV care pathway, testing is followed by assessment of eligibility for ART for those who are diagnosed with HIV. Those eligible for ART should initiate treatment, and those not yet eligible must remain in pre-ART care. Pre-ART is the time period between when a person is tested positive for HIV until when he/she becomes eligible for ART. This includes three groups: (1) those who have been tested for their CD4 count, know their result and are not yet eligible for ART, (2) those who have been tested for their CD4 count but do not know the result, and (3) those who have not yet been tested for CD4 count, but have been diagnosed with HIV. The length of the pre-ART period for the second and third groups could vary depending on the delay between testing positive for HIV infection and obtaining the CD4 count results. A later diagnosis could mean a lower CD4 count and hence a shorter pre-ART period. Those not yet eligible should be retained in care for regular monitoring until they are eligible for ART. Within the pre-ART period, Rosen et al. have described three distinct stages: testing to staging (CD4 counts); staging to ART eligibility; and ART eligibility to ART initiation (Rosen and Fox 2011).

Once a person has been tested for HIV, the barriers related to testing, as described above, have been overcome. Yet there is a significant challenge in keeping people in pre-ART care (Rosen and Fox 2011), despite the fact they have already had some point of contact with the health system, and in theory could enroll and be retained in care immediately after diagnosis. Among those who know their status, only 57% are assessed for ART eligibility—which means that over 40% of people are lost between their diagnosis and determining their eligibility for ART initiation. Of those who are assessed for eligibility, 66% start ART, and of those not yet eligible, only 45% remain in pre-ART care. Rosen et al., in their review, found this proportion to be similar (Rosen and Fox 2011). The median proportion of PLHIV completing stage 2 (staging to ART eligibility) was 46%.

In the studies examined by Kranzer et al., only four studies assessed "Pre-ART Care" interventions for reducing losses occurring in the pre-ART period. These included immediate CD4 count testing, better referral systems (Nsigaye et al. 2009), transport vouchers (Nsigaye et al. 2009), and regular visits to refill medication (Kohler et al. 2011). It is also possible that people who test for their eligibility based on CD4 never return for their results. This means that despite availability of health services (supply side), individual-level circumstances, including discomfort related to the HIV infection and/or willingness (whether socioeconomic or stigma/perception related), are playing an important role in retention in care losses. The pre-ART period is complicated from a programmatic perspective. The length of this period is extremely variable and dependent on many factors; starting with the availability of health care resources, but also strongly influenced by individual- and household-level barriers to accessing care. Significant losses are occurring in the pre-ART care period, where there is a substantial failure in linking people from diagnosis, to pre-ART care, and eventually to ART. Interventions aimed at retaining people in care during this pre-ART period could be very effective since individuals have already made some point of contact with the health care system.

ART INITIATION AND ADHERENCE

Initiation of ART largely depends on the success of retaining people in pre-ART care, although "test and treat" also provides a good model that can be effective in initiation and bypassing the issues related to pre-ART care. Once PLHIV start treatment, adherence is critical for successful outcomes. There are several demand and supply side factors that play an important role, not only for starting treatment, but also for adhering to treatment regimens; these need to be appreciated more fully by health care providers and policy makers alike. Supply side/health care facilities and treatment/medication are of prime importance and have rightly occupied a central focus in the HIV response. However, as people are on treatment for life (spanning up to decades for young people initiating therapy), adherence to treatment is equally important. Evidence shows that there are significant losses during this phase and therefore there is a need to understand demand side barriers more carefully.

At the individual level, barriers can be economic, psychological, and physical. Competing demands on scarce resources and poverty-related barriers such as food insecurity, homelessness, and lack of means of transport, all have a negative impact on adherence. Psychological preparedness, stigma, and side effects related to medications also deter individuals from adhering to treatment. Factors at the household level may serve as additional demand side barriers. These may include availability of support, inter personal relationships, attitude toward health care, knowledge of disease, food security, sharing of medication, or any form of support received through the government. The community can create an enabling environment that supports adherence. These may include provisions such as support groups, community counseling, food centers, and government safety net programs for affected households, as well as a community's knowledge, cultural beliefs, and stigma related to HIV. On the supply side, there are several aspects that can be strengthened beyond the provision of medication. Psychological support, counseling, disease management for comorbidities and side effects, emphasis on general wellness, therapeutic and supplementary nutrition support may all have an impact on supporting PLHIV to remain on treatment.

FOOD AND NUTRITION IN HIV INFECTION

NUTRITION AND HIV INFECTION

Nutrition is important at all stages of HIV infection. The vicious cycle of malnutrition and HIV is shown in Figure 4.3. HIV affects the immune system, which increases the risk of infections. In turn, infection increases nutritional needs while at the same time increasing nutrient losses and reducing their intake and absorption. The ensuing deterioration of nutritional status affects the immune system and bodily strength, and the cycle continues with disease progression and further worsening of nutritional status. This section discusses the relationship between HIV infection and nutrition, along with ways to reduce and reverse this deteriorating cycle using a combination of medical treatment (biological aspect) and food and nutrition support (biological and behavioral aspects). The focus is on resource-limited settings.

NUTRITION AND ART

In resource-limited settings, the HIV epidemic is often highest where malnutrition is already prevalent. Many patients first present to the clinic malnourished and with an advanced stage of disease, and malnutrition is also associated with high mortality in the early months of treatment (van der Sande et al. 2004; Paton et al. 2006; Zachariah et al. 2006). The faster nutritional recovery can be achieved through ART and nutritional support, the greater the possibility of reduced mortality.

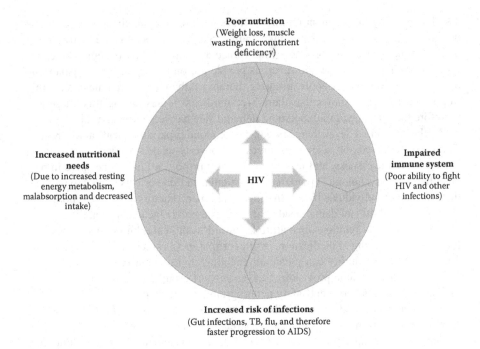

FIGURE 4.3 The vicious cycle involving HIV infection and malnutrition. (Adapted from RCQHC and FANTA Project 2003, Nutrition and HIV/AIDS: A Training Manual.)

As PLHIV stay on treatment for life, adequate nutrition remains important, but the nature of nutrition challenges change. After years on treatment, PLHIV may face high blood pressure, diabetes, increased risk of heart disease, reduced bone density, and/or dyslipidemia. Many PLHIV may have been at risk of these conditions irrespective of their HIV infection, and the suppressed infection as well as its on going treatment may further increase their risk (Fitch and Grinspoon 2011). A healthy diet can contribute to managing these conditions, and regular monitoring is important.

BOX 4.1   NUTRITIONAL NEEDS DURING MALNUTRITION

WHO recommendations for treatment of malnutrition in adults are non-HIV specific. Severely malnourished adults (BMI < 16 kg/m^2) should receive a therapeutic food nutritionally equivalent to F100 therapeutic milk. For initial treatment, people 19–75 years old should consume 40 kcal/kg/day of this therapeutic food, and people 15–18 years old should consume 50 kcal/kg/day (WHO 1999).

Moderately malnourished adults can be given supplementary foods such as fortified-blended foods, compressed bars, biscuits or lipid-based nutrient supplements (LNS) (WHO 1999, 2008, 2011; de Pee and Semba 2010). Most specialized food products for treating severe acute malnutrition (SAM) were formulated for children. For adults, it is best to use a product that is adapted to their taste preferences and has a reduced content of some nutrients (in particular, iron, zinc, copper, and vitamin A) because adults with SAM have to consume a higher absolute amount of the products than children.

It is important to note that food-insecure people in more affluent societies are at higher risk of becoming overweight, obese, or developing other related health problems than people who are food-secure. This is due to the fact that relatively cheap foods typically have a high-energy content from sugar and/or fat, but low nutritional value in terms of micronutrients, good quality protein, and so on (Drewnowski and Darmon 2005). This makes it harder for food-insecure PLHIV in these societies to manage their risk of noncommunicable disease, which is already higher both due to their HIV infection and its treatment, and due to the cost of a more healthy diet.

ART and Nutritious Foods Are Required to Restore Health and Nutritional Status of Malnourished PLHIV

Figure 4.4 summarizes how HIV and malnutrition negatively reinforce each other, and how malnutrition is also a consequence of poverty and food insecurity. It also shows how malnutrition is a consequence of HIV infection through different pathways, including HIV's impact on food intake and absorption, as well as how it alters metabolism.

As ART and specific therapies for opportunistic infections (OIs) treat the infections, nutrient absorption and metabolism will improve (although treatment may also

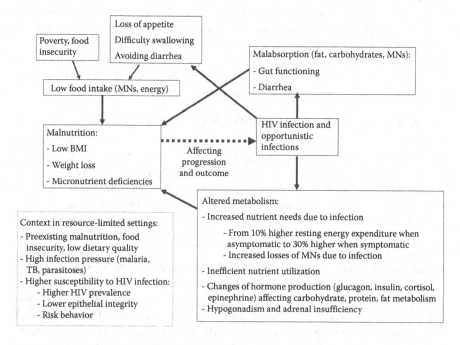

FIGURE 4.4 Relationship between HIV and malnutrition. (Reprinted with permission from the *Food and Nutrition Bulletin*, de Pee S, and Semba RD. 2010. 31(4):S313–44.)

negatively affect metabolism). However, this will only result in improved nutritional status and health when the diet provides the nutrients that are required to rebuild the body's tissues and to restore bodily functions. The more advanced the disease stage, the more challenging it is to manage HIV (including OIs), to treat factors that affect food intake (such as mouth ulcers and loss of appetite), and to restore nutritional status.

Nutritional Needs of PLHIV

A 10% increase in energy intake is recommended during asymptomatic HIV infection (World Health Organization 2003) to support the increased resting energy expenditure. However, it is important to note that weight loss during HIV infection is mainly a result of reduced food intake as a consequence of reduced appetite. Careful study (in developed countries) of the energy balance of asymptomatic PLHIV has shown that reduced physical activity usually compensates for the increased energy needs of resting metabolism (Kosmiski 2011).

However, where people are involved in physical labor and are unlikely or unable to reduce physical activity, and where meeting normal energy requirements may already be difficult, increasing energy intake by 10% during asymptomatic infection is reasonable advice. During periods of symptomatic infection, energy expenditure goes up by 20%–30%, and therefore the recommendation is to increase energy intake by 20%–30% during and shortly after symptomatic infection (convalescence period). Energy requirements of PLHIV on ART are not well known and are likely to vary according to the severity of their clinical condition. However, they are very unlikely to be lower than that of people without HIV infection, or higher than what is required during symptomatic infection. Furthermore, certain groups, according to life stage, have increased recommended energy requirements, which need to be added to the increased requirement due to HIV. In adolescence, requirements for energy are highest during the period of peak growth, particularly in boys who gain a greater amount of height and lean body mass than girls (Robinson 2001). Monitoring weight is the best way to ascertain whether energy intake meets requirements.

Purpose and Type of Food and Nutrition Support for PLHIV

As discussed above, good nutrition that provides adequate calories and nutrients is essential to all PLHIV before and during ART, and during early as well as later phases of treatment, whether in resource-adequate or resource-limited settings. For this reason, nutrition education, as well as regular assessment of nutritional status, food consumption practices, and counseling tailored to individual needs is important for all PLHIV.

While counseling on healthy dietary practices is important for all, some PLHIV may require specific food and nutrition support to treat malnutrition, that is, rebuilding tissues (muscle mass and fat mass), restoring bodily functions, and ensuring adequate nutrient intake to maintain health and nutritional status and/or support continued access and adherence to treatment and care.

Support to enable adequate nutrient intake typically comes in the form of specific nutritious commodities, including micronutrient supplements, fortified blended foods, lipid-based nutrient supplements, as well as fresh foods such as fruits, vegetables, and animal source foods. These can be provided in-kind or in the form of commodity vouchers that can be redeemed for specific products. This type of support is appropriate where PLHIV cannot access these commodities due to affordability and/ or availability constraints.

BOX 4.2 RECOMMENDED NUTRITIONAL INTAKE FOR PEOPLE LIVING WITH HIV

Protein intake: The percentage of energy intake from protein should remain the same for PLHIV as for HIV-negative people, but when energy intake is increased, the total amount of protein will also be higher. Furthermore, in order to treat malnutrition, it is important that the protein sources provide enough essential amino acids. This means that there should be different sources of protein in the diet, including some with a high PDCAAS (protein digestibility corrected amino acid score) value, such as soybeans or animal source foods, including dairy.

Fat intake: Recommendations for fat intake are the same for PLHIV as for HIV-negative people: 15%–30% of energy intake (WHO 2014) In order to increase energy intake during convalescence, eating energy-dense foods, such as fatty foods and foods with a higher sugar content (e.g., fruit), may help to keep bulk relatively low so that extra energy intake can increase. It is important to note that PLHIV should consume unsaturated rather than saturated fats. PLHIV should eat foods that are dense in a range of nutrients, not only sugar or fat but also micronutrients.

Micronutrient intake: Because micronutrients are important for the immune system and other bodily functions, maintaining an adequate intake is very important for PLHIV. So far there is no conclusive evidence on whether PLHIV, in comparison to non-HIV infected people, should increase (or reduce) their micronutrient intake, or whether there are any specific micronutrients that they should consume more (or less) of (de Pee and Semba 2010; Forrester and Sztam 2011). WHO recommends consumption of the full FAO/WHO recommended nutrient intake for normal healthy people per day (RNI/day). The South African Academy of Science recommends an intake of 1–2 RNI/day because of higher needs during infection and the likelihood of preexisting deficiencies (Karsegard et al. 2004) Many people are unlikely to meet the recommended nutrient intake, especially when their diets lack diversity and contain only small amounts of animal source foods, fortified foods, fruits, or vegetables. Micronutrient supplements may therefore be required to ensure an adequate intake.

Most care and treatment programs that include a nutrition component provide nutrition assessment and counseling and prioritize the provision of food support to malnourished PLHIV starting ART. The food provided is often fortified blended food and/or a ready-to-use therapeutic food. Apart from supporting the treatment of malnutrition, specific foods may also be required to manage side effects, including nausea and lack of appetite. So far, provision of food or micronutrient supplements for maintenance of nutritional status is rare.

Enablers play an important role in increasing ART uptake and initial adherence and, as such, are important for promoting universal access to treatment. How long food support is provided depends on improvement in nutritional status (in the case of specialized food products), the opportunity costs of accessing treatment, and the patients' ability to earn a living. Whether or not food and nutrition support have an impact on treatment success depends on many factors; such as the context, clinical status of the individual, disease progression, adherence to treatment, type of food supplement, and nutrient intake (de Pee and Semba 2010). It is important that these factors are taken into account when designing an evaluation of a program's impact on malnutrition and treatment outcome.

APPLYING THE MATRIX FRAMEWORK TO FOOD AND NUTRITION ASSISTANCE: OPPORTUNITIES FOR PROGRAMMING

As described in the beginning of the chapter, HIV in the coming years will likely be integrated in many sectors. Therefore, it is critical to look at food and nutrition interventions beyond just food assistance, and within the broader context of structural interventions. The proposed framework (Figure 4.2) provides a systematic way of thinking through nutrition and food assistance interventions in a holistic way; these could be HIV specific or sensitive. Figure 4.5 illustrates food and nutrition interventions at the community and health systems levels throughout the HIV continuum of care.

The bases for the above interventions have three main areas of focus: food security and nutrition for adherence and retention in care; social protection linkages,

Continuum of HIV care	Food and nutrition: Linkages with social protection and health systems	
	Community level	**Health systems level**
HIV Transmission	• Food as an enabler to access preventative and screening services • Nutrition messaging BCC[a] • Resilience building, e.g., food for assets • Education, including nutrition • School feeding	• Preventative health facilities • Nutrition assessment/screening • Therapeutic and supplementary foods as needed • Tracking malnourished individuals • Nutrition counseling
HIV Testing	• Food as an enabler to access screening services (e.g., food centers) • Nutrition (knowledge among community health workers	• Nutrition assessment/screening • Therapeutic and supplementary foods • Nutrition counseling • Tracking malnourished individuals

Pre-ART care
 	
ART Initiation and Adherence
	• Referral to social safety nets for PLHIV to remain in care
	  ○ Food as an enabler to remain in care/food centers
	  ○ Economic strengthening activities/resilience building linked with food and nutrition support
	• Nutrition knowledge among community health workers
	• Nutrition messaging BCC[a]
	• Focus on key populations (e.g., adolescents, IDU
		• Regular nutrition assessment
		• Referral to food and nutrition assistance
		  ○ Therapeutic and supplementary foods
		  ○ Tracking of malnourished individuals
		• Social safety nets offering food and nutrition support linked with health systems
		• Nutrition counseling
		• Prevention of mother-to-child transmission services
		  ○ Linkages with sexual and reproductive health services

[a]Behavior change communication.

FIGURE 4.5 Food and nutrition interventions at the community and health systems levels throughout the HIV continuum of care.

for example, livelihood support relevant for all stages within the HIV continuum of care; and an emphasis on linkages with sexual and reproductive health and maternal, newborn, and child health.

ROLE OF FOOD SECURITY AND NUTRITION IN ADHERENCE

Realizing that food insecurity and poverty are important barriers to seeking a diagnosis and to starting and adhering to care and treatment, several programs provide food assistance to food-insecure PLHIV (de Pee et al. 2014). This offsets the opportunity costs of accessing treatment and compensates for the loss of income and livelihood following prolonged illness. This type of support often comes in the form of foods for the family, such as staple foods, beans or lentils, and vegetable oil, but may also come in the form of vouchers for foods or transport, or as cash. It is important to note that when PLHIV receive nutritious foods for treating malnutrition, this also supports their adherence to care and treatment.

The role of food security and nutrition, as related to adherence to treatment and retention in care, has been extensively reviewed by de Pee et al. (2014). It was found that conditional food assistance among food-insecure populations is an effective strategy for improving adherence. In a number of the studies that were reviewed, food assistance was conditioned upon visits to clinic or pharmacies. As discussed by the authors, food assistance and nutrition support play a dual role for HIV: a biological intervention, and/or an enabler to modify behavior that impacts adherence to treatment. While the biological intervention aspect is covered by health systems, the enabling environment created by food assistance takes place in the communities of PLHIV (Figure 4.6). However, the interaction and overlap between health

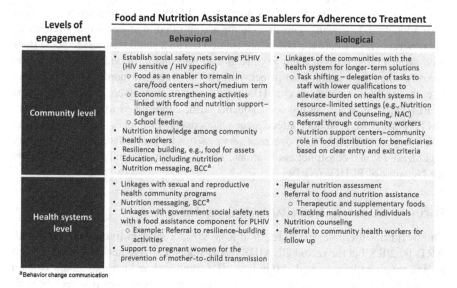

Levels of engagement	Food and Nutrition Assistance as Enablers for Adherence to Treatment	
	Behavioral	**Biological**

Community level	• Establish social safety nets serving PLHIV (HIV sensitive / HIV specific)
	  o Food as an enabler to remain in care/food centers – short/medium term
	  o Economic strengthening activities linked with food and nutrition support – longer term
	  o School feeding
	• Nutrition knowledge among community health workers
	• Resilience building, e.g., food for assets
	• Education, including nutrition
	• Nutrition messaging, BCC[a]
		• Linkages of the communities with the health system for longer-term solutions
		  o Task shifting – delegation of tasks to staff with lower qualifications to alleviate burden on health systems in resource-limited settings (e.g., Nutrition Assessment and Counseling, NAC)
		  o Referral through community workers
		  o Nutrition support centers–community role in food distribution for beneficiaries based on clear entry and exit criteria

Health systems level	• Linkages with sexual and reproductive health community programs
	• Nutrition messaging, BCC[a]
	• Linkages with government social safety nets with a food assistance component for PLHIV
	  o Example: Referral to resilience-building activities
	• Support to pregnant women for the prevention of mother-to-child transmission
		• Regular nutrition assessment
		• Referral to food and nutrition assistance
		  o Therapeutic and supplementary foods
		  o Tracking malnourished individuals
		• Nutrition counseling
		• Referral to community health workers for follow up

[a]Behavior change communication

FIGURE 4.6   Food and nutrition interventions impact adherence to treatment through behavioral and biological pathways: linkages between roles of communities and health systems.

systems and communities is imperative, since treatment is for life, and health systems are significantly underresourced and overstretched. With regard to food support and nutrition, for instance, communities or community health workers can play a role by identifying malnourished PLHIV and conducting Nutrition Assessment and Counseling (NAC) based on criteria established by clinicians. In turn, health systems can link vulnerable PLHIV to safety nets that include a food assistance component (completing the service to NACS—for Support); an example of such a program is described below.

FOCUS ON SOCIAL PROTECTION/ECONOMIC STRENGTHENING ACTIVITIES

PLHIV are often temporarily unable to earn a living, and can find themselves in a situation of economic shock associated with health care costs. The impact on the most vulnerable populations is many fold worse. This situation can quickly lead to increased food insecurity, forgoing treatment, selling off assets, or sending children to work instead of school. Food and nutrition assistance is therefore an essential part of a comprehensive HIV treatment and care package. But one of the concerns for food assistance programs has been the issue of sustainability, as food support for PLHIV and their families can be very costly. There is increasing interest in exploring options to link PLHIV with economic strengthening activities and livelihood support once they graduate from food support, which is often linked to having recovered from malnutrition. These programs could be specifically for PLHIV, or as part of general social protection schemes within a country.

In an initiative funded by multilateral donations and PEPFAR, WFP supports the Ethiopian Health Sector to conduct NACS for acutely malnourished people living with HIV in the most underdeveloped regions of the country. During the treatment period, food-insecure families of malnourished PLHIV receive monthly vouchers or cash allocation. Following recovery, clients are enrolled in an economic strengthening program (ES), where the clients are trained to run a small business to boost their food security and prevent them from relapsing into malnutrition. During the initial period of the ES program, food-insecure PLHIV also receive monthly food vouchers or cash. In addition, food-insecure HIV-positive pregnant women, as well as orphans to PLHIV, receive a monthly food voucher/cash, conditioned to the adherence to PMTCT services or school attendance, respectively. Ethiopia's national HIV and AIDS authority (F/HAPCO) oversees services run by health facilities, community organizations, and consumer associations. The food support component is funded by the Network of PLHIV (NEP+).

FOCUS ON MATERNAL, NEONATAL, AND CHILD HEALTH

The world has the potential to reach at least 90% of women living with HIV with ARTs by 2015, but the recent UNAIDS report states that "greater efforts are needed to link pregnant women and children to HIV treatment and care; pregnant women living with HIV are less likely than treatment-eligible adults overall to receive antiretroviral therapy, and treatment coverage among children living with HIV in 2012 was less than half the coverage for adults." In order to reach the goal of reducing the number of new infections by 90% among children by 2015, linkages of preventative strategies, such as family planning services, with reproductive health services (antenatal care, postnatal care), along with access to HIV testing, treatment, and counseling, and a deeper understanding of demand side barriers, will be essential.

There is an opportunity to leverage maternal, neonatal, child health (MNCH) programs and a role for community engagement in the integration of nutrition, food security, and social protection with health systems. Looking beyond traditional service delivery, an interesting example is the Philani Child Health and Nutrition Project serving the informal settlements in the Eastern Cape, South Africa; home for close to 1 million people. The community-based, non governmental organization provides basic child health and nutrition to communities wrought with poverty, unemployment, poor housing, child malnutrition, and disease. Philani programs incorporate home-based care, antenatal programs, nutrition support and counseling, and skills training (livelihood support). By 2005, there were approximately 30% HIV-positive pregnant women in Philani's target communities, and therefore all their programs have an HIV lens when providing education, care, and support.

From a perspective of community/health systems linkages, two aspects are noteworthy. First, there are opportunities in resource-limited settings to establish referral loops between communities and health facilities. Philani's mothers-to-be and mentor mothers programs provide support to women during and after their pregnancies to ensure good nutrition for them and their children. The community workers (chosen from the same communities and trained) are active in referring the women and children to appropriate health services as needed. In turn, the local health facilities/doctors may also refer discharged patients to the community workers for follow-up monitoring and provision of care. Second, despite present efforts, much more can be done for PMTCT and pediatric HIV by leveraging the outreach of community workers to actively look for pregnant women and monitor children. Philani's experience shows that often they are the first point of contact for HIV-positive children, their mothers, and HIV-positive pregnant women in the communities that they serve and they are then able to link them to local health services for treatment. Nutrition and child health are entry points for Philani's programs.

CONCLUSION

There is an opportunity to envision the world with zero AIDS-related deaths, but much remains to be done. The successes achieved and lessons learned now will pave the way for future work in the field of HIV/AIDS. Emphasis on women and key populations, in addition to integration with health systems, will have to be the focus. While treatment needs to play a central role in the response, if truly getting to zero new infections is the goal, demand side barriers such as poverty, food insecurity, stigma, and perceptions need to be carefully understood and overcome. Opportunities of integration beyond health systems—with national social protection schemes, livelihood support, and resilience building programs—are essential in ensuring sustainability and adherence to care and treatment. Partnerships have been the key to the successes achieved so far, and partnerships will be instrumental in continuing to address the epidemic going forward.

REFERENCES

de Pee, S., N. Grede, D. Mehra, and M. W. Bloem. 2014. The enabling effect of food assistance in improving adherence and/or treatment completion for antiretroviral therapy and tuberculosis treatment: A literature review. *AIDS and Behavior* 18 (Suppl 5):S459–64. doi: 10.1007/s10461-014-0870-4.

de Pee, S. and R. D. Semba. 2010. Role of nutrition in HIV infection: Review of evidence for more effective programming in resource-limited settings. *Food and Nutrition Bulletin* 31 (4):S313–44.

Deeks, S. G., S. R. Lewin, and D. V. Havlir. 2013. The end of AIDS: HIV infection as a chronic disease. *Lancet* 382 (9903):1525–33. doi: 10.1016/S0140-6736(13)61809-7.

Drewnowski, A. and N. Darmon. 2005. The economics of obesity: Dietary energy density and energy cost. *American Journal of Clinical Nutrition* 82 (1 Suppl):265S–73S.

England, R. 2011. A strategic revolution in HIV and global health. *Lancet* 378 (9787):226. doi: 10.1016/S0140-6736(11)61119-7.

Fitch, K. and S. Grinspoon. 2011. Nutritional and metabolic correlates of cardiovascular and bone disease in HIV-infected patients. *American Journal of Clinical Nutrition* 94 (6):1721S–8S. doi: 10.3945/ajcn.111.012120.

Forrester, JE and Sztam KA. 2011. Micronutrients in HIV/AIDS: Is there evidence to change the WHO 2003 recommendations? *The American Journal of Clinical Nutrition* 94(6): 1683S–9S.

Gardner, E. M., M. P. McLees, J. F. Steiner, C. Del Rio, and W. J. Burman. 2011. The spectrum of engagement in HIV care and its relevance to test-and-treat strategies for prevention of HIV infection. *Clinical Infectious Diseases* 52 (6):793–800. doi: 10.1093/cid/ciq243.

Horvath, K. J., J. M. Oakes, B. R. Rosser, G. Danilenko, H. Vezina, K. R. Amico, and J. Simoni. 2013. Feasibility, acceptability and preliminary efficacy of an online peer-to-peer social support ART adherence intervention. *AIDS and Behavior* 17 (6):2031–44. doi: 10.1007/s10461-013-0469-1.

Karim, S. S. and Q. A. Karim. 2011. Antiretroviral prophylaxis: A defining moment in HIV control. *Lancet* 378 (9809):e23–5. doi: 10.1016/S0140-6736(11)61136-7.

Kim, J. Y., P. Farmer, and M. E. Porter. 2013. Redefining global health-care delivery. *Lancet* 382 (9897):1060–9. doi: 10.1016/S0140-6736(13)61047-8.

Kohler, P. K., M. H. Chung, C. J. McGrath, S. F. Benki-Nugent, J. W. Thiga, and G. C. John-Stewart. 2011. Implementation of free cotrimoxazole prophylaxis improves clinic retention among antiretroviral therapy-ineligible clients in Kenya. *AIDS* 25 (13):1657–61. doi: 10.1097/QAD.0b013e32834957fd.

Kosmiski, L. 2011. Energy expenditure in HIV infection. *American Journal of Clinical Nutrition* 94 (6):1677S–82S. doi: 10.3945/ajcn.111.012625.

Kranzer, K., D. Govindasamy, N. Ford, V. Johnston, and S. D. Lawn. 2012. Quantifying and addressing losses along the continuum of care for people living with HIV infection in sub-Saharan Africa: A systematic review. *Journal of the International AIDS Society* 15 (2):17383. doi: 10.7448/IAS.15.2.17383.

Karsegard VL, Raguso CA, Genton L, Hirschel B, Pichard C. 2004. L-Ornithine alpha-ketoglutarate in HIV infection: effects of muscle, gastrointestinal, and immune functions. *Nutrition* 20:515–20.

Magnani, R., K. Sabin, T. Saidel, and D. Heckathorn. 2005. Review of sampling hard-to-reach and hidden populations for HIV surveillance. *AIDS* 19 (Suppl 2):S67–72.

Mugavero, M. J., W. E. Norton, and M. S. Saag. 2011. Health care system and policy factors influencing engagement in HIV medical care: Piecing together the fragments of a fractured health care delivery system. *Clinical Infectious Diseases* 52 (Suppl 2):S238–46. doi: 10.1093/cid/ciq048.

Nsigaye, R., A. Wringe, M. Roura, S. Kalluvya, M. Urassa, J. Busza, and B. Zaba. 2009. From HIV diagnosis to treatment: Evaluation of a referral system to promote and monitor access to antiretroviral therapy in rural Tanzania. *Journal of the International AIDS Society* 12 (1):31. doi: 10.1186/1758-2652-12-31.

Paton, N. I., S. Sangeetha, A. Earnest, and R. Bellamy. 2006. The impact of malnutrition on survival and the CD4 count response in HIV-infected patients starting antiretroviral therapy. *HIV Medicine* 7 (5):323–30. doi: 10.1111/j.1468-1293.2006.00383.x.

Robinson, F. 2001. Manual of dietetic practice. *Nutrition Bulletin* 26 (4):354. doi: 10.1046/j.1467-3010.2001.0173b.x.

Rosen, S. and M. P. Fox. 2011. Retention in HIV care between testing and treatment in sub-Saharan Africa: A systematic review. *PLOS Medicine* 8 (7):e1001056. doi: 10.1371/journal.pmed.1001056.

Schwartlander, B., J. Stover, T. Hallett, R. Atun, C. Avila, E. Gouws, and Group Investment Framework Study. 2011. Towards an improved investment approach for an effective response to HIV/AIDS. *Lancet* 377 (9782):2031–41. doi: 10.1016/S0140-6736(11)60702-2.

UNAIDS. 2012. Treatment 2015. Joint United Nations Programme on HIV/AIDS (UNAIDS). Accessed September 10, 2014. http://www.unaids.org/en/media/unaids/contentassets/documents/unaidspublication/2013/JC2484_treatment-2015_en.pdf.

UNAIDS. 2013. Global Report: UNAIDS report on the global AIDS epidemic 2013. Joint United Nations Programme on HIV/AIDS (UNAIDS). Accessed September 10, 2014. http://www.unaids.org/en/media/unaids/contentassets/documents/epidemiology/2013/gr2013/unaids_global_report_2013_en.pdf.

United Nations. 2013. A new global partnership: Eradicate poverty and transform economies through sustainable development: The report of the high-level panel of eminent persons on the post-2015 development agenda. [Report]. United Nations Publications. Accessed September 10, 2014. http://www.un.org/sg/management/pdf/HLP_P2015_Report.pdf.

van der Sande, M. A., M. F. Schim van der Loeff, A. A. Aveika, S. Sabally, T. Togun, R. Sarge-Njie, and H. C. Whittle. 2004. Body mass index at time of HIV diagnosis: A strong and independent predictor of survival. *JAIDS Journal of Acquired Immune Deficiency Syndromes* 37 (2):1288–94.

Weiser, S. D., K. Leiter, D. R. Bangsberg, L. M. Butler, F. Percy-de Korte, Z. Hlanze, and M. Heisler. 2007. Food insufficiency is associated with high-risk sexual behavior among women in Botswana and Swaziland. *PLOS Medicine* 4 (10):1589–97; discussion 1598. doi: 10.1371/journal.pmed.0040260.

WHO. 2008. Essential prevention and care interventions for adults and adolescents living with HIV in resource-limited settings.

WHO. 2011. IMAI district clinician manual.

WHO. 2014. Population nutrient intake goals for preventing diet-related chronic diseases.

World Health Organization. 1999. Management of severe malnutrition. A manual for physicians and other senior health workers.

World Health Organization. 2003. Nutrient requirements for people living with HIV/AIDS: Report of a technical consultation. [Technical consultation meeting]. World Health Organization. Accessed September 10, 2014. http://www.who.int/nutrition/publications/Content_nutrient_requirements.pdf.

Zachariah, R., M. Fitzgerald, M. Massaquoi, O. Pasulani, L. Arnould, S. Makombe, and A. D. Harries. 2006. Risk factors for high early mortality in patients on antiretroviral treatment in a rural district of Malawi. *AIDS* 20 (18):2355–60. doi: 10.1097/QAD.0b013e32801086b0.

5 Food Insecurity and Tuberculosis

Cara S. Guenther and Louise C. Ivers

CONTENTS

Despite the existence of a cure, tuberculosis (TB) remains one of the world's deadliest infectious diseases, second only to HIV/AIDS (Semba et al. 2010; Hood 2013; World Health Organization 2014). Currently infecting some 2 billion people, and killing a staggering 1.5 million people in 2013 alone, TB is responsible for more deaths worldwide than any other bacterial infection (Lönnroth et al. 2009; Semba et al. 2010). This death toll is particularly pronounced in resource-poor countries, where 95% of all TB deaths occur and where the disease is estimated to cause 25% of all preventable deaths (World Health Organization 2014). However, TB is indeed a global phenomenon, as middle-income and even some high-income countries face a significant prevalence of TB amongst the poor. Poverty and resource inequity are often common denominators in TB cases (Cegielski and McMurray 2004).

This unequal distribution of both TB infections and mortality due to TB, comes as little surprise given TB's many social determinants and their links to poverty. This chapter focuses on one of the most crucial of these determinants—food insecurity. For decades, studies and clinical experiences have pointed to a bidirectional additive relationship between TB, food security, and body mass. In fact, historically, the disease was referred to as "consumption" and "phthisis," precisely because of the severe weight loss its patients experience (Gauss 1936; Kennedy et al. 1996; Schwenk and Macallan 2000; Semba et al. 2010). Similarly, physicians have long noted the other side of this relationship: that food insecurity heightens the risk of developing active TB (Gauss 1936). In fact, physician David A. Stewart wrote in 1920 that, "the death rate from TB in England rises and falls with the price of bread" (Gauss 1936; Stewart 1922, pp. 130–134).

The important association between food insecurity and TB, however, has not been sufficiently acknowledged by program and policy makers, or even, for that matter, by doctors, many of whom fail to document the contribution of malnutrition to a patient's death (Hood 2013). These practices must change if TB and food insecurity are to be comprehensively addressed. Acknowledging and identifying the nature of the relationship between the two conditions is essential not only for effective treatment and disease eradication but also for the prevention and management of overlapping disease burdens. This task becomes even more important as the prevalence of both multidrug resistant (MDR-TB) and extensively drug-resistant TB (XDR-TB) continues to rise. It is estimated that in 2013, 480,000 people developed MDR-TB worldwide and that 9% of these cases were in fact cases of XDR-TB (World Health Organization 2014).

In accordance with this imperative, this chapter explores how food insecurity and TB affect each other by both directly and indirectly impacting individuals' nutrition statuses, adherence to treatment, outcomes, and coping strategies.

TUBERCULOSIS AND IMMUNE RESPONSE

The development of active TB disease involves two steps: infection and progression to active disease. *M. tuberculosis*, the mycobacterium that causes TB, is transmitted through infected aerosol droplets that are released most commonly through coughing (Schluger and Rom 1998; Semba et al. 2010). The normal immune response is complex and at the most basic level involves macrophages engulfing the mycobacterium, granuloma development, and recruiting B- and T-lymphocytes to aid in limiting the growth of, and killing the mycobacterium (Schluger and Rom 1998; Sinclair et al. 2011). Various factors may negatively impact the immune system's ability to fight the mycobacteria. When an individual comes in contact with these TB-infected droplets, three outcomes are possible: (i) the lungs' epithelial barrier protects the individual from infection, (ii) the bacteria breaks through the epithelial barrier, causing a primary infection which the body's cell-mediated immunity nonetheless contains, or (iii) active disease occurs (Schluger and Rom 1998; Semba et al. 2010; Lawn and Zumla 2011).

A primary latent infection (ii) is neither symptomatic nor contagious. It can, however, reactivate and develop into an active infection at any point when the individual's immune system can no longer contain the infection (Semba et al. 2010; Lawn and Zumla 2011). A latent infection is generally diagnosed if active TB cannot be confirmed despite a patient's positive reaction to the tuberculin skin test. However, diagnosing a latent infection through a tuberculin skin test becomes more complicated when testing a patient who received Bacillus Calmette-Guérin (BCG) vaccine as a child, because both a latent infection and the vaccine bring about an immune response, which is precisely what the tuberculin skin test detects.

In the third outcome (iii), the mycobacterium that penetrates the lungs' epithelial barrier is neither destroyed nor contained by the macrophages in the alveoli. As a result, these patients develop an active and contagious infection. When this form of infection occurs upon initial exposure, the patient is said to have primary progressive disease (Semba et al. 2010).

Patients with an active infection are said to have either pulmonary or extrapulmonary TB. A patient is diagnosed with pulmonary TB when a sputum test detects the mycobacteria in a patient's lungs. Since this type of TB is easily spread through coughing, pulmonary TB makes up 80% of all active cases (Semba et al. 2010). A patient has extrapulmonary TB when the mycobacteria attacks the body anywhere other than the lungs—most frequently at the lymph nodes, the pleura, the meninges, kidneys, bones, and joints. One to two percent of all TB cases are miliary TB, a form of the disease in which the mycobacteria infiltrates the bloodstream and is disseminated throughout the body. Since extrapulmonary TB does not affect the lungs, sputum tests usually cannot detect the presence of *M. tuberculosis*, rendering this type of TB more difficult to diagnose. Physicians can only definitively diagnose extrapulmonary TB if they find mycobacteria in lymph node specimens, pleural fluid, or another tissue.

It is not possible to determine how many people annually come in contact with TB but develop neither a latent nor an active infection. However, of the 2 billion people infected with *M. tuberculosis*, it is estimated that 95% have a latent infection and only about 5% develop primary progressive disease immediately upon exposure (Semba et al. 2010).

RELATIONSHIP BETWEEN FOOD INSECURITY AND TUBERCULOSIS

A household is considered to have food security if all members have "physical and economic access to sufficient, safe, and nutritious food that meets their dietary needs and food preferences for an active and healthy life" (Food and Agriculture Organization 2006). Lack of access to such food, on the other hand, qualifies a household as food *insecure*, which can contribute to malnutrition and impaired immune function, as well as lead to psychological stress and risky behaviors. Sustained, adequate nutrition is dependent upon, but not guaranteed by, the presence of food security in households.

For decades, studies have demonstrated an association between TB, nutritional status, and food security (Dodor 2008; Semba et al. 2010). Cochrane (1945), a physician and prisoner during World War II, noted how, in 1945, the incidence of TB was higher in patients who did not receive sufficient amounts of food. Another prisoner of war, Leyton (1946), compared TB incidence amongst British and Russian prisoners during World War II. He noted that both groups of prisoners had similar types and amounts of manual labor, living conditions, and clothing, but only the British prisoners received weekly Red-Cross rations. While British prisoners had a 1.2% TB incidence rate, Russian prisoners had one between 15% and 20%.

Other studies have shown that the majority of patients suffering from TB are malnourished (Karyadi et al. 2000; Schwenk and Macallan 2000; Madebo et al. 2003; Dodor 2008; Semba et al. 2010; Mupere et al. 2012). For example, a 2002 study in Ghana found a 51% prevalence of malnutrition (body mass index (BMI) < 18.5 kg/m^2) amongst 570 adults who had active pulmonary TB for the first time, but were not pregnant, breastfeeding, diabetic, or HIV positive (Dodor 2008). Of these patients, 24% were mildly malnourished (BMI = 17.0–18.4 kg/m^2), 12% were moderately malnourished (BMI = 16.0–16.9 kg/m^2), and 15% were severely malnourished (BMI < 16.0 kg/m^2). Similarly, a two-phase (1995–1999 and 2000–2012) retrospective cohort study of 747 adults with pulmonary TB and known HIV status living in urban Uganda found similar results (Mupere et al. 2012): 42% of the TB patients had a low BMI (<18.5 kg/m^2). Additionally, of the 311 patients whose tissue mass they measured, 33% had reduced lean tissue mass and 43% had reduced fat mass. Karyadi et al. (2000) found similar results when comparing 41 patients with active pulmonary TB to 41 controls matched for age and sex: pulmonary patients had lower BMIs and skin fold thicknesses. Similarly, Madebo et al. (2003) found TB patients in Ethiopia, regardless of HIV status, had significantly lower weight, BMI, and middle-upper arm circumference than their healthy counterparts.

In addition to noting the co-morbidity of wasting and TB, studies have demonstrated that poor nutrition status is a risk factor for mortality in TB patients (McKeown and Record 1962; Zachariah et al. 2002; Cegielski and McMurray 2004; Semba et al. 2010; Mupere et al. 2012). In fact, McKeown et al. (1962) argued that the decrease in TB death rate from 40/1000 person-years in the beginning of the nineteenth century to 14/1000 person-years at the end of the nineteenth century was caused by improvements in nutrition, rather than medical advances (Cegielski and McMurray 2004). A study conducted in Malawi in 1999 found that early mortality rate, defined as death within the first four weeks of treatment, was significantly greater for patients who were moderately or severely malnourished, regardless of age or HIV status (Zachariah et al. 2002; Semba et al. 2010). Similar findings were reported from Uganda by Mupere et al. (2012).

While these studies do not determine the direction of the relationship between malnutrition and TB, they do illustrate the co-morbidity seen in patients, the heightened risk of death in TB patients with poor nutrition status, and the need for programs to address both conditions. However, as the next two sections demonstrate, studies also show the four major ways in which food insecurity heightens the risk of TB: by causing protein–energy malnutrition and micronutrient deficiencies as well as by contributing to diabetes and tobacco use.

PROTEIN–ENERGY MALNUTRITION AND TUBERCULOSIS

Food insecurity may result in malnutrition. People with protein–energy malnutrition are deficient in protein, which the body requires for growth and regeneration.

Protein–energy malnutrition, if acute, can lead to wasting, and, if chronic, can lead to stunting (Hood 2013). In addition, protein–energy malnutrition weakens the cell-mediated immune system (Escott and Newell 2007; Semba et al. 2010)—the body's main defense mechanism against *M. tuberculosis* (Cegielski and McMurray 2004). This effect has been observed experimentally in mice. When Chan et al. (1996) infected two groups of mice with BCG, and gave one group a protein-rich diet and the other a protein-deficient diet, all of the mice with the protein-rich diets survived the infection, whereas all of the mice receiving the protein-deficient diet died within 66 days. In addition to dying earlier, the protein-deficient mice had higher bacterial burdens and worse granuloma development, as compared to the mice that received a protein-rich diet. In humans, Pelly et al. (2005) found that Peruvian patients with less muscle mass had suppressed immune reactions to TB antigens, as measured by TB skin test results.

As a result of its detrimental effect on host immune response, protein–energy malnutrition has been associated with increased risk of active TB infection, and those who are malnourished are at an increased risk of not only developing primary progressive disease, but also having a latent infection progress into an active one (Cegielski and McMurray 2004; Escott and Newell 2007; Semba et al. 2010). With an estimated 805 million people in the world facing food insecurity, the majority of whom live in the developing world, resource-poor countries house an overwhelming amount of individuals with compromised immune systems, in addition to having the highest burden of latent TB (World Food Programme 2014).

These interactions between nutrition and TB are not restricted to resource-poor settings. Tverdal (1986) followed over 1.7 million Norwegians above the age of 15 for 8–19 years and found that those with a low BMI were five times as likely of contracting TB than those in the highest BMI category. Lönnroth et al. (2010) reported similar results when they conducted a systematic review of cohort studies that used active TB as the outcome and recorded both baseline BMI and disease status. Six studies meeting these criteria were conducted at different points over the past 60 years, in four different resource-rich countries, and looked at different demographics; despite these differences, in all studies, the authors found a log-linear inverse relationship between BMI and incidence of active TB for people with a BMI between 18.5 and 30 kg/m^2. With each unit increase in BMI, TB incidence decreased by 13.8%. These studies suggest that, in the appropriate risk environment, for patients with BMIs between 18.5 and 30 kg/m^2, BMI could be a good indicator of the risk of developing active TB. The authors also found that while the inverse log-linear relationship holds true for BMIs above 25 kg/m^2, it becomes less clear for BMIs greater than or equal to 30 kg/m^2. Since only two of the included studies analyzed the relationship between TB incidence and BMI < 18.5 kg/m^2, further studies at these levels of underweight are required.

MICRONUTRIENT DEFICIENCY AND TUBERCULOSIS

Studies have demonstrated how micronutrient deficiencies may impact a person's risk of contracting TB by compromising immune response. Like protein–energy malnutrition, studies have linked specific nutrient deficiencies to an increased risk of primary progressive disease and the progression of latent TB infection into active TB (Downes

1950; Escott and Newell 2007; Semba et al. 2010). While the ways in which each micronutrient affects the cell-mediated immune response is beyond the scope of this chapter, studies explore the role of vitamin A (Sklan et al. 1994; Rwangabwoba et al. 1998; van Lettow et al. 2003; Semba et al. 2010; Sinclair et al. 2011), vitamin B (van Lettow et al. 2003), vitamin C (van Lettow et al. 2003; Bakaev and Duntau 2004; Vijayamalini and Manoharan 2004; Lamsal et al. 2007; Semba et al. 2010), vitamin D (van Lettow et al. 2003; Cegielski and McMurray 2004; Sinclair et al. 2011), vitamin E (Sinclair et al. 2011), folate, zinc (Smith et al. 1973; McMurray et al. 1990; Shankar and Prasad 1998; Karyadi et al. 2000; Cegielski and McMurray 2004; Gupta et al. 2009; Sinclair et al. 2011), and selenium (Sinclair et al. 2011) in immune function.

Vitamin A

Many of the studies investigating direct links between nutritional status and TB were in the pre-chemotherapy era, with the majority predating 1950 (van Lettow and Whalen 2008). For example, Finkelstein (1932) showed that rats who received vitamin A supplements before or upon inoculation with TB mycobacteria lived longer before succumbing to the infection, compared to the control groups, and Solotorovsky et al. (1961) illustrated that TB-infected chicks were more likely to survive if they received vitamin A supplements (van Lettow et al. 2003). Furthermore, although unable to determine the direction of the relationship, researchers have noted vitamin A deficiencies amongst individuals with TB. Madebo et al. (2003) found that TB patients in Ethiopia had lower vitamin A levels than their healthy controls, and that this deficiency was strongly associated with low anthropometric measures (Semba et al. 2010). Similarly, Van lettow et al. (2005) noted that 59% of the pulmonary TB patients in their Malawi study were vitamin A deficient.

Vitamin B

Studies have also considered the role of vitamin B levels in tuberculosis and reported mixed results. For example, a 1988 study using dietary surveys of 1187 individuals of Indian descent living in London found a TB incidence of 133/1000 in lifelong vegetarians, compared to 48/1000 in omnivores (Chanarin and Stephenson 1988). While the difference was significant ($p = 0.0016$), the flawed methodology raised some questions about the results. The study only had a 50% response rate to their surveys and never actually measured cobalamin (vitamin B12) serum levels, assuming both that vegetarians had lower cobalamin serum levels and that the difference in cobalamin, rather than other factors, was the main reason for the higher prevalence of TB amongst the vegetarian respondents (Cegielski and McMurray 2004). A study in London noted raised vitamin B12 and normal folate levels in patients with severe pulmonary tuberculosis (Morris et al. 1989; Semba et al. 2010) and a study in Nigeria did not find any difference in serum vitamin B12 levels when comparing tuberculosis patients and blood donors (Knox-Macaulay 1990).

Vitamin C

Lamsal et al. (2007) found that patients with pulmonary TB in Nepal had significantly lower mean levels of plasma vitamin C compared to healthy controls ($p < 0.0001$). Similarly, Madebo et al. (2003) noted significantly lower vitamin C levels in Ethiopian tuberculosis patients compared to healthy counterparts. Adult male pulmonary TB patients in India were also found to have lower vitamin C levels than their healthy counterparts (Vijayamalini and Manoharan 2004; Semba et al. 2010). In a study looking at Finnish male smokers aged between 50 and 69 years old, however, Hemilä et al. (1999) found that the inverse relationship between tuberculosis incidence and vitamin C intake was no longer statistically significant after adjusting for cofounders.

Vitamin D

Studies have explored vitamin D levels in patients with tuberculosis. Grange et al. (1985) and Chan et al. (1994) found normal vitamin D levels in patients with active TB (Semba et al. 2010). Davies et al. (1985) found that TB patients had significantly lower serum 25-OHD levels (p < 0.005) than their healthy counterparts. They did not, however, note any differences in 1,25 and 24,25-$(OH)_2D$ levels between patient and control groups (Davies et al. 1985). In the United Kingdom, Douglas et al. (1996) found that TB incidence is greatest in the summer, after patients had endured a cold winter with little exposure to vitamin D. The delay could be explained by slow disease progression and diagnosis (Schwenk and Macallan 2000). However, the role of vitamin D in protecting against tuberculosis infection is affected by diet, sunlight exposure, and genetic variations in receptors and thus may vary from population to population (Schwenk and Macallan 2000).

Vitamin E

Lamsal et al. (2007) found that patients with pulmonary TB had significantly lower levels of vitamin E (p < 0.001). Similarly, significantly lower serum vitamin E levels have been reported in TB patients in Ethiopia (Madebo et al. 2003) and adult male pulmonary tuberculosis patients in India (Vijayamalini and Manoharan 2004); van Lettow et al. (2004) reported that of the 500 pulmonary tuberculosis patients in their study in Malawi, 12% where vitamin E deficient.

Other Micronutrients

Van Lettow et al. (2004) noted that 80% of the pulmonary TB patients participating in their study in Malawi were zinc deficient. Similarly, when comparing 41 patients with active pulmonary TB to 41 controls matched for age and gender, the patients had significantly lower plasma zinc concentrations (Karyadi et al. 2000). Zinc deficiencies have been associated with protein–energy malnutrition. Ray et al. (1998) noted that malnourished children had lower plasma zinc levels than healthy children, but children with TB had the lowest plasma zinc levels. They did not, however, note a significant difference in plasma zinc levels between malnourished children with active TB and nutritionally healthy children with active TB. Furthermore, the authors found that plasma zinc levels of Indian children with disseminated TB were significantly lower than those of children with pulmonary TB.

Micronutrient Supplementation

In the eighteenth and nineteenth centuries, the use of cod-liver oil was a popular treatment for TB. Known to be rich in vitamins A and D, cod-liver oil was often used as a treatment for TB. It found remarkable success when compared to the alternative of symptomatic treatment (van Lettow and Whalen 2008). Studies have also illustrated the potential preventative benefits of sufficient vitamin A levels. A 1940s study conducted in Harlem, New York City, found that taking vitamin and mineral supplements reduced the risk of developing primary progressive TB; families who received the supplement had a TB attack rate of 0.16/100 person-years, whereas those families that did not receive the supplement had one of 0.91/100 person-years (Downes 1950). While this study illustrates that vitamin and mineral supplements decrease the risk of developing primary progressive TB, it does not illustrate that nutrient deficiency causes a higher TB attack rate. However, a 7-year longitudinal study also conducted in the 1940s, following 1100 low-income men living in Philadelphia who at baseline did not have TB, found that men who were vitamin A or C deficient at baseline had significantly higher risk of developing active TB (Getz et al. 1951). Despite the aforementioned studies, there is little direct evidence that routine micronutrient supplementation improves treatment outcomes or quality of life in TB patients (Sinclair et al. 2011).

DIABETES AS A RISK FACTOR FOR TUBERCULOSIS

Food insecurity, where studied, has often been associated with obesity rather than undernutrition, perhaps because the most inexpensive options for urban families in resource-rich environments are often unhealthy, processed foods (Ivers and Cullen 2011). Food insecurity is also a risk factor for diabetes mellitus, and has been associated with poor diabetes control in the United States (Seligman et al. 2007, 2010a, b, 2012). Interestingly, Lönnroth et al. (2010) found that the aforementioned inverse relationship between body mass and TB holds true for patients with a BMI between 25 and 30 kg/m^2. In other words, patients who are overweight, according to this study, had a lower risk of contracting TB. However, the relationship did not hold true for BMI > 30 kg/m^2. These results raise interesting questions about the pathways through which food insecurity and *M. tuberculosis* interact, especially given that studies have noted the co-morbidity of diabetes mellitus, a condition often linked with obesity, and TB since the early 1900s (Mugusi et al. 1990; Jeon and Murray 2008). In Indonesia, diabetes mellitus was associated with pulmonary TB. 13.2% of the 454 newly diagnosed pulmonary TB patients had diabetes, compared to 3.2% of the matched controls (Alisjahbana et al. 2006). Similar results were found in other country studies (Lienhardt et al. 2005; Jeon and Murray 2008).

Some studies have attempted to determine the directionality of the relationship between diabetes and TB. In particular, researchers have observed that diabetes weakens both innate and adaptive immune responses, thereby rendering the diabetic more vulnerable to TB infection (Stevenson et al. 2007; Jeon and Murray 2008). A comprehensive review by Jeon and Murray (2008) of three prospective cohort studies, eight case–control studies, and two other studies found that diabetes mellitus increased the risk of TB. The meta-analysis demonstrated this relationship despite the fact that the 13 studies varied in study designs, background TB incidence, and geographic region. Stevenson et al. (2007) estimated that in 2000 diabetes accounted for 14.8% of annual incident pulmonary TB in India and 80.5% of the annual incident cases of pulmonary TB amongst diabetics in India. Lönnroth et al. when looking at 22 countries with a high prevalence of TB, calculated that the population attributable fraction for diabetes is 6%. While these estimates vary, they do demonstrate the detrimental impact of diabetes on TB (Lonnroth and Raviglione 2008; Lönnroth et al. 2009). A study in Nigeria found that 42.6% of TB patients had blood glucose results that fell into either the impaired glucose tolerance or diabetes categories (Oluboyo and Erasmus 1990). Since hyperglycemia disappeared in almost all patients after 3 months of TB chemotherapy, this effect of TB infection raises questions about whether TB can increase the chances that a patient becomes diabetic.

Today, 180 million people are diabetics, a figure that is expected to double by 2030 (Jeon and Murray 2008). This rise in diabetes incidence is most troubling for countries such as India and China where the prevalence of diabetes is increasing most rapidly and the burden of TB is the greatest (Jeon and Murray 2008). Food insecurity is, of course, not associated with all cases of diabetes, but as the incidences of obesity and type 2 diabetes continue to rise in settings with high TB prevalence around the world, it is becoming all the more urgent for medical practitioners, policy makers, and program implementers to understand the role of diabetes as a risk factor for TB-infected populations and the role that food insecurity may play in these overlapping epidemics. Studies point out that given the rise in obesity and diabetes, the "typical" profile of an undernourished TB patient may no longer describe patients' disease experiences in certain countries (World Health Organization 2009; Semba et al. 2010).

TOBACCO USE AS A RISK FACTOR FOR TUBERCULOSIS

The relationship between tobacco use and TB infection has been documented since the early twentieth century (Slama et al. 2007). While beyond the scope of this chapter, the effect of smoking on the immune response to TB, at the most basic level, is that smoking both decreases the lungs' ability to clear pathogens and impairs macrophage's ability to fight the pathogens (Maurya et al. 2002).

Slama et al. (2007) found that active smokers have an odds ratio of 1.8 (95% CI 1.5–2.1) for TB infection. Furthermore, this meta-analysis showed that, when compared to people who have never smoked, current and former smokers are respectively 2.6 times and 1.6 times as likely to develop active pulmonary TB, and this association has been confirmed in a number of studies (Maurya et al. 2002; Bates et al. 2007). Exposure to second-hand smoke seems to have a similar effect. Slama et al. (2007) found that five out of the six studies that looked at effect of exposure to smoke on TB infection in children reported that children exposed to smoke were significantly more at risk of TB infection and disease than those who were not.

Relevant to the discussion in this chapter is that a number of studies have also linked smoking to food insecurity. For example, Widome et al. (2014) found that U.S. veterans facing food insecurity were more likely to smoke tobacco than those who were not. A study looking at Latino adults over the age of 20 found that a larger proportion of individuals with low or marginal food security smoke than those who were food secure (Iglesias-Rios et al. 2013). Similarly, Cutler-Triggs et al. (2008) found that smoking was an independent risk factor for household food insecurity. This relationship holds true in Indonesia as well, where Semba et al. (2011) found a significant association ($p < 0.0001$) between paternal smoking and household food insecurity.

Smoking could increase low-income families' risk of becoming food insecure by diverting funds for cigarettes that could be used for food instead (Semba et al. 2007; Widome et al. 2014). Alternatively, it is possible that food insecurity drives people to smoke. Studies have linked food insecurity to depression and anxiety, especially among women (Hadley et al. 2008; Ivers and Cullen 2011; Okechukwu et al. 2012). In fact, Okechukwu et al. (2012) found that low-wage nursing home workers in the United States who faced food insecurity were twice as likely to have depressive symptoms compared to those who did not report food insecurity, even when the authors incorporated financial strain and work–family spill over. Similarly, a study in rural Ethiopia found that houses with food insecurity were significantly more likely to report symptoms of high anxiety (65% vs. 34%) or depression (62% vs. 27%) (Hadley et al. 2008). As an additional pathway for ill health, the interaction between food insecurity, tobacco use, and TB is important to explore, and more research is needed to review the public health impact of this complex relationship.

TUBERCULOSIS AND FOOD INSECURITY PATHWAYS ARE MULTIDIRECTIONAL

The pathways between TB and food insecurity are multidirectional: while food insecurity may put a person at risk of contracting the disease, once contracted, TB may also put the patient at risk of becoming malnourished and food insecure.

Tuberculosis disease itself results in abnormal metabolic processes, increased resting energy expenditure, and decreased appetite (Cegielski and McMurray 2004; Semba et al. 2010; Sinclair et al. 2011). As a result of these effects, TB causes a patient's energy expenditure to exceed the energy available from their food intake, leading to metabolism of fat and protein reserves (Semba et al. 2010). Active TB infection also causes an "anabolic block" during which patients use more protein intake for oxidation and energy production (Gupta et al. 2009). As a result, amino acids are kept from synthesizing proteins, decreasing muscle tissue growth in patients with active TB (Macallan et al. 1998; Semba et al. 2010).

Additionally, TB can cause a household to become food insecure or drive a family deeper into preexisting conditions of food insecurity. Given the wasting effect the disease has on an affected individual, TB often renders the patient unable to contribute to the day-to-day activities of his or her household, thereby reducing the household work force (Wyss et al. 2001; Escott and Newell 2007; Sinclair et al. 2011). Tanimura et al. (2014) found in their systematic review of 49 studies that lost income often poses a greater financial burden for TB patients than medical and nonmedical treatment costs of their disease, and that poverty is intimately associated with food insecurity. Other studies have confirmed the importance of lost income for patients with TB (Wyss et al. 2001; Sinclair et al. 2011).

TB, as such, threatens to decrease not only the household income but also, in some cases, the household diversification of labor, rendering the family more vulnerable to droughts and other labor shocks. Such a reduction in labor can force a previously food-secure family into food insecurity or worsen the situation of those already dealing with food insecurity (Escott and Newell 2007). Furthermore, patients and their families often have to cover health care and transportation costs, even in countries where the government provides free TB care (Wyss et al. 2001; Tanimura et al. 2014). For example, a study examining access to TB services for Somali pastoralists in Ethiopia observed that many families had to sell livestock in order to afford treatment (Gele et al. 2010). Twelve studies included in a systematic review of 44 qualitative studies on treatment adherence reported that families were forced to choose between working and seeking treatment (Munro et al. 2007). These extra costs can drive families into food insecurity.

While studies have shown that the majority of newly diagnosed TB patients have lower BMIs (Kennedy et al. 1996; Zachariah et al. 2002; Dodor 2008; Mupere et al. 2012), suffer from macro- and micro nutrient deficiencies (Downes 1950; Getz et al. 1951; van Lettow et al. 2003; Cegielski and McMurray 2004; Pelly et al. 2005; Escott and Newell 2007; Lönnroth and Raviglione 2008; Lönnroth et al. 2009, 2010; Semba et al. 2010), and experience increased costs and decreased income (Gele et al. 2010; Wyss et al. 2001; Escott and Newell 2007; Munro et al. 2007; Sinclair et al. 2011), they have not measured food insecurity specifically, nor been able to determine the directionality of the interactions between food insecurity, undernutrition, and TB.

TUBERCULOSIS VACCINATION

Food insecurity (through malnutrition) can reduce the efficacy of the TB vaccine, Bacillus Calmette-Guérin (BCG). The vaccine's effectiveness varies considerably, and generally only children living in countries with high risk of TB receive the vaccine. Those who receive BCG often test positive by tuberculin skin test, limiting the usefulness of the test in the setting of vaccination, although reactivity to the tuberculin skin test (i.e., positive test results) has been shown to wane over time, especially if the child receives the vaccine at birth (Semba et al. 2010).

Unfortunately, studies have shown that the vaccine's already troublesome efficacy can be compounded by poor nutrition (Ziegler and Ziegler 1975; Sinha and Bang 1976; Satyanarayana et al. 1980; Semba et al. 2010). A study conducted in West Bengal found that vaccinated children with protein–energy malnutrition exhibited significantly lower reactivity to skin tests administered 6–8 weeks after vaccination than the control group (Sinha and Bang 1976). Another study in India found that vaccinated children with kwashiorkor were significantly less likely to have a positive skin result and their area of induration was significantly smaller when compared to nutritionally healthy children and children with mild, moderate, or severe protein–energy malnutrition (Satyanarayana et al. 1980). At this time, it is unclear how nutritional status at birth affects the vaccine's effectiveness. Given that BCG is usually administered at birth, understanding how birth weight and early infant nutrition affect the protective ability of the vaccine has important implications for determining the optimal use of the vaccine, and complementary support programs at the time of vaccine delivery.

The incomplete protection provided by the BCG vaccine coupled with the effects of nutrition on the vaccine's efficacy is especially problematic given the geographic overlap of TB, food insecurity, and poor nutrition status.

TUBERCULOSIS TREATMENT

Given the body of research and clinical experience surrounding TB and its relation to nutrition, it seems increasingly clear that protecting individuals from TB infection relies, at least in part, on ensuring adequate and ongoing access to safe and nutritious food—the very definition of food security. The importance of food security, however, does not end with TB prevention; once a patient has been infected, his or her relative degree of food security plays a critical role in either helping or hindering treatment and recovery. Directly observed treatment, short course (DOTS) is the primary treatment method for TB. Under this treatment plan, patients with non-drug-resistant TB receive four antimicrobial drugs for 6 months from a health care provider or a trained community health worker. The WHO estimates that DOTS has treated 56 million people since 1995 (World Health Organization 2014).

However, food insecurity threatens to undermine the success of DOTS. Food insecurity may negatively affect treatment-seeking behavior and adherence in TB patients. A study in Swaziland in 2005 that conducted 41 semi structured, recorded interviews, including 10 patients and 10 community health workers, found that patients stopped taking their medication because treatment made them hungrier and they were unable to secure the necessary amounts of food to match their appetites (Escott and Newell 2007). For example, in describing a 22-year-old female patient:

> she got tired of taking the tablets...the tablets would make her hungry, but they didn't have much food because her father died.

Similarly, regarding a 32-year-old female patient:

> they can't take the tablets on the empty stomach and so end up not taking the tablets... because the tablets make a person very hungry. (Escott and Newell 2007)

In response to these complaints, some health workers tried to provide patients with food from their own homes—an unsustainable and ineffective solution given the impoverishment of the workers themselves (Escott and Newell 2007). Similarly, a systematic review of 44 qualitative studies on treatment adherence found that seven studies mentioned that the quality of food accessible by patients impacted treatment adherence (Munro et al. 2007). In five of those studies, patients cited stopping medication or leaving the hospital when they could not access food (Munro et al. 2007). This detrimental effect that treatment-induced hunger has on treatment adherence illustrates the need for programs to address patients' food insecurity. This phenomenon is well described in the literature on HIV treatment adherence, but has received less attention in the literature on TB treatment adherence. Inconsistent and, in some cases, truncated treatment for TB delays rehabilitation, may extend the amount of time that a patient is contagious, and may increase the risk that the patient's TB will become drug-resistant.

In addition to affecting treatment adherence, food insecurity and related nutritional deprivation can also lead to a slow rehabilitation for even the most treatment-adherent patients. Poor nutrition has been linked to delayed bacilli clearance from sputum, for example (Escott and Newell 2007). This effect was ameliorated by nutritional supplements in one study; accelerated sputum clearance of TB and improvements in lesions were observed at the 2-month check-up for adult patients who received daily vitamin A and zinc supplements during TB chemotherapy (Karyadi et al. 2002; van Lettow et al. 2003). Unfortunately, the same supplements did not heal the cavities, increase hemoglobin concentrations, or continue to improve lesion areas after the first 2 months.

Researchers have also examined the effect of chemotherapy on micronutrient levels. Lamsal et al. (2007) found that after 2 months of chemotherapy, patients' vitamin C levels had increased significantly ($p = 0.0001$). Similarly, Ray et al. (1998) noted that after 6 months of therapy, Indian children had significantly increased plasma zinc levels than before therapy, regardless of the type of tuberculosis. While studies have examined the effect of treatment on serum calcium levels (Brodie et al. 1981; Perry et al. 1982; Kitrou et al. 1983) and serum vitamin D levels (Davies et al. 1985; Williams et al. 1985), results are contradictory. Finally, Visser et al. found that after one week of chemotherapy, patients had lower plasma pyridoxine levels (vitamin B6) (Visser et al. 2004).

Although studies on whether treatment directly impacts a patient's anthropometric measurements have been conducted, their results have been less conclusive, as treatment for TB is not always associated with a reestablishment of normal body mass, or even associated with weight gain. While the previously mentioned study in Ghana could not comment on the directionality of the relationship between TB and under-nutrition, the data did demonstrate improved nutritional status in patients once they started receiving chemotherapy (Dodor 2008). Following 2 months of intensive treatment, 75% of patients experienced an increase in BMI ranging anywhere from 0.01 to >3 kg/m^2. On the other hand, 25% of patients experienced a decrease in BMI. The percent of underweight patients decreased from 51% to 40% (BMI < 18.5 kg/m^2) after 2 months of treatment. However, the fact that age, marital status, employment status, educational level, monthly income, and belief in avoiding certain food types were significantly associated with increased BMI during treatment, but sputum smear type, sex, duration of symptoms, and family size were not significantly associated, suggested that food security and related socioeconomic factors, rather than the administering of anti-TB treatment, were responsible for the increase in BMI. Another study found that patients had improved weight, muscle mass and function, subcutaneous fat, and serum albumin levels at 4 and 8 weeks after the start of chemotherapy (Harries et al. 1988).

A study in Tanzania demonstrates just how important access to sufficient quality and quantity of food is to weight gain in patients receiving TB treatment. While all patients gained weight during the study, Kennedy et al. (1996) noticed that those patients who required a longer hospital stay, either because they had not yet exhibited bacilli-free sputum or because they had relapsed, gained more weight than those requiring shorter hospital stays. There was a significant association between month of discharge and weight gain while hospitalized ($p < 0.0001$), meaning that those patients who remained sick for a longer period actually experienced more, not less, weight gain. This relationship between length of hospital stay and weight gain was observed for both male and female patients, with women gaining more weight than men. While all patients lost weight once they returned home, those who were discharged earliest from the hospital experienced the least weight gain not only while hospitalized but also during the entire 12-month study. Multiple factors could have accounted for these findings. Although the study did not measure food access at the hospital compared to that available at the patients' homes, the fact that length of stay was the determinant most positively associated with weight gain suggests that the food provided by the hospital more adequately met the patients' caloric and nutritional needs than the food they obtained at home. However, patients are, in all likelihood, more active at home than in the hospital, so the increase in energy expenditure and subsequent increase in caloric demands at home could also have contributed to the patients' weight loss after leaving the hospital (Kennedy et al. 1996). These results illustrate just how crucial nutritional support and assessment of food security can be for both ambulatory patients and their families, many of whom are unable to cope with the recently released patient's increased caloric demands due to increased energy expenditure and the return of healthy appetites. Patients who lack access to adequate nutrition to sustain them throughout treatment, and who therefore are at risk of stopping treatment, would benefit greatly from food assistance (Escott and Newell 2007).

Despite the wealth of research emphasizing the importance of nutrition in TB treatment, TB patients, and doctors alike, continue to experience a dearth of evidence-based recommendations for nutritional guidelines for TB patients (Hood 2013). Furthermore, there is a lack of information on how to address the structural and economic aspects of food insecurity that may give rise to undernutrition in this population.

SPECIAL POPULATIONS

Given the synergistic relationship between TB and food insecurity, and the many, complicated ways in which the two affect each other, special attention—both academically and programmatically—needs to be paid to those who are most at risk of being both food insecure and developing active TB infection: children, and people living with HIV infection.

CHILDREN

WHO estimated in 2013 that TB killed 80,000 HIV-negative children and that half a million of the annual new cases of TB are in children (World Health Organization 2014), but insufficient attention is paid to this important issue. Children constitute an at-risk population because they are more likely to develop active TB than adults (Newton et al. 2008). In children with healthy immune systems, age is the main predictor of whether TB infection progresses to active disease (Marais et al. 2006), having the highest risk of developing active TB during the first 2 years of life (Marais et al. 2004, 2006; Newton et al. 2008; Semba et al. 2010; Narasimhan et al. 2013). The risk for immunocompromised children remains consistently high throughout life and does not seem to change with the child's age (Marais et al. 2006). The risk of developing active TB is heightened in children under the age of two and immunocompromised children because their cell-mediated immune responses are not as developed as older children or adults (Marais et al. 2006; Newton et al. 2008). For the same reason, young and immunocompromised children are also more at risk of developing miliary and extrapulmonary TB (Marais et al. 2006; Newton et al. 2008; Semba et al. 2010). Children are also more likely than adults to succumb to their TB infections (Newton et al. 2008), with the highest risk of TB mortality in infants (Narasimhan et al. 2013).

The bidirectional, synergistic relationship between nutrition and TB holds true for children as well as for adults (Shimeles and Lulseged 1994; Semba et al. 2010). Although the directionality of the association was not determined, a study in Ethiopia found that 25% of children between 4 and 60 months old hospitalized for severe protein–energy malnutrition also suffered from TB (Shimeles and Lulseged 1994). However, while poor nutrition is cited as a risk factor of TB in children, the ways in which these two conditions interact have yet to be fully understood (Jaganath and Mupere 2012). Studies have shown that breast milk contains nutrients and immune factors that control inflammation and boost innate immunity. Given the immune properties in breast milk, it is possible that children who are weaned prematurely are less protected against TB, especially since studies show that not exclusively breastfeeding children increases their risk of contracting other respiratory infections (Wayse et al. 2004; Coles et al. 2005; Dornelles et al. 2007; Jaganath and Mupere 2012).

According to the United Nations Fund for Children, 25% of all children in 2012 are stunted, a sign of chronic malnutrition (UNICEF 2014), and half a million cases of pediatric TB were diagnosed in 2013 (World Health Organization 2013). Given the high rates of pediatric malnutrition and the high burden of TB in children, special consideration in both policy and programmatic work needs to be paid to children when it comes to TB prevention and treatment.

People Living with HIV Infection

As discussed in more detail in Chapter 4, HIV, like poor nutrition, weakens the immune system. As a result, HIV-infected individuals are the most at risk of TB infection. Specifically, HIV infection alters the cell-mediated immunity, the body's main defense against TB infection. As a result, HIV increases the risk of both primary infection and reactivation of latent TB (Sharma et al. 2005; DeRiemer et al. 2007; Narasimhan et al. 2013). In addition to increasing the risk of active TB infection, the weakened immune systems in HIV-positive individuals also cause TB infection to progress and spread further (Sharma et al. 2005; DeRiemer et al. 2007; Semba et al. 2010; Narasimhan et al. 2013). Individuals with HIV-TB coinfection are more likely to die of both diseases. Given that up to 50% of adults in the Indian subcontinent, Southeast Asia, and sub-Saharan Africa have latent TB infection (World Health Organization 2014), the detrimental effects of HIV on the body's ability to contain the TB infection pose a serious threat to public health.

The relationship between food insecurity, TB, and HIV is complex and compounding, and requires both better understanding and better programmatic interventions. People coinfected with HIV and TB experience a heightened risk of food insecurity. Illness, inability to work, competing priorities for household spending (e.g., on health care versus food), are compounded when diseases coexist. Social discrimination may prevent families affected by HIV, or coinfected by HIV and TB, from relying on community members for food assistance (Deribew et al. 2010). Additionally, over 50% of maternal mortality during pregnancy in mothers with TB is due to coinfection with HIV (Loto and Awowole 2012). The loss of a caretaker, especially one with an important role in the household for food acquisition and meal preparation, as well as reduction in the available household workforce, renders the remaining members of family even more vulnerable to food insecurity. Food insecurity, in turn, increases the risk that family members will be infected with TB, prolongs the length of treatment, and worsens treatment outcomes should such infection occur. Inability to work or attend school due to illness and increased expenditures on health care contribute to food insecurity amongst households affected by HIV.

Coinfection with TB and HIV has become increasingly prevalent around the world and are major causes of mortality (DeRiemer et al. 2007). Program managers and policy makers must acknowledge the importance of their interactions with food insecurity to attempt to avoid the negative additive effects.

SUMMARY

Food insecurity is a critically important factor in TB prevention, care, and treatment. Through diverse and interacting pathways such as malnutrition, tobacco use, adherence to treatment, and reduced immune function, food insecurity negatively impacts both public health efforts to control TB, and individual patients' treatment course. Given that TB remains a major public health crisis, more attention should be placed on these important interactions in an effort to more effectively address both the global epidemic of TB and the crisis of food insecurity.

REFERENCES

Alisjahbana, B., R. van Crevel, E. Sahiratmadja, M. den Heijer, A. Maya, E. Istriana, and J. W. van der Meer. 2006. Diabetes mellitus is strongly associated with tuberculosis in Indonesia. *International Journal of Tuberculosis and Lung Disease* 10 (6):696–700.

Bakaev, V. V. and A. P. Duntau. 2004. Ascorbic acid in blood serum of patients with pulmonary tuberculosis and pneumonia. *International Journal of Tuberculosis and Lung Disease* 8 (2):263–6.

Bates, M. N., A. Khalakdina, M. Pai, L. Chang, F. Lessa, and K. R. Smith. 2007. Risk of tuberculosis from exposure to tobacco smoke: A systematic review and meta-analysis. *Archives of Internal Medicine* 167 (4):335–42. doi: 10.1001/archinte.167.4.335.

Brodie, M. J., A. R. Boobis, C. J. Hillyard, G. Abeyasekera, I. MacIntyre, and B. K. Park. 1981. Effect of isoniazid on vitamin D metabolism and hepatic monooxygenase activity. *Clinical Pharmacology & Therapeutics* 30 (3):363–7.

Cegielski, J. P. and D. N. McMurray. 2004. The relationship between malnutrition and tuberculosis: Evidence from studies in humans and experimental animals. *International Journal of Tuberculosis and Lung Disease* 8 (3):286–98.

Chan, J., Y. Tian, K. E. Tanaka, M. S. Tsang, K. Yu, P. Salgame, and B. R. Bloom. 1996. Effects of protein calorie malnutrition on tuberculosis in mice. *Proceedings of the National Academy of Sciences of the United States of America* 93 (25):14857–61.

Chan, T. Y., P. Poon, J. Pang, R. Swaminathan, C. H. Chan, M. Nisar, and P. D. Davies. 1994. A study of calcium and vitamin D metabolism in Chinese patients with pulmonary tuberculosis. *Journal of Tropical Medicine and Hygiene* 97 (1):26–30.

Chanarin, I. and E. Stephenson. 1988. Vegetarian diet and cobalamin deficiency: Their association with tuberculosis. *Journal of Clinical Pathology* 41 (7):759–62.

Cochrane, A. L. 1945. Tuberculosis among prisoners of war in Germany. *British Medical Journal* 2 (4427):656–8.

Coles, C. L., D. Fraser, N. Givon-Lavi, D. Greenberg, R. Gorodischer, J. Bar-Ziv, and R. Dagan. 2005. Nutritional status and diarrheal illness as independent risk factors for alveolar pneumonia. *American Journal of Epidemiology* 162 (10):999–1007. doi: 10.1093/aje/kwi312.

Cutler-Triggs, C., G. E. Fryer, T. J. Miyoshi, and M. Weitzman. 2008. Increased rates and severity of child and adult food insecurity in households with adult smokers. *Archives of Pediatrics & Adolescent Medicine* 162 (11):1056–1062. doi: 10.1001/archpediatrics.2008.2.

Davies, P. D., R. C. Brown, and J. S. Woodhead. 1985. Serum concentrations of vitamin D metabolites in untreated tuberculosis. *Thorax* 40 (3):187–90.

de Pee, S. and R. D. Semba. 2010. Role of nutrition in HIV infection: Review of evidence for more effective programming in resource-limited settings. *Food and Nutrition Bulletin* 31 (4):S313–44.

Deribew, A., G. Abebe, L. Apers, C. Jira, M. Tesfaye, J. Shifa, and R. Colebunders. 2010. Prejudice and misconceptions about tuberculosis and HIV in rural and urban communities in Ethiopia: A challenge for the TB/HIV control program. *BMC Public Health* 10:400. doi: 10.1186/1471-2458-10-400.

DeRiemer, K., L. M. Kawamura, P. C. Hopewell, and C. L. Daley. 2007. Quantitative impact of human immunodeficiency virus infection on tuberculosis dynamics. *American Journal of Respiratory and Critical Care Medicine* 176 (9):936–44. doi: 10.1164/rccm.200603-440OC.

Dodor, E. 2008. Evaluation of nutritional status of new tuberculosis patients at the Effia-Nkwanta regional hospital. *Ghana Medical Journal* 42 (1):22–8.

Dornelles, C. T., J. P. Piva, and P. J. Marostica. 2007. Nutritional status, breastfeeding, and evolution of infants with acute viral bronchiolitis. *Journal of Health, Population and Nutrition* 25 (3):336–43.

Douglas, A. S., D. P. Strachan, and J. D. Maxwell. 1996. Seasonality of tuberculosis: The reverse of other respiratory diseases in the UK. *Thorax* 51 (9):944–6.

Downes, J. 1950. An experiment in the control of tuberculosis among Negroes. *Milbank Mem Fund Q* 28 (2):127–59.

Escott, S. and J. Newell. 2007. Don't forget the bigger picture: The impact of societal issues on a community-based TB programme, Swaziland. *Journal of Health Organization and Management* 21 (6):506–18.

Finkelstein, M. H. 1932. Effect of carotene on course of *B. tuberculosis* infection of mice fed on a vitamin A deficient diet. *Experimental Biology and Medicine* 29 (8):969–71.

Food and Agriculture Organization. 2006. Food security. Agriculture and Development Economics Division (ESA). Accessed September 10, 2014. http://www.fao.org/forestry/13128-0e6f36f27e0091055bec28ebe830f46b3.pdf.

Gauss, H. 1936. Nutrition and tuberculosis. *CHEST Journal* 2 (7):20–4. doi: 10.1378/chest.2.7.20.

Gele, A. A., M. Sagbakken, F. Abebe, and G. A. Bjune. 2010. Barriers to tuberculosis care: A qualitative study among Somali pastoralists in Ethiopia. *BMC Research Notes* 3:86. doi: 10.1186/1756-0500-3-86.

Getz, H. R., E. R. Long, and H. J. Henderson. 1951. A study of the relation of nutrition to the development of tuberculosis; influence of ascorbic acid and vitamin A. *American Review of Tuberculosis* 64 (4):381–93.

Grange, J. M., P. D. Davies, R. C. Brown, J. S. Woodhead, and T. Kardjito. 1985. A study of vitamin D levels in Indonesian patients with untreated pulmonary tuberculosis. *Tubercle* 66 (3):187–91.

Gupta, K. B., R. Gupta, A. Atreja, M. Verma, and S. Vishvkarma. 2009. Tuberculosis and nutrition. *Lung India* 26 (1):9–16. doi: 10.4103/0970-2113.45198.

Hadley, C., A. Tegegn, F. Tessema, J. A. Cowan, M. Asefa, and S. Galea. 2008. Food insecurity, stressful life events and symptoms of anxiety and depression in east Africa: Evidence from the Gilgel Gibe growth and development study. *Journal of Epidemiology and Community Health* 62 (11):980–6.

Harries, A. D., W. A. Nkhoma, P. J. Thompson, D. S. Nyangulu, and J. J. Wirima. 1988. Nutritional status in Malawian patients with pulmonary tuberculosis and response to chemotherapy. *European Journal of Clinical Nutrition* 42 (5):445–50.

Hemilä, H., J. Kaprio, P. Pietinen, D. Albanes, and O. P. Heinonen. 1999. Vitamin C and other compounds in vitamin C rich food in relation to risk of tuberculosis in male smokers. *American Journal of Epidemiology* 150 (6):632–41.

Hood, M. L. 2013. A narrative review of recent progress in understanding the relationship between tuberculosis and protein energy malnutrition. *European Journal of Clinical Nutrition* 67 (11):1122–8. doi: 10.1038/ejcn.2013.143.

Iglesias-Rios, L., J. E. Bromberg, R. P. Moser, and E. M. Augustson. 2013. Food insecurity, cigarette smoking, and acculturation among Latinos: Data from NHANES 1999–2008. *Journal of Immigrant and Minority Health*. doi: 10.1007/s10903-013-9957-7.

Ivers, L. C. and K. A. Cullen. 2011. Food insecurity: Special considerations for women. *American Journal of Clinical Nutrition* 94 (6):1740s–4s. doi: 10.3945/ajcn.111.012617.

Jaganath, D. and E. Mupere. 2012. Childhood tuberculosis and malnutrition. *Journal of Infectious Diseases* 206 (12):1809–15. doi: 10.1093/infdis/jis608.

Jeon, C. Y. and M. B. Murray. 2008. Diabetes mellitus increases the risk of active tuberculosis: A systematic review of 13 observational studies. *PLOS Medicine* 5 (7):e152. doi: 10.1371/journal.pmed.0050152.

Karyadi, E., W. Schultink, R. H. Nelwan, R. Gross, Z. Amin, W. M. Dolmans, and C. E. West. 2000. Poor micronutrient status of active pulmonary tuberculosis patients in Indonesia. *Journal of Nutrition* 130 (12):2953–8.

Karyadi, E., C. E. West, W. Schultink, R. H. Nelwan, R. Gross, Z. Amin, and J. W. van der Meer. 2002. A double-blind, placebo-controlled study of vitamin A and zinc supplementation in persons with tuberculosis in Indonesia: Effects on clinical response and nutritional status. *American Journal of Clinical Nutrition* 75 (4):720–7.

Kennedy, N., A. Ramsay, L. Uiso, J. Gutmann, F. I. Ngowi, and S. H. Gillespie. 1996. Nutritional status and weight gain in patients with pulmonary tuberculosis in Tanzania. *Transactions of the Royal Society of Tropical Medicine and Hygiene* 90 (2):162–6.

Kitrou, M. P., A. Phytou-Pallikari, S. E. Tzannes, K. Virvidakis, and T. D. Mountokalakis. 1983. Serum calcium during chemotherapy for active pulmonary tuberculosis. *European Journal of Respiratory Diseases* 64 (5):347–54.

Knox-Macaulay, H. H. 1990. Serum cobalamin concentration in tuberculosis. A study in the Guinea savanna of Nigeria. *Tropical and Geographical Medicine* 42 (2):146–50.

Lamsal, M., N. Gautam, N. Bhatta, B. D. Toora, S. K. Bhattacharya, and N. Baral. 2007. Evaluation of lipid peroxidation product, nitrite and antioxidant levels in newly diagnosed and two months follow-up patients with pulmonary tuberculosis. *Southeast Asian Journal of Tropical Medicine and Public Health* 38 (4):695–703.

Lawn, S. D. and A. I. Zumla. 2011. Tuberculosis. *Lancet* 378 (9785):57–72.

Leyton, G. B. 1946. Effects of slow starvation. *Lancet* 2 (6412):73–9.

Lienhardt, C., K. Fielding, J. S. Sillah, B. Bah, P. Gustafson, D. Warndorff, and K. McAdam. 2005. Investigation of the risk factors for tuberculosis: A case–control study in three countries in West Africa. *International Journal of Epidemiology* 34 (4):914–23. doi: 10.1093/ije/dyi100.

Lonnroth, K., E. Jaramillo, B. G. Williams, C. Dye, and M. Raviglione. 2009. Drivers of tuberculosis epidemics: The role of risk factors and social determinants. *Social Science & Medicine* 68 (12):2240–6. doi: 10.1016/j.socscimed.2009.03.041.

Lonnroth, K. and M. Raviglione. 2008. Global epidemiology of tuberculosis: Prospects for control. *Seminars in Respiratory and Critical Care Medicine* 29 (5):481–91. doi: 10.1055/s-0028-1085700.

Lonnroth, K., B. G. Williams, P. Cegielski, and C. Dye. 2010. A consistent log-linear relationship between tuberculosis incidence and body mass index. *International Journal of Epidemiology* 39 (1):149–55. doi: 10.1093/ije/dyp308.

Loto, O. M. and I. Awowole. 2012. Tuberculosis in pregnancy: A review. *Journal of Pregnancy* 2012:379271. doi: 10.1155/2012/379271.

Macallan, D. C., M. A. McNurlan, A. V. Kurpad, G. de Souza, P. S. Shetty, A. G. Calder, and G. E. Griffin. 1998. Whole body protein metabolism in human pulmonary tuberculosis and undernutrition: Evidence for anabolic block in tuberculosis. *Clinical Science* 94 (3):321–31.

Madebo, T., B. Lindtjorn, P. Aukrust, and R. K. Berge. 2003. Circulating antioxidants and lipid peroxidation products in untreated tuberculosis patients in Ethiopia. *American Journal of Clinical Nutrition* 78 (1):117–22.

Marais, B. J., R. P. Gie, H. S. Schaaf, N. Beyers, P. R. Donald, and J. R. Starke. 2006. Childhood pulmonary tuberculosis: Old wisdom and new challenges. *American Journal of Respiratory and Critical Care Medicine* 173 (10):1078–90. doi: 10.1164/rccm.200511-1809SO.

Marais, B. J., R. P. Gie, H. S. Schaaf, A. C. Hesseling, C. C. Obihara, J. J. Starke, and N. Beyers. 2004. The natural history of childhood intra-thoracic tuberculosis: A critical review of literature from the pre-chemotherapy era. *International Journal of Tuberculosis and Lung Disease* 8 (4):392–402.

Maurya, V., V. K. Vijayan, and A. Shah. 2002. Smoking and tuberculosis: An association overlooked. *International Journal of Tuberculosis and Lung Disease* 6 (11):942–51.

McKeown, T, and R. G. Record. 1962. Reasons for the decline of mortality in England and Wales during the nineteenth century. *Population Studies* 16 (2):94–122. doi: 10.1080/00324728.1962.10414870.

McMurray, D. N., R. A. Bartow, C. L. Mintzer, and E. Hernandez-Frontera. 1990. Micronutrient status and immune function in tuberculosis. *Annals of the New York Academy of Sciences* 587:59–69.

Morris, C. D., A. R. Bird, and H. Nell. 1989. The haematological and biochemical changes in severe pulmonary tuberculosis. *Quarterly Journal of Medicine* 73 (272):1151–9.

Mugusi, F., A. B. Swai, K. G. Alberti, and D. G. McLarty. 1990. Increased prevalence of diabetes mellitus in patients with pulmonary tuberculosis in Tanzania. *Tubercle* 71 (4):271–6.

Munro, S. A., S. A. Lewin, H. J. Smith, M. E. Engel, A. Fretheim, and J. Volmink. 2007. Patient adherence to tuberculosis treatment: A systematic review of qualitative research. *PLOS Medicine* 4 (7):e238. doi: 10.1371/journal.pmed.0040238.

Mupere, E., L. Malone, S. Zalwango, A. Chiunda, A. Okwera, I. Parraga, and C. C. Whalen. 2012. Lean tissue mass wasting is associated with increased risk of mortality among women with pulmonary tuberculosis in urban Uganda. *Annals of Epidemiology* 22 (7):466–73. doi: 10.1016/j.annepidem.2012.04.007.

Narasimhan, P., J. Wood, C. R. Macintyre, and D. Mathai. 2013. Risk factors for tuberculosis. *Pulmonary Medicine* 2013:828939. doi: 10.1155/2013/828939.

Newton, S. M., A. J. Brent, S. Anderson, E. Whittaker, and B. Kampmann. 2008. Paediatric tuberculosis. *Lancet Infectious Diseases* 8 (8):498–510. doi: 10.1016/S1473-3099(08)70182-8.

Okechukwu, C. A., A. M. El Ayadi, S. L. Tamers, E. L. Sabbath, and L. Berkman. 2012. Household food insufficiency, financial strain, work-family spillover, and depressive symptoms in the working class: The work, family, and health network study. *American Journal of Public Health* 102 (1):126–33. doi: 10.2105/AJPH.2011.300323.

Oluboyo, P. O. and R. T. Erasmus. 1990. The significance of glucose intolerance in pulmonary tuberculosis. *Tubercle* 71 (2):135–8.

Pelly, T. F., C. F. Santillan, R. H. Gilman, L. Z. Cabrera, E. Garcia, C. Vidal, and C. A. Evans. 2005. Tuberculosis skin testing, anergy and protein malnutrition in Peru. *International Journal of Tuberculosis and Lung Disease* 9 (9):977–84.

Perry, W., M. A. Erooga, J. Brown, and T. C. Stamp. 1982. Calcium metabolism during rifampicin and isoniazid therapy for tuberculosis. *Journal of the Royal Society of Medicine* 75 (7):533–6.

Ray, M., L. Kumar, and R. Prasad. 1998. Plasma zinc status in Indian childhood tuberculosis: Impact of antituberculosis therapy. *International Journal of Tuberculosis and Lung Disease* 2 (9):719–25.

Rwangabwoba, J. M., H. Fischman, and R. D. Semba. 1998. Serum vitamin A levels during tuberculosis and human immunodeficiency virus infection. *International Journal of Tuberculosis and Lung Disease* 2 (9):771–3.

Satyanarayana, K., P. Bhaskaram, V. C. Seshu, and V. Reddy. 1980. Influence of nutrition on postvaccinial tuberculin sensitivity. *American Journal of Clinical Nutrition* 33 (11):2334–7.

Schluger, N. W. and W. N. Rom. 1998. The host immune response to tuberculosis. *American Journal of Respiratory and Critical Care Medicine* 157 (3 Pt 1):679–91. doi: 10.1164/ajrccm.157.3.9708002.

Schwenk, A. and D. C. Macallan. 2000. Tuberculosis, malnutrition and wasting. *Current Opinion in Clinical Nutrition and Metabolic Care* 3 (4):285–91.

Seligman, H. K., A. B. Bindman, E. Vittinghoff, A. M. Kanaya, and M. B. Kushel. 2007. Food insecurity is associated with diabetes mellitus: Results from the National Health Examination and Nutrition Examination Survey (NHANES) 1999–2002. *Journal of General Internal Medicine* 22 (7):1018–23. doi: 10.1007/s11606-007-0192-6.

Seligman, H. K., B. A. Laraia, and M. B. Kushel. 2010a. Food insecurity is associated with chronic disease among low-income NHANES participants. *Journal of Nutrition* 140 (2):304–10. doi: 10.3945/jn.109.112573.

Seligman, H. K, T. C. Davis, D. Schillinger, and M. S. Wolf. 2010b. Food insecurity is associated with hypoglycemia and poor diabetes self-management in a low-income sample with diabetes. *Journal of Health Care for the Poor and Underserved* 21 (4):1227. doi: 10.1353/hpu.2010.0921.

Seligman, H. K., E. A. Jacobs, A. López, J. Tschann, and A. Fernandez. 2012. Food insecurity and glycemic control among low-income patients with type 2 diabetes. *Diabetes Care* 35 (2):233–8.

Semba, R. D., A. A. Campbell, K. Sun, S. de Pee, N. Akhter, R. Moench-Pfanner, and M. W. Bloem. 2011. Paternal smoking is associated with greater food insecurity among poor families in rural Indonesia. *Asia Pacific Journal of Clinical Nutrition* 20 (4):618–23.

Semba, R. D., I. Darnton-Hill, and S. de Pee. 2010. Addressing tuberculosis in the context of malnutrition and HIV coinfection. *Food and Nutrition Bulletin* 31 (4):S345–64.

Semba, R. D., L. M. Kalm, S. de Pee, M. O. Ricks, M. Sari, and M. W. Bloem. 2007. Paternal smoking is associated with increased risk of child malnutrition among poor urban families in Indonesia. *Public Health Nutrition* 10 (1):7–15. doi: 10.1017/s136898000722292x.

Shankar, A. H. and A. S. Prasad. 1998. Zinc and immune function: The biological basis of altered resistance to infection. *American Journal of Clinical Nutrition* 68 (2 Suppl): 447S–63S.

Sharma, S. K., A. Mohan, and T. Kadhiravan. 2005. HIV-TB co-infection: Epidemiology, diagnosis & management. *Indian Journal of Medical Research* 121 (4):550–67.

Shimeles, D. and S. Lulseged. 1994. Clinical profile and pattern of infection in Ethiopian children with severe protein-energy malnutrition. *East African Medical Journal J* 71 (4):264–7.

Sinclair, D., K. Abba, L. Grobler, and T. D. Sudarsanam. 2011. Nutritional supplements for people being treated for active tuberculosis. *Cochrane Database of Systematic Reviews* (11):Cd006086. doi: 10.1002/14651858.CD006086.pub3.

Sinha, D. P. and F. B. Bang. 1976. Protein and calorie malnutrition, cell-mediated immunity, and B.C.G. vaccination in children from rural West Bengal. *Lancet* 2 (7985):531–4.

Sklan, D., D. Melamed, and A. Friedman. 1994. The effect of varying levels of dietary vitamin A on immune response in the chick. *Poultry Science* 73 (6):843–7.

Slama, K., C. Y. Chiang, D. A. Enarson, K. Hassmiller, A. Fanning, P. Gupta, and C. Ray. 2007. Tobacco and tuberculosis: A qualitative systematic review and meta-analysis. *International Journal of Tuberculosis and Lung Disease* 11 (10):1049–61.

Smith, J. C., Jr., E. G. McDaniel, F. F. Fan, and J. A. Halsted. 1973. Zinc: A trace element essential in vitamin A metabolism. *Science* 181 (4103):954–5.

Solotorovsky, M., R. Gala, H. Siegel, R. L. Squibb, and G. N. Wogan. 1961. Effect of dietary fat and vitamin A on avian tuberculosis in chicks. *American Review of Respiratory Disease* 84 (2):226–35.

Stewart, D.A. 1922. Modern facts and phases of tuberculosis. *The American Journal of Nursing* 23(2):130–34.

Stevenson, C. R., N. G. Forouhi, G. Roglic, B. G. Williams, J. A. Lauer, C. Dye, and N. Unwin. 2007. Diabetes and tuberculosis: The impact of the diabetes epidemic on tuberculosis incidence. *BMC Public Health* 7:234. doi: 10.1186/1471-2458-7-234.

Tanimura, T., E. Jaramillo, D. Weil, M. Raviglione, and K. Lonnroth. 2014. Financial burden for tuberculosis patients in low- and middle-income countries: A systematic review. *European Respiratory Journal* 43 (6):1763–75. doi: 10.1183/09031936.00193413.

Tverdal, A. 1986. Body mass index and incidence of tuberculosis. *European Journal of Respiratory Diseases* 69 (5):355–62.

UNICEF. 2014. Nutrition. [web page]. Accessed September 10, 2014. http://www.unicef.org/nutrition/.

van Lettow, M., W. W. Fawzi, and R. D. Semba. 2003. Triple trouble: The role of malnutrition in tuberculosis and human immunodeficiency virus co-infection. *Nutrition Reviews* 61 (3):81–90.

van Lettow, M., A. D. Harries, J. J. Kumwenda, E. E. Zijlstra, T. D. Clark, T. E. Taha, and R. D. Semba. 2004. Micronutrient malnutrition and wasting in adults with pulmonary tuberculosis with and without HIV co-infection in Malawi. *BMC Infectious Diseases* 4 (1):61. doi: 10.1186/1471-2334-4-61.

van Lettow, M., C. E. West, J. W. van der Meer, F. T. Wieringa, and R. D. Semba. 2005. Low plasma selenium concentrations, high plasma human immunodeficiency virus load and high interleukin-6 concentrations are risk factors associated with anemia in adults presenting with pulmonary tuberculosis in Zomba district, Malawi. *European Journal of Clinical Nutrition* 59 (4):526–32. doi: 10.1038/sj.ejcn.1602116.

van Lettow, M. and C. C. Whalen. 2008. Tuberculosis. In *Nutrition and Health in Developing Countries*. R. D. Semba and M. W. Bloem, eds. Humana Press, Totowa, NJ.

Vijayamalini, M. and S. Manoharan. 2004. Lipid peroxidation, vitamins C, E and reduced glutathione levels in patients with pulmonary tuberculosis. *Cell Biochemistry and Function* 22 (1):19–22. doi: 10.1002/cbf.1039.

Visser, M. E., C. Texeira-Swiegelaar, and G. Maartens. 2004. The short-term effects of anti-tuberculosis therapy on plasma pyridoxine levels in patients with pulmonary tuberculosis. *International Journal of Tuberculosis and Lung Disease* 8 (2):260–2.

Wayse, V., A. Yousafzai, K. Mogale, and S. Filteau. 2004. Association of subclinical vitamin D deficiency with severe acute lower respiratory infection in Indian children under 5 y. *European Journal of Clinical Nutrition* 58 (4):563–7. doi: 10.1038/sj.ejcn.1601845.

Widome, R., A. Jensen, A. Bangerter, and S. S. Fu. 2014. Food insecurity among veterans of the US wars in Iraq and Afghanistan. *Public Health Nutrition* 1–6. doi: 10.1017/s136898001400072x.

Williams, S. E., A. G. Wardman, G. A. Taylor, M. Peacock, and N. J. Cooke. 1985. Long term study of the effect of rifampicin and isoniazid on vitamin D metabolism. *Tubercle* 66 (1):49–54.

World Food Programme. 2014. Hunger statistics. World Food Programme. Accessed February 8, 2014. http://www.wfp.org/hunger/stats.

World Health Organization. 2009. *2009 Update Tuberculosis Facts.*

World Health Organization. 2013. *Roadmap for Childhood Tuberculosis.*

World Health Organization. 2014. Tuberculosis. WHO, Last modified March 2014. Accessed January 29, 2014. http://www.who.int/mediacentre/factsheets/fs104/en/.

Wyss, K., P. Kilima, and N. Lorenz. 2001. Costs of tuberculosis for households and health care providers in Dar es Salaam, Tanzania. *Tropical Medicine & International Health* 6 (1):60–8.

Zachariah, R., M. P. Spielmann, A. D. Harries, and F. M. Salaniponi. 2002. Moderate to severe malnutrition in patients with tuberculosis is a risk factor associated with early death. *Transactions of the Royal Society of Tropical Medicine and Hygiene* 96 (3):291–4.

Ziegler, H. D. and P. B. Ziegler. 1975. Depression of tuberculin reaction in mild and moderate protein-calorie malnourished children following BCG vaccination. *Johns Hopkins Medical Journal* 137 (2):59–64.

6 Food Insecurity and Noncommunicable Diseases among the Poorest

Gene Bukhman

CONTENTS

INTRODUCTION

The literature on food insecurity, as it relates to noncommunicable diseases (NCDs), has focused primarily on drivers of overweight, obesity, and ultimately death from diabetes, hypertension, and vascular disease in middle and older ages. The perspective of this chapter is that, for the most part, this discussion has failed to adequately capture the specific issues around NCDs and food insecurity in the poorest populations in the world, where deaths due to NCDs are more concentrated at younger ages, and are often due to a different set of diseases and underlying risk factors than in low- and middle-income countries more generally. Those living in extreme poverty are more rarely overweight or obese. Food insecurity in these populations is pervasive and needs to be a major consideration in the programming of health interventions. The chapter will review the existing general literature on NCDs, food insecurity, and poverty. The chapter will then propose some directions for future research into the role of food insecurity as a risk factor for the high incidence and case fatality rates for NCDs in settings of extreme poverty. The chapter will also examine the likely role of NCDs as a driver of food insecurity. Finally, the chapter will discuss policy implications.

DEFINITIONAL ISSUES

One of the challenges in discussing this set of topics is that the definitions of NCDs, poverty, and food insecurity are complicated. Each of these terms covers a spectrum of issues. The term NCDs encompasses a range of disorders; from heart attacks in the elderly due to overweight and tobacco use, to rheumatic heart disease in children due to untreated streptococcal pharyngitis. In the case of poverty, the populations concerned range from those living with so few resources that they can barely survive (extreme poverty) to those living with less than half of the resources available to others in a generally affluent society (relative poverty). In the case of food insecurity, the problem includes both those who are frankly malnourished, as well as those who are not underweight, but do not have reliable access to nutritious foods.

The majority of the literature on NCDs, food insecurity, and poverty has focused on the particular issue of food insecurity as a driver of unhealthy diets and obesity in populations living in relative poverty. Here, we highlight the less commonly analyzed issue of food insecurity as it relates to NCDs among those populations that are not meeting even their most basic needs. Although the NCDs endemic to these populations are not well enough studied, there is reason to think that they are comprised of a different set of pathologies, with a different set of risk factors, than those NCDs more common in developing countries in general, or among the poor in wealthy countries (Figure 6.1).

DEFINING FOOD INSECURITY

The concept of food insecurity attempts to capture the broad effects of lack of reliable access to healthy food. The field of food insecurity has struggled with measurement issues and there is, at present, no standard instrument (Coates et al. 2006).

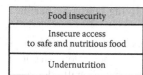

Food insecurity	Poverty	NCDs
Insecure access to safe and nutritious food	Extreme income poverty (≤$1.25 per day)	Cause unknown, genetic, or driven by infectious diseases, indoor air pollution
Undernutrition	Acute poverty (multidimensional poverty index)	e.g., rheumatic heart disease, type 1 diabetes, asthma, cervical cancer, most breast cancer, leukemias and lymphomas, sickle-cell anemia, mental illness, epilepsy
	≤$2 per day	
	Relative poverty (e.g., ≤$4, $5 per day)	
		Unhealthy diets, tobacco, lack of physical activity
		e.g., coronary heart disease, type 2 diabetes, some chronic obstructive lung disease, some cancers

FIGURE 6.1 Definitions of food insecurity, poverty, and NCD. *The intersecting subset of issues highlighted in this chapter are outlined in a thicker stroke.*

(See Chapter 3 for more detailed discussion of the measurement of food insecurity.) For the most part, the literature on NCDs and food insecurity has focused on populations that have normal body mass for height, but lack dependable access to good food, rather than those that are actually underweight. This chapter extends this analysis to include populations that are currently thin.

DEFINING POVERTY

Since the end of World War II, there has been a significant focus of national governments and the United Nations on reducing or eliminating poverty as defined by an unacceptable deprivation of resources. National income poverty lines, controlled for purchasing power parity (PPP), vary significantly between countries and tend to increase along with overall per capita income. Most recently, the World Bank defined an international poverty line for extreme poverty as an annual income of less than $1.25 PPP 2005 dollars per day (Chen and Ravallion 2008). This is based on the mean national poverty lines for the 13 poorest countries in 2005.

There are significant limitations to income-based measures of poverty, but this chapter will not explore this issue extensively (Anand et al. 2010). One example of an effort to use an alternative approach is the Oxford Poverty and Human Development Initiative's multidimensional poverty index (MPI) (Alkire and Santos 2013). This index measures poverty based on 10 kinds of deprivations in three dimensions (health, education, and living standards), often based on data from demographic and health surveys (DHS) and subject to the limitations of those surveys. Some deprivations are weighted more heavily than others. For example, a household is considered nutritionally deprived if at least one child or adult in the household is malnourished. Nutritional deprivation has a 17% weight. All individuals in a household are considered poor if the household has more than 33% of weighted deprivations. The percent of the population in countries that is MPI-poor tends to be higher than the fraction living below the international poverty line of $1.25 per day, and somewhat lower than the fraction living below $2 per day, although there are some exceptions.

In the context of the discussion in this chapter on food insecurity and poverty, it is interesting to look at the relationship between the percent of the population in a country that is MPI-poor and the fraction of the poor who live in nutritionally deprived households (Velasquez-Melendez et al. 2011, Alkire et al. 2013). A major limitation of this kind of analysis appears to be that the DHS surveys often look at nutritional status for only a particular subset of the population. This could lead to underestimation of nutritional deprivation in otherwise MPI-poor households. Nevertheless, there is a general trend that in countries where more than 15% of the population is MPI-poor, 19% of the poor live in nutritionally deprived households. In contrast, in countries where less than 15% of the population is MPI-poor, a median of only 0.9% of poor live in nutritionally deprived households (see Figure 6.2). It would theoretically be possible to look at the prevalence of obesity in MPI-poor households using the same demographic and health survey data, although this has not been done to our knowledge (see discussion below).

DEFINITION OF NCDs OF POVERTY

NCDs are defined by the Global Burden of Disease (GBD) study as all those conditions (including mental illness) that cause death and suffering with the exception of injuries, communicable, maternal, neonatal, and nutritional disorders (Chen and Ravallion 2008, Murray et al. 2013). More narrowly, the World Health Organization (WHO) defines NCDs as principally those diseases (cardiovascular disease, diabetes, chronic respiratory disease, and cancer) that share four common risk factors: physical inactivity, unhealthy diets, tobacco use, and harmful use of alcohol (Blakely et al. 2005, World Health Organization 2008). It was this second definition (used by WHO) that formed the basis of a high-level meeting of the United Nations on NCDs held in September of 2011 (Chen and Ravallion 2007, Assembly 2011). However, the first, broader definition will be the focus of this chapter because of its better relevance for the poorest populations.

The data on NCDs are rarely disaggregated by income level. Most of the data on the prevalence of these conditions, even in the developing world, comes from

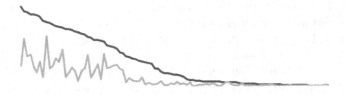

FIGURE 6.2 Rank order list of countries by percent of the population that is poor by the multidimensional poverty index (black line). Percent of the poor in the same countries who live in households where at least one child or adult was nutritionally deprived in a demographic and health survey (gray line). (Data from Alkire, S., A. Conconi, and J. M. Roche. 2013. *Multidimensional Poverty Index 2013: Brief Methodological Note and Results*. Oxford Poverty and Human Development Initiative (OPHI).)

middle-income countries or from urban areas of low-income countries that are generally less poor. Even given these limitations, there are ways of looking at the NCD burden among the poorest. Increasing evidence is showing that NCDs in this population are distributed among a broader range of causes with no single disease being dominant (a "long-tail distribution") (Binagwaho et al. 2014, Central Statistical Office Swaziland and Macro International Inc. 2008, Bukhman and Kidder 2011). Additionally, it appears that the risk factors for these diseases are more likely to be either idiopathic, genetically determined, or have links to nontraditional risk factors, such as infectious diseases or indoor air pollution, than they are to classic lifestyle risk factors (Commerford and Mayosi 2006, de Martel et al. 2012).

The GBD study models death, disability, and risk factors for all major diseases in all countries (Institute for Health Metrics and Evaluation 2013). Sub-Saharan Africa is the region with the largest number of low-income countries and has the highest concentration of extreme poverty. For sub-Saharan African countries in the 2010 GBD study, two-thirds of the years of life lost and disability-adjusted life years due to NCDs and injuries were in those under the age of 40. This age distribution alone suggests that the specific conditions involved must be different that those typically thought of as NCDs in wealthy settings, which primarily cause deaths at middle and older ages. Although it is not possible to look at the poorest populations across countries in the GBD data set, it is possible to look at countries that have a very high concentration of extreme poverty. It is beyond the scope of this chapter to look at the NCD risk factor profile in every low-income country, however. To take just one example, Liberia in 2010 was a country where 84% of the population lived on less than $1.25 per day (84% MPI-poor) (Alkire and Santos 2010). In the GBD study, only 10% of the NCD burden in Liberia was explained by traditional lifestyle risk factors such as salt consumption, overweight and obesity, physical inactivity, alcohol, and tobacco use.

FOOD INSECURITY AS A RISK FACTOR FOR NCDs AMONG THE POOR: TRADITIONAL HYPOTHESES

The literature on the role of food insecurity as a risk factor for NCDs has traditionally focused on two hypotheses. First, there is the hypothesis that nutritional deprivation *in utero* leads to overweight, diabetes, hypertension, and vascular disease in adulthood. Second, there is a hypothesis that unreliable access to food in general might lead to use of cheaper and more caloric foods that contribute to obesity (see Figure 6.3). At times, these hypothesized connections between food insecurity and overweight have been seen as drivers of nutritional transitions and epidemics of obesity in developing countries (Popkin 1994, Popkin et al. 2012).

In this chapter, we do not assess the quality of evidence linking food insecurity with obesity in general, but briefly lay out the arguments for the traditional hypotheses and then move on to examine the relationship between food insecurity and NCDs among those living in extreme poverty who are *not* overweight or obese. Food insecurity is an important outcome worth preventing in and of itself (Campbell 1991). Similarly, overweight and obesity are common among the poor in high-income countries and increasingly in middle-income countries and are linked to poor health

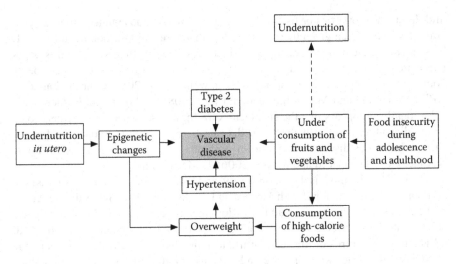

FIGURE 6.3   Most commonly hypothesized mechanisms for an association between food insecurity and NCDs. *These are probably not the mechanisms most relevant for populations living in extreme and acute poverty.*

outcomes (Collaboration et al. 2009, Pan et al. 2012). The limitation of the current literature is that it focuses almost exclusively on obesity to the exclusion of other NCDs and risk factors that are more common among the poorest.

FETAL ORIGINS OF ADULT NCDS (THE BARKER HYPOTHESIS)

Leadership on the hypothesis on the fetal origins of vascular disease and diabetes is often attributed to British physician and epidemiologist David Barker (Cooper 2013). In a 1986 paper in the *Lancet*, Barker and his statistician colleague Clive Osmond observed that the regions of England and Wales with the highest mortality from ischemic heart disease during the 1970s were also the parts of the country that had the highest infant (particularly neonatal) mortality rates from 1921 to 1925 (Barker and Osmond 1986). Barker suggested that fetal and infant undernutrition may play a strong role in the development of ischemic heart disease later in life. He also coined the term "thrifty phenotype" to describe the hypothesis that fetal malnutrition could lead to islet cell dysfunction and subsequent diabetes when calories are more abundant (Hales and Barker 1992). Since that time, epigenetic changes have been proposed as a mechanism linking poor nutrition *in utero* with adult diseases (Hadley and Patil 2006, Maes et al. 2010, Wang et al. 2013). Although the Barker hypothesis focused primarily on metabolic disease, obesity, diabetes, hypertension, and vascular disease, there has also been interest in other NCDs such as osteoporosis (Gluckman et al. 2008).

We do not examine the validity of the hypothesis on the developmental origins of NCDs in this chapter. It is important to note, however, that this field is controversial. An important analysis published in the *Lancet* in 2002, for example, found publication bias and flawed adjustment in studies on the relationship between low birth weight and increased blood pressure in adulthood, concluding that "birth weight is of little relevance to blood pressure levels in later life" (Huxley et al. 2002). A more recent meta-analysis on low birth weight and adult overweight and obesity actually found an inverse relationship between the two (Schellong et al. 2012).

Regardless of the evidence on the developmental origins of NCDs in adults, it is an important field of inquiry, and in the global health context, it has been used to argue for the collateral benefits of improved maternal and child nutrition. It has also been used to predict a coming epidemic of metabolic disease in developing countries (Robinson 2001).

Hypothesis on Food Insecurity and Obesity

The second major hypothesis on food insecurity and NCDs has linked childhood and adult food insecurity with overweight, obesity, and ultimately diabetes, metabolic syndromes, and vascular disease. The mechanisms for this association have been thought to be consumption of less-expensive, higher-calorie foods rather than fruits and vegetables (Dietz 1995, Drewnowski and Darmon 2005). The evidence to support this hypothesis is conflicted and comes mainly from high-income countries, although it is increasingly being investigated in middle-income and low-income countries as well (Olson 1999, Adams et al. 2003, Chaput et al. 2007, Mohamadpour et al. 2012, Santos 2013). Cross-sectional studies in low- and middle-income countries have not found a consistent relationship between food insecurity and overweight (Isanaka et al. 2007). One major limitation of this research is a failure to look specifically at those living in absolute poverty (e.g., income less than $1.25 per day) as opposed to relative poverty. For example, demographic and health surveys in Brazil have found a trend of increased obesity among the poorest quintile of the population (Santos 2013). However, the prevalence of extreme poverty is low in Brazil (6.1% between 2002 and 2012), so even within the poorest quintile, only 30% will be living with an income less than $1.25 per day (United Nations Development Program 2014). One study found a positive relationship between mild—but not moderate or severe— food insecurity and overweight among Brazilian women (Velasquez-Melendez et al. 2011). But even this relationship disappeared when looking at the poorest quintile of the population, let alone those living in extreme poverty.

IS THE DOUBLE BURDEN OF OBESITY AND UNDERNUTRITION AMONG THE (EXTREME) POOR A MYTH?

As discussed, the literature on food insecurity and NCDs has been focused on explaining the prevalence of overweight and obesity among those in relative (but rarely extreme) poverty. Before moving on to the relationship between food insecurity and NCDs among the poor who are not overweight or obese, it is worth exploring how common overweight and obesity actually are among those living in extreme poverty. It is clear that overweight and obesity are increasingly common among the relatively poor in high-, middle-, and even low-income countries, particularly among women. In low- and middle-income countries, however, the increase in overweight and obesity is likely a reflection of the fact that parts of the population are moving out of extreme poverty. Demographic and health surveys (the main source of data on population biometrics for low- and middle-income countries) typically report rates of obesity by relative wealth quintile. This means that over the past two decades, the fraction of the population in developing countries living in extreme poverty in the lower quintiles has decreased because the rate of extreme poverty in these populations has fallen from 52% in 1981 to 34% in 2000 and to 25% in 2005 (Chen and Ravallion 2008).

While there are populations of people living in extreme poverty who also have high rates of obesity, this phenomenon is largely restricted to poor women in parts of Southern Africa (particularly Lesotho and Swaziland), as well as Latin America and the Middle East (Blakely et al. 2005). The populations of these regions only accounted for around 10% of the world's poor in 2004 (Chen and Ravallion 2007). The rate of obesity in Swaziland within the poorest quintile was only 13% among women and 1% among men (Bukhman et al. 2008, Central Statistical Office Swaziland and Macro International Inc. 2008, Nzwalo and Cliff 2011). Meanwhile, the rate of overweight and obesity among the poorest quintile continue to be extremely low in South Asia and most of Africa (where most of the poor live). This kind of rough analysis strongly suggests that much less than 5% of the world's extreme poor are obese.

Two examples are worth considering: Haiti and Uganda. The 2012 Demographic and Health survey (DHS) for Haiti shows that among women aged 15–49, around 8% were obese (Birbeck and Kalichi 2003, Cayemittes et al. 2012). However, among the poorest quintile of this population, only 1% were obese, while 17% were underweight (4% severely). Similarly, overweight and obesity were more common in urban (31%) rather than rural areas (20%), and there was a strong, positive relationship between economic status and body mass index (BMI) overall. Similarly, a geographical analysis of obesity and overweight in Uganda found that high BMI among women and children was clustered in urban areas, among those in the highest wealth class and in the south-west of the country (Bukhman and Kidder 2011, Cheng et al. 2013, Turi et al. 2013). Only 1% of those in the poorest quintile were obese (4.3% overweight), while 34% in highest quintile were overweight or obese (Gelberg et al. 1997, Uganda Bureau of Statistics UBOS and ICF International 2012).

Analysis of the data for all the DHS studies conducted between 1991 and 2008 showed a consistent relationship over time between higher wealth and higher BMI (Weiser et al. 2010, 2012, Neuman et al. 2011). Mean BMI among the poorest quintile remained low within low-income countries. Geographical analysis of the DHS data set from 1994 and 2008 also showed that underweight and overweight tended not to coexist in the same neighborhood, reflecting the concentration of overweight in urban areas (Corsi et al. 2011).

Thus, while overweight and obesity are significant issues in low- and middle-income countries, this is not the dominant problem among the poorest segments of these societies. Therefore, the rest of this chapter focuses on other aspects of the NCD burden and its relationship to food insecurity among the poorest.

Before continuing on, however, it is important to note that consumption of fruits and vegetables can be quite low among those living in extreme poverty because of their higher cost to produce or purchase relative to other foods (Ruel et al. 2005, Hall et al. 2009, Karthikeyan et al. 2012, Sharma et al. 2013). To a large extent, increasing fruit and vegetable consumption (which may be feasible with relatively low-cost strategies) has not been a priority for global health policy because key micronutrients (vitamin A and iron) can be supplied independently (Ali and Tsou 1997, World Health Organization 2003, Pomerleau et al. 2005, Kanungsukkasem et al. 2009, Ludwig et al. 2012, Rich et al. 2012). However, low fruit and vegetable consumption is a significant risk factor for vascular disease, and there have not been any replaceable micronutrients identified to substitute for that consumption (Lock et al. 2005). Ironically, for populations living in extreme poverty—who are otherwise low risk for vascular disease—the NCD policy community is the group most likely to advocate for a focus on fruits and vegetables as part of agriculture policy and school-feeding programs (Nugent 2011).

FOOD INSECURITY AS A RISK FACTOR FOR DEVELOPING AND DYING FROM NCDs AMONG THE POOREST

As discussed, the nature of the NCD burden among those living in acute and extreme poverty is not dominated by classic lifestyle risk factors. There has been little integrated analysis of the role of food insecurity as risk factor for the NCD incidence and death in this population. Here, we examine several categories of possible relationships that deserve further research and give examples of work that has already been done (Table 6.1).

UNCERTAINTY AND HUNGER LEADING TO MENTAL ILLNESS

Mental illness is a major aspect of the NCD burden among the poorest, accounting for probably about 3%–4% of disability-adjusted life years in these populations (DALYs) (Institute for Health Metrics and Evaluation 2013). Food insecurity in and of itself is an inherently terrible state for households. It almost goes without saying that food insecurity is associated with anxiety and depression and possibly more severe mental illness among the poorest, the vast majority of whom are living in a state of food insecurity most of the time. There have been a number of studies looking at food insecurity as a risk factor for mental illness (Hadley and Patil 2006, Birbeck et al. 2007, Crepin et al. 2007, Hadley et al. 2008, Maes et al. 2010, Cole and Tembo 2011, Partners In Health 2011, Tsai et al. 2012, Vaid et al. 2012, Cheng et al. 2013, Garcia et al. 2013, Teferra et al. 2013). One study in Brazil observed a link between food insecurity and asthma exacerbations (Weiser et al. 2007, Ribeiro-Silva et al. 2014). One hypothesis was that food insecurity led to anxiety that could, in turn, trigger asthma exacerbations. To our knowledge, there has not been an attempt to quantify what fraction of mental illness is explained by food insecurity among those living in extreme poverty.

FETAL MICRONUTRIENT DEFICIENCIES LEADING TO CONGENITAL DEFECTS

Congenital defects probably account for 1%–2% DALYs among the poorest and occur at significantly higher rates than in high-income populations. Some of these congenital abnormalities are due to fetal micronutrient deficiencies and can be

TABLE 6.1

Alternative Mechanism for Food Insecurity as a Risk Factor for Incidence and Case Fatality of Endemic NCDs among the Poorest

	Mechanism	Probable Disease Impact	Examples — Possible Disease Impact
Uncertainty, hunger	n/a	Anxiety, depression (Weaver and Hadley 2009)	Asthma exacerbations (Ribeiro-Silva et al. 2014)
In utero micronutrient deficiencies	Folate deficiency	Congenital heart disease (Jenkins et al. 2007); Neural-tube defects (Blencowe et al. 2010)	
Childhood undernutrition	Unknown, pancreatic calcification		Malnutrition-associated diabetes (Fekadu et al. 2010)
Poor food quality	Cyanogen exposure: poor cassava root processing	Konzo (Nzwalo and Cliff 2011)	Endomyocardial fibrosis (Bukhman et al. 2008)
	Aflatoxin exposure: poor storage and drying of maize and groundnuts	Hepatocellular carcinoma (Liu and Wu 2010)	
Medication interactions	Hypoglycemia with insulin and sulfonylureas; Antiepileptic drug toxicity	Epilepsy (Birbeck and Kalichi 2003)	Diabetes (Bukhman and Kidder 2011, Cheng et al. 2013)
Adverse changes in healthcare-related behavior	Late presentation		Breast cancer (Sharma et al. 2013)
	Poor adherence to medical therapy		Rheumatic heart disease (Musoke et al. 2013), diabetes (Bukhman and Kidder 2011, Cheng et al. 2013), epilepsy (Birbeck et al. 2007, Vaid et al. 2012, Crepin et al. 2007), schizophrenia (Teferra et al. 2013)
High-risk sexual behavior	HIV infection leading to HIV-associated NCDs		Heart failure, HIV-associated malignancies (Weiser et al. 2007)
Trade-offs	Lack of investment in improved cooking stoves or fuels		Chronic lung disease (Salvi and Barnes 2009)

prevented through nutritional interventions as part of prenatal care. These interventions are rarely discussed in the context of NCD control, but include folate supplementation to prevent congenital heart disease and neural tube defects (Jenkins et al. 2007, Blencowe et al. 2010, Casper 2011). There is a need for better quantification of the burden of congenital disease avertable through nutritional interventions.

CHILDHOOD MALNUTRITION LEADING TO MALNUTRITION-RELATED ATYPICAL DIABETES MELLITUS

Diabetes mellitus is less common in populations living in extreme poverty than in other populations, with a prevalence of approximately 1%–2% in those over the age of 15 (McLarty et al. 1989, Salvi and Barnes 2009). This reflects the lower prevalence of overweight and obesity in these populations. Additionally, there is a greater proportion of the disease that is type 1, although this still remains a rare condition (10% of diabetes prevalence at the very most) (Elamin et al. 1989, Kim and Chan 2013). Of the remaining patients with diabetes, a greater proportion is young and malnourished than is typical in other settings (Abdulkadir 2005, Gill et al. 2009, Weaver and Hadley 2009, Gill et al. 2010). Although these patients require insulin for glucose control, they do not develop ketoacidosis, and present at later ages than is typical for type 1 diabetes.

As discussed, there has been much written about the possible relationship between fetal undernutrition, overweight, and type 2 diabetes in adulthood. But there is also another line of investigation linking persistent undernutrition and the so-called atypical, tropical, or malnutrition-associated diabetes mellitus (Abu-Bakare et al. 1986, Nwokolo 1986, Ribeiro-Silva et al. 2014). This entity has been described since at least the 1950s (Hugh-Jones 1955, van der Werf et al. 1987, Jenkins et al. 2007). Suggested mechanisms have included pancreatic injury, as well as auto-immunity (Kanungo et al. 2002, Blencowe et al. 2010, Nabunnya and Nakwagala 2011). The issue has been explored particularly well in Ethiopia due to interest on part of researchers there, but is likely relevant in other parts of the world where the majority of patients with diabetes requiring insulin are found in rural areas (Alemu et al. 2009, Fekadu et al. 2010).

INADEQUATE FOOD PROCESSING LEADING TO AFLATOXIN AND CYANOGEN TOXICITY

Food quality in the context of NCDs is usually discussed in terms of lack of fruits or vegetables. Although this is important, it is probably not a dominant mechanism for NCDs among the poorest as shown, for example, by risk factor analysis in the GBD study Institute for Health Metrics and Evaluation 2013). Another aspect of food quality that may be significant is the role of inadequate food processing resulting in exposure to toxins (Nzwalo and Cliff 2011). As discussed above, the NCD burden among the poorest is dispersed among many different conditions with no single disease dominating. Liver cancer is one of the most common malignancies affecting populations living in extreme poverty (although it is likely to account for less than 0.5% of DALYs). There is substantial literature linking poor processing of groundnuts and maize with fungal growth and aflatoxin exposure (Liu and Wu 2010).

Aflatoxin exposure, an independent risk factor for hepatocellular carcinoma, is particularly dangerous in the setting of hepatitis B and hepatitis C infection.

Another example of inadequate food processing leading to an NCD is cyanogen exposure from cassava roots. This mechanism has been relatively well established for the upper-motor neuron disease Konzo (Liu and Wu 2010, Nzwalo and Cliff 2011). There is also a putative relationship that has not been as well established in the case of endomyocardial fibrosis, a significant cause of heart failure among the poor in some parts of the world (Bukhman et al. 2008, Nzwalo and Cliff 2011, Cheng et al. 2013).

Discussions on NCD policy may be an opportunity for countries to refocus on interventions to improve food processing.

INTERMITTENT UNDERNUTRITION LEADING TO MEDICATION TOXICITY

Another less commonly discussed effect of food insecurity on poor outcomes from NCDs is the impact of intermittent undernutrition on medication absorption. This has been described in rural Zambia, where famine led to overdose of antiepileptic medications (Birbeck and Kalichi 2003). Another less well-documented example is in the case of diabetes, where lack of access to food can lead to hypoglycemia in those taking insulin (Bukhman and Kidder 2011, Cheng et al. 2013, Sharma et al. 2013).

Further documentation of this issue in other disease entities is important in terms of advocating for nutritional support as an integral part of therapy, as described below.

ADVERSE CHANGES IN HEALTHCARE-RELATED BEHAVIOR: LATE PRESENTATION AND POOR ADHERENCE TO THERAPY

It has been documented in the United States that food insecurity causes individuals to prioritize their activities in a way that can have negative consequences for their health (Gelberg et al. 1997). Because accessing healthcare has opportunity costs in terms of transportation and loss of time, a patient's focus on meeting their more basic needs may lead to late presentation and poor adherence to therapy. This phenomenon is discussed in more detail in Chapter 2 (Weiser et al. 2010, 2012).

The effect of food insecurity on late presentation and poor adherence to therapy is very likely to be equally relevant for NCDs of poverty, although it is not as well documented (Bukhman and Kidder 2011). Understanding the structural barriers to early presentation for care may lead to greater emphasis on active case finding as treatment programs are established for rheumatic heart disease or breast cancer, for example (Karthikeyan et al. 2012, Sharma et al. 2013).

The need for nutritional support has been a commonly acknowledged part of HIV interventions (World Health Organization 2003, Rich et al. 2012). It is critical to document the role of food insecurity in NCD treatment in order to argue for nutritional services in those conditions as well. To date, the best-studied conditions have been epilepsy, schizophrenia, and diabetes. A group working in Zambia, for example, found a trend toward higher rates of food insecurity among those living with epilepsy (Birbeck et al. 2007). Another team working in Benin found high rates of malnutrition among those with epilepsy when compared to the general population (Crepin et al. 2007). Inadequate availability of food was found to be a significant factor in nonadherence to treatment for schizophrenia in Ethiopia (Teferra et al. 2013). Groups working in Kenya and Rwanda have discussed how food insecurity presents a danger of hypoglycemia to those taking insulin for diabetes (Birbeck et al. 2007, Crepin et al. 2007, Bukhman and Kidder 2011, Vaid et al. 2012, Cheng et al. 2013, Teferra et al. 2013).

HIGH-RISK SEXUAL BEHAVIOR LEADING TO HIV-ASSOCIATED NCDs

Food insecurity has been documented as a risk factor for high-risk sexual behavior in women in Botswana and Swaziland (Weiser et al. 2007). HIV is an underlying cause of several NCDs, including cardiomyopathies and HIV-associated malignancies, such as Kaposi's sarcoma and some lymphomas (Casper 2011).

TRADE-OFFS LEADING TO INCREASED EXPOSURE TO OTHER RISK FACTORS FOR NCDs

Exposure to household air pollution due to poor stoves and biomass fuels is a major driver of cardiovascular and chronic lung disease among the poorest populations (Salvi and Barnes 2009). It is likely that food insecurity makes it less likely for households to prioritize purchasing of improved stoves or fuels.

NCDs, FINANCIAL RISK, AND FOOD INSECURITY

There needs to be more research on NCDs as a driver of food insecurity through two mechanisms. First, NCDs can be debilitating and lead to loss of income by a previously productive family member. Second, the cost of obtaining healthcare to treat NCDs—which are least likely to be covered by prepayment schemes in low-income countries—can also lead to food insecurity.

CONCLUSIONS AND IMPLICATIONS FOR POLICY

In this chapter, we have argued that the nature of the relationship between food insecurity and NCDs among the poorest has little to do with overweight and obesity (the dominant concern of much of literature in other settings). Instead, food insecurity is a risk factor for NCDs of poverty through other mechanisms, such as anxiety (mental illness), fetal micronutrient deficiencies (congenital disorders), malnutrition, (malnutrition-associated) diabetes, and toxin exposure due to inadequate food preparation (e.g., konzo and endomyocardial fibrosis). Additionally, we noted the possible effect of food insecurity on medication dosage, late presentation, poor adherence, high-risk sexual behavior, and trade-offs with other protective purchases, such as improved cook stoves and fuels. Finally, we noted the risk of NCDs leading to household food insecurity through a number of mechanisms. There is need for further research to verify these relationships.

The policy implications of this perspective need to be placed in the context of both global NCD targets and also the movement for universal health coverage (World Health Organization 2013, Binagwaho et al. 2014, World Bank and World Health Organization 2014).

1. Universal health coverage schemes in low-income countries should include NCD treatment early in order to protect households from financial risk and from falling into extreme poverty and food insecurity (Kim and Chan 2013). Although NCDs are not the dominant cause of death and disability in low-income countries, their economic impact on household is increasingly being demonstrated.
2. Current global NCD monitoring frameworks have focused on prevention of premature deaths due to NCDs, both through risk factor modification and treatment access. Healthcare interventions for NCDs in settings of extreme poverty should consider nutritional interventions as part of treatment packages depending on the nature of the disease, and these interventions should be appropriately costed in national NCD strategies.
3. Interventions to improve population food security will likely have the collateral benefit of preventing some NCDs.

REFERENCES

Abdulkadir, J. 2005. Malnutrition-related diabetes mellitus in Africa. *International Journal of Diabetes in Developing Countries* 13:22–28.

Abu-Bakare, A., R. Taylor, G. V. Gill, and K. G. Alberti. 1986. Tropical or malnutrition-related diabetes: A real syndrome? *Lancet* 1 (8490):1135–1138.

Adams, E. J., L. Grummer-Strawn, and G. Chavez. 2003. Food insecurity is associated with increased risk of obesity in California women. *Journal of Nutrition* 133 (4):1070–1074.

Alemu, S., A. Dessie, E. Seid, E. Bard, P. T. Lee, E. R. Trimble, and E. H. O. Parry. 2009. Insulin-requiring diabetes in rural Ethiopia: Should we reopen the case for malnutrition-related diabetes? *Diabetologia* 52 (9):1842–1845.

Ali, M. and S. Tsou. 1997. Combating micronutrient deficiencies through vegetables—A neglected food frontier in Asia. *Food Policy* 22 (1): 17–38.

Alkire, S., A. Conconi, and J. M. Roche. 2013. *Multidimensional Poverty Index 2013: Brief Methodological Note and Results*. Oxford: Oxford Poverty and Human Development Initiative (OPHI).

Alkire, S. and M. E. Santos. 2010. *Liberia Country Briefing. Oxford Poverty and Human Development Initiative (OPHI) Multidimensional Poverty Index Country Briefing Series*. Oxford: Oxford Poverty and Human Development Initiative (OPHI).

Alkire S. and M. E. Santos. 2013. A Multidimensional Approach: Poverty Measurement & Beyond. *Soc Indic Res* 112: 239–57.

Anand, S., P. Segal, and J. E. Stiglitz. 2010. *Debates on the Measurement of Global Poverty*. Oxford University Press, USA.

Assembly, United Nations General. 2011. *Political Declaration of the High-Level Meeting of the General Assembly on the Prevention and Control of NonCommunicable Diseases*. New York: United Nations.

Barker, D. J. and C. Osmond. 1986. Infant mortality, childhood nutrition, and ischaemic heart disease in England and Wales. *Lancet* 327 (8489):1077–1081.

Binagwaho, A., M. A. Muhimpundu, G. Bukhman, and for the NCD Synergies Group. 2014. 80 under 40 by 2020: An equity agenda for NCDs and injuries. *Lancet* 383 (9911):3–4.

Birbeck, G., E. Chomba, M. Atadzhanov, and E. Mbewe. 2007. The social and economic impact of epilepsy in Zambia: A cross-sectional study. *Lancet* 6:39–44.

Birbeck, G. L. and E. M. N. Kalichi. 2003. Famine-associated AED toxicity in rural Zambia. *Epilepsia* 44 (8):1127.

Blakely, T., S. Hales, C. Kieft, N. Wilson, and A. Woodward. 2005. The global distribution of risk factors by poverty level. *Bulletin of the World Health Organization* 83 (2):118–126.

Blencowe, H., S. Cousens, B. Modell, and J. Lawn. 2010. Folic acid to reduce neonatal mortality from neural tube disorders. *International Journal of Epidemiology* 39:i110–i121.

Bukhman, G., J. Ziegler, and E. Parry. 2008. Endomyocardial fibrosis: Still a mystery after 60 years. *PLOS Neglected Tropical Diseases* 2 (2):e97.

Bukhman, G. and A. Kidder (eds). 2011. The PIH guide to chronic care integration for endemic noncommunicable diseases. Rwanda Edition. Cardiac, Renal, Diabetes, Pulmonary, and Palliative Care: Partners In Health. http://act.pih.org/ncdguide (accessed September 10, 2014).

Campbell, C. C. 1991. Food insecurity: A nutritional outcome or a predictor variable? *Journal of Nutrition* 121 (3):408–415.

Casper, C. 2011. The increasing burden of HIV-associated malignancies in resource-limited regions. *Annual Review of Medicine* 62:157–170.

Cayemittes, M., M. F. Busangu, J. de Dieu Bizimana, B. Barrère, B. Sévère, and V. Cayemittes. 2012. Haiti: Enquête Mortalité, Morbidité et Utilisation des Services 2012. EMMUS-V. Ministère de la Santé Publique et de la Population (MSPP), République d'Haïti. Accessed September 10, 2014. http://www.measuredhs.com/pubs/pdf/FR273/FR273.pdf.

Central Statistical Office Swaziland, and Macro International Inc. 2008. Swaziland. Demographic and Health Survey. 2006–07. Central Statistical Office and Macro International Inc. Accessed September 10, 2014. http://dhsprogram.com/pubs/pdf/FR202/FR202.pdf.

Chaput, J.-P., J.-A. Gilbert, and A. Tremblay. 2007. Relationship between food insecurity and body composition in Ugandans living in urban Kampala. *Journal of the American Dietetic Association* 107 (11):1978–1982.

Chen, S. and M. Ravallion. 2007. Absolute poverty measures for the developing world, 1981–2004. *Proceedings of the National Academy of Sciences* 104 (43):16757–16762.

Chen, S. and M. Ravallion. 2008. The developing world is poorer than we thought, but no less successful in the fight against poverty. *Quarterly Journal of Economics* 125 (4):1577–1625. doi: 10.1162/qjec.2010.125.4.1577.

Cheng, S., J. Kamano, N. K. Kirui, E. Manuthu, V. Buckwalter, K. Ouma, and S. D. Pastakia. 2013. Prevalence of food insecurity in patients with diabetes in western Kenya. *Diabetic Medicine* 30 (6):e215–e222.

Coates, J., E. A. Frongillo, B. L. Rogers, P. Webb, P. E. Wilde, and R. Houser. 2006. Commonalities in the experience of household food insecurity across cultures: What are measures missing? *Journal of Nutrition* 136 (5):1438S–1448S.

Cole, S. M. and G. Tembo. 2011. The effect of food insecurity on mental health: Panel evidence from rural Zambia. *Social Science & Medicine* 73 (7):1071–1079.

Collaboration, Prospective Studies, G. Whitlock, S. Lewington, P. Sherliker, R. Clarke, J. Emberson, and R. Peto. 2009. Body-mass index and cause-specific mortality in 900 000 adults: Collaborative analyses of 57 prospective studies. *Lancet* 373 (9669):1083–1096.

Commerford, P. and B. Mayosi. 2006. An appropriate research agenda for heart disease in Africa. *Lancet* 367 (9526):1884–1886.

Cooper, C. 2013. David Barker obituary: Epidemiologist who proposed the idea that common chronic diseases result from poor nutrition in the womb. *The Guardian*. Accessed September 10, 2014. http://www.theguardian.com/society/2013/sep/11/david-barker.

Corsi, D. J., J. E. Finlay, and S. V. Subramanian. 2011. Global burden of double malnutrition: Has anyone seen it? *PLOS ONE* 6 (9):e25120.

Crepin, S., D. Houinato, B. Nawana, G. D. Avode, P.-M. Preux, and J.-C. Desport. 2007. Link between epilepsy and malnutrition in a rural area of Benin. *Epilepsia* 48 (10):1926–1933.

de Martel, C., J. Ferlay, S. Franceschi, J. Vignat, F. Bray, D. Forman, and M. Plummer. 2012. Global burden of cancers attributable to infections in 2008: A review and synthetic analysis. *Lancet Oncology* 13 (6):607–615.

Dietz, W. H. 1995. Does hunger cause obesity? *Pediatrics* 95 (5):766–767.

Drewnowski, A. and N. Darmon. 2005. The economics of obesity: Dietary energy density and energy cost. *American Journal of Clinical Nutrition* 82 (1 Suppl):265S–273S.

Elamin, A., M. I. A. Omer, Y. Hofvander, and T. Tuvemo. 1989. Prevalence of IDDM in schoolchildren in Khartoum, Sudan. *Diabetes Care* 12 (6):430–432.

Fekadu, S., M. Yigzaw, S. Alemu, A. Dessie, H. Fieldhouse, T. Girma, and E. H. O. Parry. 2010. Insulin-requiring diabetes in Ethiopia: Associations with poverty, early undernutrition and anthropometric disproportion. *European Journal of Clinical Nutrition* 64 (10):1192–1198.

Garcia, J., A. Hromi-Fiedler, R. E. Mazur, G. Marquis, D. Sellen, A. Lartey, and R. Pérez-Escamilla. 2013. Persistent household food insecurity, HIV, and maternal stress in periurban Ghana. *BMC Public Health* 13:215.

Gelberg, L., T. C. Gallagher, R. M. Andersen, and P. Koegel. 1997. Competing priorities as a barrier to medical care among homeless adults in Los Angeles. *American Journal of Public Health* 87 (2):217–220.

Gill, G., P. English, and C. Price. 2010. The variable African diabetic phenotype: Tales from the north and the south. *African Journal of Diabetes* 18 (2):12–14.

Gill, G. V., J. C. Mbanya, K. L. Ramaiya, and S. Tesfaye. 2009. A sub-Saharan African perspective of diabetes. *Diabetologia* 52:8–16.

Gluckman, P. D., M. A. Hanson, C. Cooper, and K. L. Thornburg. 2008. Effect of in utero and early-life conditions on adult health and disease. *New England Journal of Medicine* 359 (1):61–73.

Hadley, C. and C. L. Patil. 2006. Food insecurity in rural Tanzania is associated with maternal anxiety and depression. *American Journal of Human Biology* 18 (3):359–368.

Hadley, C, A. Tegegn, F. Tessema, J. A. Cowan, M. Asefa, and S. Galea. 2008. Food insecurity, stressful life events and symptoms of anxiety and depression in east Africa: Evidence from the Gilgel Gibe growth and development study. *Journal of Epidemiology and Community Health* 62 (11):980–986.

Hales, C. N. and D. J. P. Barker. 1992. Type 2 (non-insulin-dependent) diabetes mellitus: The thrifty phenotype hypothesis. *Diabetologia* 35:595–601.

Hall, J. N., S. Moore, S. B. Harper, and J. W. Lynch. 2009. Global variability in fruit and vegetable consumption. *American Journal of Preventive Medicine* 36 (5):402–409.e5.

Hugh-Jones, P. 1955. Diabetes in Jamaica. *Lancet* 269 (6896):891–897.

Huxley, R., A. Neil, and R. Collins. 2002. Unravelling the fetal origins hypothesis: Is there really an inverse association between birthweight and subsequent blood pressure? *Lancet* 360 (9334):659–665.

Institute for Health Metrics and Evaluation. 2013. *Global Burden of Disease Data Visualizations.* Seattle: Institute for Health Metrics and Evaluation.

Isanaka, S., Mora-Plazas, M., Lopez-Arana, S., Baylin, A., and Villamor, E. 2007. Food insecurity is highly prevalent and predicts underweight but not overweight in adults and school children from Bogotá, Colombia. *Journal of Nutrition* 237 (12):2747–55.

Jenkins, K. J., A. Correa, J. A. Feinstein, L. Botto, A. E. Britt, S. R. Daniels, and American Heart Association Council on Cardiovascular Disease in the Young. 2007. Noninherited risk factors and congenital cardiovascular defects: Current knowledge: A scientific statement from the American Heart Association Council on Cardiovascular Disease in the Young: Endorsed by the American Academy of Pediatrics. *Circulation* 116 (17):1882–1887.

Kanungo, A., K. C. Samal, and C. B. Sanjeevi. 2002. Molecular mechanisms involved in the etiopathogenesis of malnutrition-modulated diabetes mellitus. *Annals of the New York Academy of Sciences* 958:138–143.

Kanungsukkasem, U., N. Ng, H. Van Minh, A. Razzaque, A. Ashraf, S. Juvekar, and T. H. Bich. 2009. Fruit and vegetable consumption in rural adults population in INDEPTH HDSS sites in Asia. *Global Health Action* 2: 35–43.

Karthikeyan, G., L. Zühlke, M. Engel, S. Rangarajan, S. Yusuf, K. Teo, and B. M. Mayosi. 2012. Rationale and design of a global rheumatic heart disease registry: The REMEDY study. *American Heart Journal* 163 (4):535–40.e1.

Kim, J. Y. and M. Chan. 2013. Poverty, health, and societies of the future. *JAMA* 310 (9):901–902.

Liu, Y. and F. Wu. 2010. Global burden of aflatoxin-induced hepatocellular carcinoma: A risk assessment. *Environmental Health Perspectives* 118 (6):818–24.

Lock, K. K., J. J. Pomerleau, L. L. Causer, D. R. Altmann, and M. M. McKee. 2005. The global burden of disease attributable to low consumption of fruit and vegetables: Implications for the global strategy on diet. *Bulletin of the World Health Organization* 83 (2):100–108.

Ludwig, C., G. B. Keding, J. M. Msuya, and M. B. Krawinkel. 2012. Introduction of fruits and vegetables into children's diets in the Iringa Region, Tanzania. *Journal of Tropical Pediatrics* 58 (3):241–243.

Maes, K. C., C. Hadley, F. Tesfaye, and S. Shifferaw. 2010. Food insecurity and mental health: Surprising trends among community health volunteers in Addis Ababa, Ethiopia during the 2008 food crisis. *Social Science & Medicine* 70 (9):1450–1457.

McLarty, D. G., A. B. Swai, H. M. Kitange, G. Masuki, B. L. Mtinangi, P. M. Kilima, and K. G. Alberti. 1989. Prevalence of diabetes and impaired glucose tolerance in rural Tanzania. *Lancet* 1 (8643):871–875.

Mohamadpour, M., Z. M. Sharif, and M. A. Keysami. 2012. Food insecurity, health and nutritional status among sample of palm-plantation households in Malaysia. *Journal of Health, Population, and Nutrition* 30 (3):291–302.

Murray, C. J. L., T. Vos, R. Lozano, M. Naghavi, A. D. Flaxman, C. Michaud, and B. Grant. 2013. Disability-adjusted life years (DALYs) for 291 diseases and injuries in 21 regions, 1990–2010: A systematic analysis for the Global Burden of Disease Study 2010. *Lancet* 380 (9859):2197–2223.

Musoke, C., C. K. Mondo, E. Okello, W. Zhang, B. Kakande, W. Nyakoojo, and J. Freers. 2013. Benzathine penicillin adherence for secondary prophylaxis among patients affected with rheumatic heart disease attending Mulago Hospital. *Cardiovasc J Afr* 24 (4):124–129.

Nabunnya, Y. and F. Nakwagala. 2011. Chronic tropical pancreatitis with diabetes in a resource-limited setting. *African Journal of Diabetes Medicine* 19 (1):21–22.

Neuman, M., J. E. Finlay, G. D. Smith, and S. Subramanian. 2011. The poor stay thinner: Stable socioeconomic gradients in BMI among women in lower- and middle-income countries. *American Journal of Clinical Nutrition* 94 (5):1348–1357.

Nugent, R. A. 2011. *Bringing Agriculture to the Table. How Agriculture and Food Can Play a Role in Preventing Chronic Disease.* Chicago: Chicago Council on Global Affairs.

Nwokolo, C. 1986. Tropical diabetes. *Lancet* 2 (8509):755.

Nzwalo, H. and J. Cliff. 2011. Konzo: From poverty, cassava, and cyanogen intake to toxico-nutritional neurological disease. *PLOS Neglected Tropical Diseases* 5 (6):e1051.

Olson, C. M. 1999. Nutrition and health outcomes associated with food insecurity and hunger. *Journal of Nutrition* 129 (suppl):521S–524S.

Pan, L., H. M. Blanck, B. Sherry, K. Dalenius, and L. M. Grummer-Strawn. 2012. Trends in the prevalence of extreme obesity among US preschool-aged children living in low-income families, 1998–2010. *JAMA* 308 (24):2563–2565.

Pomerleau, J. J., K. Lock, C. Knai, and M. McKee. 2005. Effectiveness of interventions and programmes promoting fruit and vegetable intake. Joint FAO/WHO Workshop on Fruit and Vegetables for Health, Kobe, Japan, September 1–3, 2004.

Popkin, B. M. 1994. The nutrition transition in low-income countries: An emerging crisis. *Nutrition Reviews* 52 (9):285–298.

Popkin, B. M., L. S. Adair, and S. W. Ng. 2012. Global nutrition transition and the pandemic of obesity in developing countries. *Nutrition Reviews* 70 (1):3–21.

Ribeiro-Silva, R. C., A. M. Oliveira-Assis, S. B. Junqueira, R. L. Fiaccone, S. M. Dos Santos, M. L. Barreto, E. de Jesus Pinto, L. A. da Silva, L. C. Rodrigues, and N. M. Alcantara-Neves. 2014. Food and nutrition insecurity: A marker of vulnerability to asthma symptoms. *Public Health Nutrition*: 17 (1):14–19.

Rich, M. L., A. C. Miller, P. Niyigena, M. F. Franke, J. B. Niyonzima, A. Socci, and A. Binagwaho. 2012. Excellent clinical outcomes and high retention in care among adults in a community-based HIV treatment program in rural Rwanda. *Journal of Acquired Immune Deficiency Syndromes* 59 (3):e35–42.

Robinson, R. 2001. The fetal origins of adult disease: No longer just a hypothesis and may be critically important in south Asia. *British Medical Journal* 322 (7283):375.

Ruel, M. T., N. Minot, and L. Smith. 2005. Patterns and determinants of fruit and vegetable consumption in sub-Saharan Africa: A multicountry comparison. World Health Organization. Accessed September 10, 2014. http://www.who.int/dietphysicalactivity/publications/f%26v_africa_economics.pdf.

Salvi, S. S. and P. J. Barnes. 2009. Chronic obstructive pulmonary disease in non-smokers. *Lancet* 374 (9691):733–743.

Santos, L. M. P. 2013. Obesity, poverty, and food insecurity in Brazilian males and females. *Cad Saude Publica* 29 (2):237–239.

Schellong, K., S. Schulz, T. Harder, and A. Plagemann. 2012. Birth weight and long-term overweight risk: Systematic review and a meta-analysis including 643,902 persons from 66 studies and 26 countries globally. *PLOS ONE* 7 (10):e47776.

Sharma, K., A. Costas, R. Damuse, J. Hamiltong-Pierre, J. Pyda, C. T. Ong, and J. G. Meara. 2013. The Haiti breast cancer initiative: Initial findings and analysis of barriers-to-care delaying patient presentation. *Journal of Oncology* 2013:1–6.

Teferra, S., C. Hanlon, T. Beyero, L. Jacobsson, and T. Shibre. 2013. Perspectives on reasons for non-adherence to medication in persons with schizophrenia in Ethiopia: A qualitative study of patients, caregivers and health workers. *BMC Psychiatry* 13:168.

Tsai, A. C., D. R. Bangsberg, E. A. Frongillo, P. W. Hunt, C. Muzoora, J. N. Martin, and S. D. Weiser. 2012. Food insecurity, depression and the modifying role of social support among people living with HIV/AIDS in rural Uganda. *Social Science & Medicine* 74 (12):2012–2019.

Turi, K. N., M. J. Christoph, and D. S. Grigsby-Toussaint. 2013. Spatial distribution of underweight, overweight and obesity among women and children: Results from the 2011 Uganda Demographic and Health Survey. *International Journal of Environmental Research and Public Health* 10 (10):4967–4981.

Uganda Bureau of Statistics UBOS, and ICF International. 2012. Uganda Demographic and Health Survey 2011. In *The DHS Program: Demographic and Health Surveys*. Kampala, Uganda and Calverton, Maryland: UBOS and ICF International Inc.

United Nations Development Program. 2014. *Human Development Report 2014. Sustaining Human Progress: Reducing Vulnerabilities and Building Resilience*. New York: United Nations Development Program.

Vaid, N. N., S. S. Fekadu, S. S. Alemu, A. A. Dessie, G. G. Wabe, D. I. W. D. I. Phillips, and M. M. Prevett. 2012. Epilepsy, poverty and early under-nutrition in rural Ethiopia. *Seizure* 21 (9):734–739.

van der Werf, T., S. Zwart, and R. Steenstra. 1987. Diabetes in rural West Africa. *Lancet* 2 (8559):638–639.

Velasquez-Melendez, G., M. M. Schlussel, A. S. Brito, A. A. M. Silva, J. D. Lopes-Filho, and G. Kac. 2011. Mild but not light or severe food insecurity is associated with obesity among Brazilian women. *Journal of Nutrition* 141 (5):898–902.

Wang, G., S. O. Walker, X. Hong, and T. R. Bartell. 2013. Epigenetics and early life origins of chronic noncommunicable diseases. *Journal of Adolescent Health* 52(suppl):S14–S21.

Weaver, L. J. and C. Hadley. 2009. Moving beyond hunger and nutrition: A systematic review of the evidence linking food insecurity and mental health in developing countries. *Ecology of Food and Nutrition* 48 (4):263–284. doi: 10.1080/03670240903001167.

Weiser, S. D., K. Leiter, D. R. Bangsberg, L. M. Butler, F. Percy-de Korte, Z. Hlanze, and M. Heisler. 2007. Food insufficiency is associated with high-risk sexual behavior among women in Botswana and Swaziland. *PLOS Medicine* 4 (10):1589–97; discussion 1598. doi: 10.1371/journal.pmed.0040260.

Weiser, S. D., A. C. Tsai, R. Gupta, E. A. Frongillo, A. Kawuma, J. Senkungu, and D. R. Bangsberg. 2012. Food insecurity is associated with morbidity and patterns of health-care utilization among HIV-infected individuals in a resource-poor setting. *AIDS* 26 (1):67–75. doi: 10.1097/QAD.0b013e32834cad37.

Weiser, S. D., D. M. Tuller, E. A. Frongillo, J. Senkungu, N. Mukiibi, and D. R. Bangsberg. 2010. Food insecurity as a barrier to sustained antiretroviral therapy adherence in Uganda. *PLOS ONE* 5 (4):e10340. doi: 10.1371/journal.pone.0010340.

World Bank, and World Health Organization. 2014. *Monitoring Progress towards Universal Health Coverage at Country and Global Levels: Framework, Measures and Targets.* World Health Organization, World Bank Group. Accessed September 10, 2014. http://apps.who. int/iris/bitstream/10665/112824/1/WHO_HIS_HIA_14.1_eng.pdf?ua=1&ua=1.

World Health Organization. 2003. *Nutrient Requirements for People Living with HIV/AIDS: Report of a Technical Consultation. [Technical Consultation Meeting].* World Health Organization. Accessed September 10, 2014. http://www.who.int/nutrition/publications/ Content_nutrient_requirements.pdf.

World Health Organization. 2008. 2008–2013 *Action Plan for the Global Strategy for the Prevention and Control of Noncommunicable Diseases.* Geneva: World Health Organization.

World Health Organization. 2013. Draft comprehensive global monitoring framework and targets for the prevention and control of noncommunicable diseases. Sixty-Sixth World Health Assembly Provisional agenda item 13.1. World Health Organization.

7 Food Insecurity
Special Considerations for Women's Health

Jessica E. Teng, Kimberly A. Cullen,
and Louise C. Ivers

CONTENTS

INTRODUCTION

The concept of being food secure, defined at the 1996 United Nations World Food Summit as "when all people, at all times, have physical, social, and economic access to sufficient, safe, nutritious food which meets their dietary needs and food preferences for an active and healthy life" (Food and Agriculture Organization 1996), is a complex and multidimensional issue that rests on three pillars: (1) food availability,

(2) food access, and (3) food use. Though each of these three pillars can stand on its own, all three are necessary to form a solid foundation upon which individuals, households, and communities can build. Each pillar consists of a series of interconnected fibers of gender, age, education, health, and other factors that affect an individual's ability to achieve and maintain a food-secure state. See Chapter 1 for a detailed review of the concepts of food security.

Addressing issues specific to women is critical in discussions of food insecurity. Although they contribute to half of the world's food production, women have more difficulty than men in accessing resources such as land, credit, and agricultural inputs and services (Lubbock and Borquia 1998, Food and Agriculture Organization 2010), and make up 70% of the worlds' poor (United Nations Development Fund for Women 2010). Women's traditional role in society as caregivers and food preparers, and the increasing recognition of their role as heads of households, further supports the consideration of women as a special group in which to evaluate the impact and consequences of food insecurity. The U.N. special rapporteur on the Right to Food, Olivier De Schutter, recently went so far as to say that gender equality is "the single most important determinant of food security" (De Schutter 2013).

The evidence described in this chapter supports the supposition that women require special consideration in discussions of food insecurity and its impact on health.

FOOD INSECURITY AND MICRONUTRIENT ADEQUACY

Women of childbearing age and children under five years old are at particular risk of poor health outcomes due to undernutrition and micronutrient deficiencies. Food security does not guarantee a nutritious diet, but these deficiencies can often be a consequence of food insecurity.

A number of studies have documented a relationship between food insecurity and inadequate nutrient uptake in women in the United States and Canada. In a study of 3744 women in the United States, Rose and Oliveira (1997) found that food insecurity was associated with reduced micronutrient intake among women of childbearing age, based on 24-hour recall. Women from food-insufficient households had mean intakes that were below two-thirds of the recommended daily allowance for calcium, iron, vitamin E, magnesium, and zinc, and were more likely to consume less than 50% of recommended energy intake compared to the mean nutrient and energy intakes of those from food-sufficient households. A study of food insecurity and nutrient adequacy of 153 women in families receiving emergency food assistance in Canada found a high prevalence of inadequacies, in excess of 15%, for vitamin A, folate, iron, and magnesium in severely food-insecure households (Tarasuk and Beaton 1999). McIntyre et al. (2007) used a merged data set of 226 Canadian food-insecure women and found prevalence of inadequacy in excess of 25% for iron, magnesium, thiamin, vitamin A, B6, B12, C, and zinc. Similar findings were reported in the United States of lower intakes of calcium, folate, and vitamin E, in addition to these aforementioned nutrients by food-insecure women compared to food-secure women (Cristofar and Basiotis 1992, Dixon et al. 2001). Consumption of less than the recommended daily allowance for vitamin C was also found in a cohort of women in rural New York, in addition to declining frequency of fruit and vegetable consumption with increasing food insecurity (Kendall et al. 1996).

By contrast, one study, with a cohort of 916 refugees recently resettled in Australia, showed no significant association between gender and low vitamin B12 levels (Benson et al. 2013). Overall, 16.5% of newly arrived refugees had vitamin B12 deficiency, but contrary to the authors' hypothesis, low levels were more prevalent in males than females, and in older age groups compared to younger refugees. The highest prevalence of vitamin B12 deficiency was amongst refugees from Bhutan, Iran, and Afghanistan. Despite high prevalence of food insecurity in the African countries represented in the study cohort, refugees from Africa demonstrated less vitamin B12 deficiency than refugees from other countries. The authors note that the United Nations World Food Program (WFP) and the United Nations High Commissioner for Refugees (UNHCR) had supplemental nutrition programs in place in the source country of some of the African refugees and that these programs may explain the lower rates of vitamin B12 deficiency in this group (United Nations World Food Programme and United Nations High Commissioner for Refugees 2009). Low maternal levels of vitamin B12 may be a risk factor for neural tube defects in children (Wang et al. 2012). This finding has led to an ongoing discussion on whether vitamin B12 should be supplemented along with folic acid to pregnant women.

A detailed review of the medical consequences of micronutrient deficiency is beyond the scope of this chapter, but on a broad level, insufficient micronutrient intake has been linked with a variety of poor health outcomes. Additionally, nutrient deficiencies that can result from food insecurity and inadequate consumption of certain foods can be exacerbated by other medical conditions. HIV infection, for example, increases resting energy expenditure, while also impairing the metabolic functions in absorption, storage, and utilization of nutrients (Piwoz 2004, Katona and Katona-Apte 2008). See Chapter 4 for more information on the intersection of HIV, nutrition, and food insecurity.

FOOD INSECURITY AND WEIGHT

If food security were to be considered only in terms of access to food in sufficient quantity, it might follow logically that food insecurity would be associated with being underweight. However, the relationship between food insecurity and weight is complex and not yet clearly defined. In cross-sectional studies conducted in the United States, food insecurity has been consistently associated with obesity among women (Olson 1999, Townsend et al. 2001, Adams et al. 2003, Hanson et al. 2007), but the direction of causality and association is unclear. In a review of the literature, Franklin et al. (2012) concluded that women who experience food insecurity are more likely to be overweight or obese compared to those who are food secure; however, over time, food insecurity did not appear to promote increased weight gain. Dinour et al. (2007) proposed a conceptual framework for this "Food Insecurity–Obesity Paradox," in which they hypothesize that negative coping strategies in response to food insecurity, including physiological, economical and food choices, psychological stress, parental protection of children from hunger, and physical adaptation to the feast/famine cycle, all may contribute to obesity. Meanwhile, few data exist to define the association between food insecurity and weight among individuals in resource-poor settings.

FOOD INSECURITY AND WEIGHT IN THE UNITED STATES AND OTHER HIGH-INCOME COUNTRIES

Much of the current evidence from high-income countries suggests an association between food insecurity and overweight or obesity in women, with few results and inconsistent findings in men. A cross-sectional study using data from the 1994, 1995, and 1996 "Continuing Survey of Food Intakes by Individuals" showed that food insecurity was related to overweight status in women in the United States (but not in men), with the prevalence of overweight status in women increasing as food insecurity increased. Mildly food-insecure women were 30% more likely to be overweight than those who were food secure (Townsend et al. 2001). In a randomly selected sample of 8169 women in California, obesity was more prevalent in food-insecure (31.0%) than in food-secure women (16.2%), with a greater likelihood in non-White women (Adams et al. 2003). In a population-based sample of 193 women of child-bearing age in rural New York, women in food-insecure households were on average 2 body mass index (BMI) units heavier than women in households that were food secure after controlling for income level, educational level, single parent status, and employment status (Olson 1999). Consistent with these findings, in an analysis of 4172 women who participated in the 1999–2002 National Health and Nutrition Examination Survey (NHANES), marginal food security was associated with being overweight, and low food security was associated with being obese among women (Hanson et al. 2007). More recently, in a population-based cohort of adults in Paris, France, women with very low food security were twice as likely to be obese as their food-secure counterparts, even when controlling for confounding factors. No association was found between food insecurity and obesity in men (Martin-Fernandez et al. 2014).

In an analysis of 1909 women and 2117 men from the 1999 to 2002 NHANES, Tayie and Zizza (2009) found that there was a significant interaction between food security and height in the association between food insecurity and BMI, meaning that the trends in the association between food insecurity and BMI were different for different levels of height. Shorter height was associated with lower socioeconomic status and may result from chronic undernutrition: the authors proposed including height as an interaction term in analyses of food insecurity and BMI.

As cross-sectional studies cannot determine causality, longitudinal analyses have been performed to attempt to better define the relationship between food security and weight in women. In a prospective cohort study of 1707 urban women in 20 U.S. cities, Whitaker and Sarin (2007) found a positive association between food security status at baseline and obesity at baseline and follow-up. This association lost statistical significance after adjusting for sociodemographic factors. The authors concluded that changes in food security status were not significantly associated with changes in weight over the 2-year study period, and that food insecurity does not have a causal relationship with weight gain or obesity.

Two studies analyzed longitudinal data from the Panel Study of Income Dynamics (PSID), a nationally representative sample focused on economic dynamics of households in the United States. Using data from the 1999 and 2001 PSID surveys, Jones and Frongillo (2007) found no statistically significant association between food insecurity and subsequent weight gain in U.S. women over 2 years. However, the relationship between food security status and weight gain did differ by baseline weight group: among overweight women, those who were food secure gained 2.2 kg more over the 2-year study period than their food-insecure counterparts, suggesting some relationship. Martin and Lippert (2012) used 1999, 2001, and 2003 PSID data for a sample of 7931 adults to evaluate the hypothesis that gendered expectations of child rearing are responsible for the association between food insecurity and obesity or overweight in women. They examined the impact of motherhood and children in the household on the association between food insecurity and weight. They found that food-insecure mothers were more likely to be overweight or obese, and more likely to gain weight over time than both women without children and their male counterparts. Martin and Lippert included only those who had a documented body weight, and those aged 18–55 in 1999 in their study, and excluded foreign-born women (as the PSID is not a representative sample of immigrants living in the United States). As food insecurity was not associated with being overweight or obese or gaining excess weight among fathers or child-free women and men, the authors highlighted the importance of considering mothers' adaptive responses to the threat of food insecurity in the household, which appears to result in their own ill-health, while attempting to protect children from the effects. Although not specifically designed to address the issue, the previously mentioned study by Hanson et al. (2007) found that food insecurity was related to a greater likelihood of obesity among married women, those living with partners, and widows, when compared with never-married women. Both of these studies highlight the potential importance of relationships—to children or partners—in the associations between food insecurity and weight in women.

Dubois et al. (2011) examined this issue from the perspective of whether household-level food insecurity impacted the weight of the children in the household in a cohort of 1190 Canadian and 1674 Jamaican families. Girls aged 10–11 in Québec, Canada, who lived in food-insecure homes, were five times as likely to be overweight or obese when compared to girls living in food-secure homes; there was no difference among boys in the same age group. The authors noted that a greater proportion of overweight/obese children were from single-parent households. Interestingly, this association was reversed in the Jamaican population studied, where children living in food-insecure homes were less likely to be obese compared to children living in food-secure homes. Furthermore, no gender disparity was found between Jamaican boys and girls, suggesting the relationship between weight and food insecurity is multifactorial in nature.

Most studies evaluating food insecurity and weight are cross-sectional and causal inference is not possible. However, one study found a directional relationship between obesity and food insecurity. Using data from the Bassett Mothers Health Project for a prospective cohort study of 622 childbearing women living in rural upstate New York, Olson and Strawderman (2008) determined that obesity may lead to food insecurity. Women who were obese early on during their pregnancies were highly likely to be food insecure 2 years later, while there was no significant association between being food insecure at pregnancy and being obese 2 years later. Another significant finding was that obesity combined with food insecurity presented the greatest risk for major weight gain. In a qualitative study, Bove and Olson (2006) conducted in-depth interviews with 28 women living in rural New York to provide some insights into the relationship of overweight with food insecurity and identified several factors contributing to obesity, including transportation difficulties, physical inactivity, social isolation, food insecurity, emotional eating, and disordered eating, often around time of fluxes in household food supplies.

In contrast to the studies conducted in North America, in a study in Trinidad & Tobago, which is considered a high-income economy by the World Bank, women with moderate food insecurity were more likely to be underweight when compared to food-secure women (Gulliford et al. 2003).

FOOD INSECURITY AND WEIGHT IN LOWER-INCOME SETTINGS

In resource-poor settings where food availability is often limited, few data exist to define relationships between food insecurity and body weight. A conventional assumption may be that in settings where access to food (even low-nutrient food) is limited, food insecurity might result in insufficient calorie intake, causing food-insecure individuals to be underweight. However, studies are inconsistent in their findings.

In Nepal, women living with moderate food insecurity were more likely to be underweight compared to food-secure women (Gulliford et al. 2003, Singh et al. 2014). By contrast, a cross-sectional study conducted in urban Uganda to determine the relationship between food insecurity and body composition found that, in univariate analysis, food-insecure women (but not men) were more likely to be overweight or to have at-risk waist circumference compared to those who were food secure. After adjusting for potentially confounding effects, however, there were no significant differences between the two gender groups (Chaput et al. 2007).

Studies conducted in countries that are World Bank-defined "upper middle income" economies also have mixed findings. In rural Malaysia in 2005, among a sample of 200 women, 58% of food-insecure women were overweight or obese compared to 38% of food-secure women, and after controlling for confounding variables, food-insecure women were still significantly more likely to have an at-risk waist circumference than food-secure, but not obese women (Shariff and Khor 2005). More recently in 2013, in a survey of 223 low-income households with mothers in rural Malaysia, there were no significant associations between food insecurity status, BMI, and waist circumference, despite high prevalence of food insecurity (84%), obesity (52%), and at-risk waist circumference (47%) (Ihabi et al. 2013). In Colombia, household hunger was significantly associated with underweight in both mothers and children; food insecurity was not a predictor of overweight in women (Isanaka et al. 2007). A recent study conducted in Tehran, Iran, found a significant association between severe food insecurity and abdominal obesity in women (in this study, abdominal obesity was classified as having a waist circumference greater than or equal to 88 cm). Mohammadi et al. (2013) found that women from food-insecure households were 2.8 times more likely than their food-secure counterparts to be at risk for abdominal obesity.

Thailand and Brazil are examples of middle-income countries in the midst of a "nutrition transition," a shift in diet that often occurs in tandem with development, from traditional foods toward a more "Western diet" with increased animal protein, dairy, and processed foods. Building on the observations of Hawkes (2006), Kelly et al. (2010) describe a convergence toward the Western diet in Thailand. The ubiquity of energy-dense, calorie-rich processed foods is followed by a divergence, whereby educated and often wealthier consumers who understand the negative health effects of this energy-dense diet are demanding healthier choices. These healthier choices come at a premium out of reach for many, setting the stage for health inequity. Recent research shows a similar phenomenon occurring in Thai women and women living in high-income countries—there is a growing inverse relationship between education level, socioeconomic status, and body weight (Aekplakorn et al. 2007, Seubsman et al. 2010).

Published studies of Brazilian women of reproductive age and adolescent girls do suggest that mild and severe food insecurity, respectively, are associated with obesity or excessive weight (Velasquez-Melendez et al. 2011, Kac et al. 2012), which may represent a "divergence phase." Schlüssel et al. (2013) provide supporting evidence of the association between obesity and household food insecurity in women and adolescents in Brazil; however, the association did not hold among children (either boys or girls).

The collection of studies mentioned here shows the varied nature of findings in different settings, illuminating the complexities of intersection of food insecurity and weight, which is at once affected by biology, behavior, relationships, adaptive strategies in the face of food insecurity, and nation- and world-wide food production, supply, and distribution.

FOOD INSECURITY, HOUSEHOLD ECONOMICS, AND RISKY COPING STRATEGIES

Implied in the concept of food insecurity is the vulnerability resulting from lack of reliable access to food. This vulnerability lies in part in the fact that individuals may use coping strategies to deal with food insecurity (or to avoid it) that are either risky to their health and well-being, or unsustainable. See Chapter 2 for a detailed discussion on the behavioral pathways that may lead to ill-health in food insecurity. When there is limited or uncertain ability to acquire acceptable foods in "socially acceptable ways," a variety of coping strategies may be used. These can include withdrawing children from school, decreasing intake of certain foods, sale of assets to purchase food, theft, or exchange of sex for food or money (Kendall et al. 1996, Weiser et al. 2007, Salaam-Blyther and Hanrahan 2009). Women are particularly vulnerable to resorting to risky coping strategies and their consequences, especially since they are often primary caretakers of children, and have food preparation responsibilities, low education levels, and/or few economic opportunities.

HIGH-RISK SEXUAL BEHAVIOR

The geographic epidemics of food insecurity and HIV overlap to such an extent that it has been referred to as a "syndemic" whereby the disease and the social condition serve to exacerbate one another (Young et al. 2014), creating a vicious feedback loop. In countries where the rights and economic status of women increase their vulnerability, this feedback loop is even more detrimental. Weiser et al. (2007) found that food insecurity was associated with high-risk sexual behavior, such as increased sex acts and a lack of control in sexual relationships, among women in Botswana and Swaziland. In Lagos, Nigeria, a survey of 320 female commercial sex workers found that 35% identified poverty and difficulty accessing food daily as the reason for joining that industry (Oyefara 2007). In qualitative interviews with women living with HIV in Uganda, Miller et al. (2011) found that food insecurity was associated with transactional sex, with lack of control over condom use, and with a likelihood of staying in abusive relationships. Food insecurity was associated with increased alcohol use, increased male sexual partners, and increased sexual acts with protection in women living in South African townships (Eaton et al. 2014). In Brazil, Tsai et al. (2012a) analyzed data on 12,684 sexually active women and found that those who were severely food insecure were less likely to use condoms consistently, and were less likely to have used a condom at last sexual intercourse. These factors fit into the pathways linking food insecurity to increased risk for sexually transmitted diseases and HIV infection. Food insecurity has also been shown to be both a barrier to initiation of antiretroviral therapy as well as to contribute to nonadherence to antiretroviral therapy (Weiser et al. 2010), which can lead to worse health outcomes.

EXPOSURE TO VIOLENCE

Food insecurity is linked with exposure to violence (Wehler et al. 2004, Chilton and Booth 2007, Melchior et al. 2009). In a qualitative study of 44 mothers from low-income families in Philadelphia, Chilton et al. (2013) found that 34 of 44 (77%) women reported experiencing violence in their current life stage, with the proportion rising to be 88% for those who had severe food insecurity. The 17 mothers who had severe food insecurity described experiences of rape and sexual assault, child abuse, being a perpetrator of violence, and attempted suicide. Ten (59%) of the severely food insecure reported being a perpetrator of violence; by food security status, this was much higher than the proportions reported among those with low food security and those who were food secure. Of the participants, 21 mothers, or almost half (19 of whom were in the very low and low food security groups, and 2 in the food-secure group) reported depressive symptoms, and were more likely than their non depressed counterparts to have longer-lasting and life-changing impacts of violence. Exposure to violence consequently affected the participants' mental health status and ability to continue their education or professions.

ECONOMIC STATUS

In the United States and Canada, lower socioeconomic status and poverty have been shown to be associated with food insecurity. In the United States, in a cohort of 606 pregnant women with incomes ≤400% of the poverty level, women from marginally food-secure or food-insecure households had significantly less income, education, and were older than food-secure women. Socioeconomic and demographic predictors of food insecurity included income, black race, and age (Laraia et al. 2006).

Food insecurity is also associated with lower household economic status in developing countries. In rural communities in Malaysia, food-insecure women had less education, lower household income, and a greater number of children, and mothers were more likely to be housewives (as opposed to have other economic activities) than women from food-secure households (Shariff and Khor 2005). Among a cohort of 3267 Bangladeshi mother–infant pairs, mothers with severe food insecurity were less wealthy than those who were food secure or occasionally to moderately food insecure (Frith et al. 2012). In Northern Jordan, in a cross-sectional study of 500 women, those with income below the poverty level were four times more likely than their wealthier counterparts to be food insecure. Illiteracy or low level of education, renting a home (rather than owning), and living in a female-led household were also risk factors for increased food insecurity among women (Bawadi et al. 2012). In Tanzania, McCoy et al. (2014) examined the complex relationship between a woman's individual food security and the likelihood of engaging in risky sexual behaviors when categorized by living in a male-headed household versus a female-headed household. An association was found between severe food insecurity in women living in a male-headed household and staying in a relationship longer than desired for material goods, though this was not statistically significant. The results of this study highlight the importance of future research on the nuanced impact of economic power on individual food security and risky behavior.

FOOD INSECURITY AND MATERNAL AND CHILD HEALTH

Laraia et al. (2006) proposed three potential reasons why food insecurity might have particular importance for women during pregnancy: (i) nutrient demands are higher, (ii) effort required for food preparation may be more difficult, and (iii) pregnant women may be obliged to leave the workforce, especially in later pregnancy, leading to financial strain. Food insecurity in pregnant women can also negatively affect children, as maternal nutrition status and weight may have long-lasting effects on fetal development that can increase the child's risk of obesity and other diseases in adulthood (Catalano 2003, Mcmillen and Robinson 2005).

MATERNAL HEALTH AND PREGNANCY OUTCOMES

Food insecurity in women during pregnancy has been associated with economic hardship for the mother and with poor pregnancy outcomes, including gestational diabetes (Borders et al. 2007, Laraia et al. 2010). A population-based postpartum survey from California's Maternal and Infant Health Assessment to study income levels and hardships before or during pregnancy found that nearly 35% of poor women and 20% of near-poor women reported food insecurity, compared with 8%, 4%, and 0.6% of women in the successively higher-income groups (Braveman et al. 2010). A prospective cohort study of 810 pregnant women in the United States with incomes ≤400% of the income/poverty ratio found 14% to be from marginally food-secure households, and 10% from food-insecure households. Food insecurity was associated with several negative health consequences, including severe pre-gravid obesity, higher gestational weight gain, and a higher adequacy of weight gain ratio. Gestational diabetes mellitus was significantly associated with those marginally food secure (Laraia et al. 2010). Food insecurity has also been associated with inability to return to pre-gravid weight status, although causality has not been determined (Olson and Strawderman 2003).

Food insecurity in pregnant women has also been associated with poor pregnancy outcomes and negative health outcomes for children, including low birth weight, birth defects, and increased risk of vertical transmission of HIV. In a random sample of women receiving welfare in the United States, 294 delivered between 1999 and 2004. Among this cohort, food insecurity was significantly associated with low birth weight delivery after adjusting for maternal age. Other factors associated with low birth weight included having a child with a chronic illness at home, increased crowding in the home, unemployment, and poor coping skills (Borders et al. 2007). A case–control study by Carmichael et al. (2007) with 1189 case mothers and 695 control mothers in the United States demonstrated that maternal food insecurity was associated with increased risk of certain birth defects such as increased risk of cleft palate, d-transposition of the great arteries, tetralogy of Fallot, spina bifida, and anencephaly, but not with cleft lip with or without cleft palate, after adjusting for maternal race-ethnicity, education, BMI, intake of folic acid-containing supplements, dietary intake of folate and energy, neighborhood crime, and stressful life events. Prenatal zinc deficiency in pregnant women has been linked to a wide range of serious complications in pregnancy, including hypertension, prolonged labor, postpartum hemorrhage, low birth weight, and congenital malformations (Shah and Sachdev 2001). For HIV-infected pregnant women, poor nutritional status that can result from being food insecure may increase the risk of vertical transmission of HIV to the child (Gillespie and Kadiyala 2005).

In addition to potentially negative consequences for pregnancy outcomes, food insecurity during the prenatal period can negatively impact maternal nutrition and mental health, as well as maternal–infant interaction. It can also be a mental stressor and lead to depression, fatigue, loss of interest, and can reduce a mother's ability to be a responsive caretaker (Frith et al. 2012). The mental health associations with food insecurity are discussed in more detail in the next section, "Food Insecurity and Mental Health." Maternal–infant interaction has been identified as an important part of child-rearing and reflects the quality of the mother–child relationship (Richter 2004). Poor maternal–infant interaction can lead to poor child development and health. In a cohort of Bangladeshi women, Frith et al. (2012) found that the quality of maternal–infant interaction was significantly improved in the group that was invited earlier to a prenatal food supplementation program, compared with the group that was invited at the standard time. The authors suggest that earlier initiation into this food supplementation program created more opportunities for social interaction and support, which could, in turn, lead to better emotional well-being. A healthier emotional state in mothers is associated with better fetal development (Collins et al. 1993, Feldman et al. 2000).

CHILD HEALTH

Several groups have studied the relationship between household food insecurity and stunted growth in children. Studies in Pakistan, Bangladesh, and Colombia found an association between childhood stunting among those with food insecurity (Baig-Ansari et al. 2006, Hackett et al. 2009, Saha et al. 2009). Three studies came to the opposite conclusion within their cohorts in Southern Ethiopia, Nepal, and Honduras, and found that household food insecurity was not associated with stunting of children, despite the high prevalence of food insecurity reported in these communities (Gray et al. 2006, Osei et al. 2010, Tessema et al. 2013). These disparate findings highlight the need for further research to study the relationship between food insecurity and childhood stunting, as well as the adaptive responses undertaken by households threatened with food insecurity.

FOOD INSECURITY AND MENTAL HEALTH

WOMEN, MOTHERS, AND THEIR CHILDREN

Food insecurity is associated with important factors related to women's mental health and well-being. See Chapter 2 for a more detailed discussion on how mental health pathways can lead to ill-health. Mothers of 3-year-old children in a cross-sectional survey of 2870 mothers in 18 U.S. cities were categorized as fully food secure (71%), marginally food secure (17%), and food insecure (12%). After adjusting for socio demographic factors, the percentage of mothers with either major depressive episode or generalized anxiety disorder increased as food insecurity category worsened, with 30.3% of food-insecure mothers suffering from one of these conditions (Whitaker et al. 2006). In cohort of 456 adults living with HIV in rural Uganda, Tsai et al. (2012b) found a significant association between food insecurity and depressive symptoms in HIV-infected women, but not men. In peri-urban Ghana, in a cohort of 232 women, those living in persistently food-insecure households were 2.8 times as likely as their food-secure counterparts to experience stress (Garcia et al. 2013). There was also a significant association between maternal stress and HIV status, by which HIV-infected women were twice as likely as non-HIV-infected women to experience maternal stress. These are findings from a multivariate model; another model, when testing the simultaneous effect of both HIV infection and persistent household food insecurity, found a staggering 15-fold chance of experiencing maternal stress compared to when neither issue was presented.

Hadley and Patil (2006) studied 449 female caretakers in rural Tanzania and found a strong positive correlation between food insecurity and anxiety and depression, which maintained true across the four ethnic groups in the sample. The authors propose three explanations for the association: first, that food insecurity can lead to poor diet, which can then influence anxiety and depression; second, that food insecurity can lead to feelings of inequality that could then elevate anxiety and depression; and third, that women may use expressions of food insecurity as a way to express their anxiety and depression.

Decreased mental health status in pregnant and postnatal women and mothers is also associated with food insecurity. In a sample of 5306 mothers in the United

States, maternal depression was associated with household food insecurity (Casey et al. 2004). Perceived stress, trait anxiety, depressive symptoms, and a locus of control attributed to chance in pregnant women were all positively correlated with household food insecurity, showing a "dose–response" as food insecurity increased. Traits such as self-esteem were inversely associated with food insecurity (Laraia et al. 2006). Dewing et al. (2013) found that food insecurity was significantly associated with postnatal depression, suicidality, and hazardous drinking in a cohort of 249 women who had given birth 3 months prior. One-third of the women who were interviewed at their 3-month postnatal visit met criteria for probable depression. For each point on the food insecurity scale, there was a 5% risk of probable depression, a 12% increased risk of having suicidal thoughts, and a 4% increased risk of hazardous drinking.

In addition to mothers suffering from mental health consequences, children in food-insecure households are also impacted. In a prospective birth cohort study, Melchior et al. (2012) showed that family food insecurity predicts high levels of children's mental health symptoms, particularly hyperactivity and inattention. Belsky et al. (2010) had similar results, and found a significant association of increased behavioral and emotional issues, and lower IQs among children with food insecurity in a bivariate model. After adjusting for household income, however, the association between food insecurity and lower child IQ was no longer significant. In all analysis models, after adjusting for household income, and material and nonmaterial household features, emotional problems in children remained significantly associated with food insecurity.

REFUGEES

Refugees are a vulnerable population and have disproportionately high prevalence of both physical (Kinzie et al. 2008, Sorkin et al. 2008) and mental health (Mollica et al. 1993, Marshall et al. 2005, Ringold et al. 2005) issues, which can be exacerbated by food insecurity. In a study of Cambodian refugee women relocated to Massachusetts, Peterman et al. (2013) conducted focus groups with 11 women about their experiences resettling in the United States, and then a survey developed from focus group themes was administered to 150 women who had lived in the states for at least 5 years. Women who were classified as food insecure (including marginal, low, and very low food security) were 3.7 times more likely to be depressed and 4.8 times more likely to be widowed than those who were food secure. Consistent with studies discussed in the "Food Insecurity, Household Economics, and Risky Coping Strategies" section of this chapter, there was a negative association between food security and poverty—the food-insecure women were less than one-third likely to have a higher income-to-poverty ratio compared with their food-secure counterparts.

INTERVENTIONS

The body of evidence regarding food insecurity and its varied associations with psychosocial and demographic determinants of health and wealth continues to grow rapidly. With this comes, at times, seemingly contradictory findings in the literature.

However, while these gaps in knowledge and in the science surrounding food insecurity are filled in, and amidst the challenges in standardizing measurement, programs exist that attempt to address the issue with a goal of improving the outcomes of individuals, households, and communities. It is helpful to think of programs with regard to the three pillars of food security: availability, access, and use to evaluate if and/ or how each of these components is addressed. Here, we select diverse examples of programs, in addition to the others detailed in Chapters 8 and 10 of the book, that are making strides in the field addressing the issue of food insecurity, with a specific emphasis on gender equity.

UNITED STATES FEDERAL FOOD PROGRAMS

Two of the largest federal food and nutrition assistance programs in the United States are the Supplemental Nutrition Assistance Program (SNAP) and the Special Supplemental Nutrition Program for Women, Infants and Children, widely known as WIC. In part due to the increasing enrollment in these programs, as well as the known association between lower socioeconomic status and obesity, a significant number of studies have been conducted to evaluate the impact of these programs on food security and weight.

The WIC program focuses on healthcare and nutrition of low-income pregnant women, breastfeeding women, and infants and children under the age of 5. Metallinos-Katsaras et al. (2011) performed a longitudinal study of WIC program participants in Massachusetts from 2001 to 2006 and measured the duration of program participation and its impact on household food insecurity. Postpartum household food insecurity was reduced in the households that reported food insecurity with hunger prenatally and most significantly impacted those who entered the program early in their pregnancy with a 39% difference between entering during the first versus third trimester.

The Supplemental Nutrition Assistance Program (SNAP), formerly called the Food Stamp Program (FSP), is a federal assistance program providing support to low-income individuals and families. Many studies have found a positive association between SNAP participation and weight gain in women (Townsend et al. 2001, Gibson 2003, 2006, Meyerhoefer and Pylypchuk 2008, Webb et al. 2008, Zagorsky and Smith 2009), and this research suggests that long-term participation in this program may cumulatively increase the risk for excess weight gain among women. It has been suggested that one factor contributing to this association is an adaptive physiological response to episodic food insecurity, which has been shown to occur in SNAP recipients called the "food stamp cycle." This refers to a cyclical pattern of overeating while food stamps and money is available, followed by abrupt food restriction once these resources have been depleted toward the end of the month (Dinour et al. 2007). Groups finding a significant association between food stamp participation and weight gain have called for the importance of investigating dietary choices of SNAP participants, as well as SNAP policies to enable participants to make healthy choices and reduce food insecurity without gaining unhealthy weight.

The majority of studies of SNAP show no association between men receiving stamps and obesity (Gibson 2003, Cole and Fox 2004, Chen et al. 2005, Ver Ploeg et al. 2007, Meyerhoefer and Pylypchuk 2008, Zagorsky and Smith 2009). However, in contrast, Leung et al. (2012) found that SNAP participation was positively associated with overweight and obesity in both men and women—both genders were at-risk for elevated waist circumference.

One study from 2007 shows that the weight gap between those who receive SNAP food assistance and those who are eligible but do not participate has lessened over the past three decades (Ver Ploeg et al. 2007), suggesting that SNAP is not in fact the cause of the weight gain found in many other cross-sectional studies. The authors caution against drawing conclusions from strictly cross-sectional data; while they conducted their analysis using data from a longer time span than many of their colleagues (NHANES surveys from 1976 to 2002), they admit that using multiple cross-sections of data can also not determine causality. The authors note that the SNAP program has not changed drastically over the study period and therefore would not be the cause for the diminished weight gap. A possible explanation is that the characteristics of those eligible for SNAP, and either choosing to participate or not participate, may be changing with time. Finally, supporting the work of colleagues Chang and Lauderdale (2005), Ver Ploeg et al. believe that overweight and obesity are affecting a larger proportion of Americans.

Next steps for these federal programs include further research and improved programmatic policies. In their review of studies conducted between 2000 and 2010 examining the effect of SNAP on weight, Larson and Story (2011) outline a series of recommendations, consistent with conclusions from the current body of literature, on future areas of research to better understand the relationship between food insecurity and overweight/obesity, as well as how SNAP can better address these overlapping health issues. Longitudinal studies are the only way to get a better understanding of causality of the relationship between food insecurity and weight, and SNAP and weight. More quantitative and qualitative studies to understand dietary practice among these populations can play an important role to understanding individuals' experience of food insecurity and weight gain. One such study by Leung et al. (2012) showed that while both SNAP participants and nonparticipants had low dietary quality scores, SNAP participants had lower quality diets than their nonparticipating counterparts. This finding highlights the need for increased nutrition education for participants, as well as programmatic policy changes to increase access to healthy foods, such as vegetables and fruit, to those receiving SNAP benefits. In accordance with the new Food Insecurity Nutrition Incentive program that is embedded in the recently passed "farm bill" (Economic Research Service 2014), SNAP participants will be able to double the value of their benefits at participating local farmer's markets. With initiatives like this, SNAP will have the potential to have an immense, nutritious impact on over 47 million participants (Food and Nutrition Service 2014).

CASH FOR WORK

In Bangladesh, Mascie-Taylor et al. (2010) evaluated the impact of a cash-for-work program on the nutritional status of 895 households enrolled during the season where food insecurity is most dire. They found those households had greater food expenditure and consumption, and women and children aged less than 5 years had improved nutritional status. It should be noted that in both intervention and control groups, many children remained malnourished despite this improvement in the intervention group. This suggests that targeting seasonality of food insecurity in some settings may be a reasonable approach.

NUTRITION EDUCATION

Nutrition education also has a role to play in impacting food security. A U.S. study of 219 female heads of households receiving food stamps randomized to receive education regarding food insecurity and nutrition or not, food security improved significantly in the intervention group (Eicher-Miller et al. 2009). Though evidence is limited on interventions with proven impact on food insecurity in women with HIV, food assistance, livelihoods programs, education, and intergenerational support show evidence of success (Eicher-Miller et al. 2009, Mamlin et al. 2009). In addition, a prospective observational cohort study of 600 adults in rural Haiti found that food assistance was associated with improved BMI, food security, and attendance at monthly clinic visits for both men and women living with HIV (Ivers et al. 2010).

CONCLUSION

Food insecurity, independent of its association with poverty and low income, has important implications for the health of women. Given the unique mechanisms by which physical, biological, mental, emotional, and behavioral factors interact and manifest differently in women than they do in men, and given that childcare and household food preparation are typically gendered, special considerations are required to understand how food insecurity impacts women and their families. Finally, due to the increasing number of female-headed households worldwide, and their disproportionately poor economic status, women in many communities would benefit from programs designed to empower women with the resources and skills necessary to provide for their households and communities.

Food insecurity in women has been significantly associated with nutrient deficiency, over- and underweight, mental health issues, risky sexual behavior, poor coping strategies, and negative pregnancy outcomes. Conclusive findings on the direction and causality of the associations between food insecurity, weight status, mental and physical health, however, are not well established. These relationships may continue to be investigated in both developed and developing settings in longitudinal studies, differentiated by weight status, behavior, and other factors before and after periods of food insecurity to try to tap into the complex relationship of these covariates. A gap in the literature remains around understanding the impacts of food insecurity on women in resource-poor settings, including impact on weight, nutrition, and pregnancy outcomes, as well as on the progression of diseases such as HIV infection; such data are also lacking for men in these settings. More research is needed to guide efficient interventions addressing food insecurity among women. It is clear, however, that a multifaceted approach is needed. Practical experience suggests that both short-term assistance to women with food insecurity, as well as longer-term strategies to improve livelihoods, address behavioral and coping strategies, acknowledge mental health components of food insecurity, and promote women's access to land and economic opportunities, play a crucial role. Rigorous monitoring and evaluation of existing programs, disaggregation of existing data by gender and standardization of a food security measurement tool can help to add to this body of evidence.

REFERENCES

Adams, E. J., L. Grummer-Strawn, and G. Chavez. 2003. Food insecurity is associated with increased risk of obesity in California women. *Journal of Nutrition* 133 (4):1070–1074.

Aekplakorn, W., M. C. Hogan, V. Chongsuvivatwong, P. Tatsanavivat, S. Chariyalertsak, A. Boonthum, and S. S. Lim. 2007. Trends in obesity and associations with education and urban or rural residence in Thailand. *Obesity* 15 (12):3113–3121. doi: 10.1038/oby.2007.371.

Baig-Ansari, N., M. H. Rahbar, Z. A. Bhutta, and S. H. Badruddin. 2006. Child's gender and household food insecurity are associated with stunting among young Pakistani children residing in urban squatter settlements. *Food and Nutrition Bulletin* 27 (2):114–127.

Bawadi, H. A., R. F. Tayyem, A. N. Dwairy, and N. Al-Akour. 2012. Prevalence of food insecurity among women in northern Jordan. *Journal of Health, Population, and Nutrition* 30 (1):49.

Belsky, D. W., T. E. Moffitt, L. Arseneault, M. Melchior, and A. Caspi. 2010. Context and sequelae of food insecurity in children's development. *American Journal of Epidemiology*. 172 (7): 809–818. doi: 10.1093/aje/kwq201.

Benson, J., C. Phillips, M. Kay, M. T. Webber, A. J. Ratcliff, I. Correa-Velez, and M. F. Lorimer. 2013. Low vitamin B12 levels among newly-arrived refugees from Bhutan, Iran and Afghanistan: A multicentre Australian study. *PLOS ONE* 8 (2):e57998. doi: 10.1371/journal.pone.0057998.

Borders, A. E., W. A. Grobman, L. B. Amsden, and J. L. Holl. 2007. Chronic stress and low birth weight neonates in a low-income population of women. *Obstetrics & Gynecology* 109 (2 Part 1):331–338. doi: 10.1097/01.AOG.0000250535.97920.b5.

Bove, C. F. and C. M. Olson. 2006. Obesity in low-income rural women: Qualitative insights about physical activity and eating patterns. *Women and Health* 44 (1):57–78. doi: 10.1300/J013v44n01_04.

Braveman, P., K. Marchi, S. Egerter, S. Kim, M. Metzler, T. Stancil, and M. Libet. 2010. Poverty, near-poverty, and hardship around the time of pregnancy. *Maternal and Child Health Journal* 14 (1):20–35. doi: 10.1007/s10995-008-0427-0.

Carmichael, S. L., W. Yang, A. Herring, B. Abrams, and G. M. Shaw. 2007. Maternal food insecurity is associated with increased risk of certain birth defects. *Journal of Nutrition* 137 (9):2087–2092.

Casey, P., S. Goolsby, C. Berkowitz, D. Frank, J. Cook, D. Cutts, and Children's Sentinel Nutritional Assessment Program Study Group. 2004. Maternal depression, changing public assistance, food security, and child health status. *Pediatrics* 113 (2):298–304.

Catalano, P. M. 2003. Obesity and pregnancy—The propagation of a viscous cycle? *Journal of Clinical Endocrinology & Metabolism* 88 (8):3505–3506.

Chang, V. W. and D. S. Lauderdale. 2005. Income disparities in body mass index and obesity in the United States, 1971-2002. *Archives of Internal Medicine* 165 (18):2122–2128.

Chaput, J.-P., J.-A. Gilbert, and A. Tremblay. 2007. Relationship between food insecurity and body composition in Ugandans living in urban Kampala. *Journal of the American Dietetic Association* 107 (11):1978–1982.

Chen, Z., S. T. Yen, and D. B. Eastwood. 2005. Effects of food stamp participation on body weight and obesity. *American Journal of Agricultural Economics* 87 (5):1167–1173.

Chilton, M. and S. Booth. 2007. Hunger of the body and hunger of the mind: African American women's perceptions of food insecurity, health and violence. *Journal of Nutrition Education and Behavior* 39 (3):116–125.

Chilton, M. M., J. R. Rabinowich, and N. H. Woolf. 2013. Very low food security in the USA is linked with exposure to violence. *Public Health Nutrition* 17 (01):73–82. doi: 10.1017/S1368980013000281.

Cole, N. and M. K. Fox. 2004. Nutrition and health characteristics of low-Income populations, Volume II: WIC participants and nonparticipants. US Department of Agriculture, Economic Research Service, Electronic publication number E-FAN-04-010-2.

Collins, N. L., C. Dunkel-Schetter, M. Lobel, and S. C. Scrimshaw. 1993. Social support in pregnancy: Psychosocial correlates of birth outcomes and postpartum depression. *Journal of Personality and Social Psychology* 65 (6):1243.

Cristofar, S. P. and P. P. Basiotis. 1992. Dietary intakes and selected characteristics of women ages 19–50 years and their children ages 1–5 years by reported perception of food sufficiency. *Journal of Nutrition Education* 24 (2):53–58.

De Schutter, O. 2013. Gender equality and food security: Women's empowerment as a tool against hunger. Asian Development Bank. Accessed September 10, 2014. http://www.adb.org/sites/default/files/pub/2013/gender-equality-and-food-security.pdf.

Dewing, S., M. Tomlinson, I. M. le Roux, M. Chopra, and A. C. Tsai. 2013. Food insecurity and its association with co-occurring postnatal depression, hazardous drinking, and suicidality among women in peri-urban South Africa. *Journal of Affective Disorders* 150 (2):460–465. doi: 10.1089/apc.2007.0102.

Dinour, L. M., D. Bergen, and M.-C. Yeh. 2007. The food insecurity-obesity paradox: A review of the literature and the role food stamps may play. *Journal of the American Dietetic Association* 107 (11):1952–1961.

Dixon, L. B., M. A. Winkleby, and K. L. Radimer. 2001. Dietary intakes and serum nutrients differ between adults from food-insufficient and food-sufficient families: Third National Health and Nutrition Examination Survey, 1988–1994. *Journal of Nutrition* 131 (4):1232–1246.

Dubois, L., D. Francis, D. Burnier, F. Tatone-Tokuda, M. Girard, G. Gordon-Strachan, and R. Wilks. 2011. Household food insecurity and childhood overweight in Jamaica and Quebec: A gender-based analysis. *BMC Public Health* 11:199. doi: 10.1186/1471-2458-11-199.

Eaton, L. A., D. N. Cain, E. V. Pitpitan, K. B. Carey, M. P. Carey, V. Mehlomakulu, and S. C. Kalichman. 2014. Exploring the relationships among food insecurity, alcohol use, and sexual risk taking among men and women living in South African Townships. *Journal of Primary Prevention* 35 (4):255–265.

Economic Research Service. 2014. Agricultural Act of 2014: Highlights and Implications. United States Department of Agriculture, http://www.ers.usda.gov/agricultural-act-of-2014-highlights-and-implications/nutrition.aspx#.U_-Y07xdUjw.

Eicher-Miller, H. A., A. C. Mason, A. R. Abbott, G. P. McCabe, and C. J. Boushey. 2009. The effect of Food Stamp Nutrition Education on the food insecurity of low-income women participants. *Journal of Nutrition Education and Behavior* 41 (3):161–168.

Feldman, P. J., C. Dunkel-Schetter, C. A. Sandman, and P. D. Wadhwa. 2000. Maternal social support predicts birth weight and fetal growth in human pregnancy. *Psychosomatic Medicine* 62 (5):715–725.

Food and Agriculture Organization. 1996. *Rome Declaration on World Food Security, World Food Summit.* Food and Agriculture Organization, Rome.

Food and Agriculture Organization. 2010. The State of Food Insecurity in the World 2010: Addressing food insecurity in protracted crises. Food and Agriculture Organization. Accessed September 10, 2014. http://www.fao.org/docrep/013/i1683e/i1683e.pdf.

Food and Nutrition Service. 2014. Supplemental Nutrition Assistance Program (SNAP): Average Monthly Participation (persons). United States Department of Agriculture. Accessed September 10, 2014. http://www.fns.usda.gov/sites/default/files/pd/15SNAPpartPP.pdf.

Franklin, B., A. Jones, D. Love, S. Puckett, J. Macklin, and S. White-Means. 2012. Exploring mediators of food insecurity and obesity: A review of recent literature. *Journal of Community Health* 37 (1):253–264.

Frith, A. L., R. T. Naved, L. A. Persson, K. M. Rasmussen, and E. A. Frongillo. 2012. Early participation in a prenatal food supplementation program ameliorates the negative association of food insecurity with quality of maternal–infant interaction. *Journal of Nutrition* 142 (6):1095–1101.

Garcia, J., A. Hromi-Fiedler, R. E. Mazur, G. Marquis, D. Sellen, A. Lartey, and R. Pérez-Escamilla. 2013. Persistent household food insecurity, HIV, and maternal stress in peri-urban Ghana. *BMC Public Health* 13:215.

Gibson, D. 2003. Food stamp program participation is positively related to obesity in low income women. *Journal of Nutrition* 133 (7):2225–2231.

Gibson, D. 2006. Long-term food stamp program participation is positively related to simultaneous overweight in young daughters and obesity in mothers. *Journal of Nutrition* 136 (4):1081–1085.

Gillespie, S. and S. Kadiyala. 2005. *HIV/AIDS and Food and Nutrition Security: From Evidence to Action.* Vol. 7, *Food Policy Reviews.* Washington, DC: International Food Policy Research Institute.

Gray, V. B., J. S. Cossman, and E. L. Powers. 2006. Stunted growth is associated with physical indicators of malnutrition but not food insecurity among rural school children in Honduras. *Nutrition Research* 26 (11):549–555.

Gulliford, M. C., D. Mahabir, and B. Rocke. 2003. Food insecurity, food choices, and body mass index in adults: Nutrition transition in Trinidad and Tobago. *International Journal of Epidemiology* 32 (4):508–516.

Hackett, M., H. Melgar-Quiñonez, and M. C. Álvarez. 2009. Household food insecurity associated with stunting and underweight among preschool children in Antioquia, Colombia. *Revista Panamericana de Salud Pública* 25 (6):506–510.

Hadley, C. and C. L. Patil. 2006. Food insecurity in rural Tanzania is associated with maternal anxiety and depression. *American Journal of Human Biology* 18 (3):359–368.

Hanson, K. L., J. Sobal, and E. A. Frongillo. 2007. Gender and marital status clarify associations between food insecurity and body weight. *Journal of Nutrition* 137:1460–1465.

Hawkes, C. 2006. Uneven dietary development: Linking the policies and processes of globalization with the nutrition transition, obesity and diet-related chronic diseases. *Globalization and Health* 2 (1):4.

Ihabi, A. N., A. J. Rohana, W. M. Wan Manan, W. N. Wan Suriati, M. S. Zalilah, and A. M. Rusli. 2013. Nutritional outcomes related to household food insecurity among mothers in rural Malaysia. *Journal of Health, Population and Nutrition* 31 (4):480–489.

Isanaka, S., M. Mora-Plazas, S. Lopez-Arana, A. Baylin, and E. Villamor. 2007. Food insecurity is highly prevalent and predicts underweight but not overweight in adults and school children from Bogota, Colombia. *Journal of Nutrition* 137 (12):2747–2755.

Ivers, L. C., Y. Chang, J. G. Jerome, and K. A. Freedberg. 2010. Food assistance is associated with improved body mass index, food security and attendance at clinic in an HIV program in central Haiti: A prospective observational cohort study. *AIDS Research and Therapy* 7:33.

Jones, S. J. and E. A. Frongillo. 2007. Food insecurity and subsequent weight gain in women. *Public Health Nutrition* 10 (2):145–151.

Kac, G., G. Velasquez-Melendez, M. M. Schlussel, A. M. Segall-Correa, A. A. Silva, and R. Perez-Escamilla. 2012. Severe food insecurity is associated with obesity among Brazilian adolescent females. *Public Health Nutrition* 15 (10):1854–1860. doi: 10.1017/s1368980011003582.

Katona, P. and J. Katona-Apte. 2008. The interaction between nutrition and infection. *Clinical Infectious Diseases* 46:1582–1588.

Kelly, M., C. Banwell, J. Dixon, S.-A. Seubsman, V. Yiengprugsawan, and A. Sleigh. 2010. Nutrition transition, food retailing and health equity in Thailand. *Australasian Epidemiological Association* 17 (3):4.

Kendall, A., C. M. Olson, and E. A. Frongillo Jr. 1996. Relationship of hunger and food insecurity to food availability and consumption. *Journal of the American Dietetic Association* 96 (10):1019–1024.

Kinzie, J. D., C. Riley, B. McFarland, M. Hayes, J. Boehnlein, P. Leung, and G. Adams. 2008. High prevalence rates of diabetes and hypertension among refugee psychiatric patients. *Journal of Nervous and Mental Disease* 196 (2):108–112.

Laraia, B. A., A. M. Siega-Riz, C. Gundersen, and N. Dole. 2006. Psychosocial factors and socioeconomic indicators are associated with household food insecurity among pregnant women. *Journal of Nutrition* 136 (1):177–182.

Laraia, B. A., A. M. Siega-Riz, and C. Gundersen. 2010. Household food insecurity is associated with self-reported pregravid weight status, gestational weight gain, and pregnancy complications. *Journal of the American Dietetic Association* 110 (5):692–701.

Larson, N.I. and M.T. Story. 2011. Food insecurity and weight status among US children and families: A review of the literature. *American Journal of Preventive Medicine* 40 (2):166–173.

Leung, C. W., W. C. Willett, and E. L. Ding. 2012. Low-income Supplemental Nutrition Assistance Program participation is related to adiposity and metabolic risk factors. *American Journal of Clinical Nutrition* 95 (1):17–24.

Lubbock, A. and R. Borquia. 1998. Survival, change and decision-making in rural households: Three village case studies from eastern Morocco. International Fund for Agricultural Development.

Mamlin, J., S. Kimaiyo, S. Lewis, H. Tadayo, F. K. Jerop, C. Gichunge, and R. Einterz. 2009. Integrating nutrition support for food-insecure patients and their dependents into an HIV care and treatment program in western Kenya. *American Journal of Public Health* 99 (2):215–221.

Marshall, G. N., T. L. Schell, M. N. Elliott, S. M. Berthold, and C.-A. Chun. 2005. Mental health of Cambodian refugees 2 decades after resettlement in the United States. *JAMA* 294 (5):571–579.

Martin-Fernandez, J., F. Caillavet, A. Lhuissier, and P. Chauvin. 2014. Food insecurity, a determinant of obesity?-an analysis from a population-based survey in the Paris metropolitan area, 2010. *Obesity Facts* 7 (2):120–129.

Martin, M. A. and A. M. Lippert. 2012. Feeding her children, but risking her health: The intersection of gender, household food insecurity and obesity. *Social Science & Medicine* 74 (11): 1754–1764.

Mascie-Taylor, C. G., M. K. Marks, R. Goto, and R. Islam. 2010. Impact of a cash-for-work programme on food consumption and nutrition among women and children facing food insecurity in rural Bangladesh. *Bulletin of the World Health Organization* 88 (11):854–860. doi: 10.2471/blt.10.080994.

McCoy, S. I., L. J. Ralph, P. F. Njau, M. M. Msolla, and N. S. Padian. 2014. Food insecurity, socioeconomic status, and HIV-related risk behavior among women in farming households in Tanzania. *AIDS and Behavior* 18 (7):1224–1236.

McIntyre, L., V. Tarasuk, and T. J. Li. 2007. Improving the nutritional status of food-insecure women: First, let them eat what they like. *Public Health Nutrition* 10 (11): 1288–1298.

Mcmillen, I. C. and J. S. Robinson. 2005. Developmental origins of the metabolic syndrome: Prediction, plasticity, and programming. *Physiological Reviews* 85 (2):571–633.

Melchior, M., A. Caspi, L. M. Howard, A. P. Ambler, H. Bolton, N. Mountain, and T. E. Moffitt. 2009. Mental health context of food insecurity: A representative cohort of families with young children. *Pediatrics* 124 (4):e564–e572.

Melchior, M., J.-F. Chastang, B. Falissard, C. Galéra, R. E. Tremblay, S. M. Côté, and M. Boivin. 2012. Food insecurity and children's mental health: A prospective birth cohort study. *PLOS ONE* 7 (12):e52615.

Metallinos-Katsaras, E., K. S. Gorman, P. Wilde, and J. Kallio. 2011. A longitudinal study of WIC participation on household food insecurity. *Maternal and Child Health Journal* 15 (5):627–633.

Meyerhoefer, C. D. and Y. Pylypchuk. 2008. Does participation in the food stamp program increase the prevalence of obesity and health care spending? *American Journal of Agricultural Economics* 90 (2):287–305.

Miller, C. L., D. R. Bangsberg, D. M. Tuller, J. Senkungu, A. Kawuma, E. A. Frongillo, and S. D. Weiser. 2011. Food insecurity and sexual risk in an HIV endemic community in Uganda. *AIDS and Behavior* 15 (7):1512–1519.

Mohammadi, F., N. Omidvar, G. G. Harrison, M. Ghazi-Tabatabaei, M. Abdollahi, A. Houshiar-Rad, and A. R. Dorosty. 2013. Is household food insecurity associated with overweight/obesity in women? *Iranian Journal of Public Health* 42 (4):380.

Mollica, R. F., K. Donelan, S. Tor, J. Lavelle, C. Elias, M. Frankel, and R. J. Blendon. 1993. The effect of trauma and confinement on functional health and mental health status of Cambodians living in Thailand-Cambodia border camps. *JAMA* 270 (5):581–586.

Olson, C. M. 1999. Nutrition and health outcomes associated with food insecurity and hunger. *Journal of Nutrition* 129(suppl):521S–524S.

Olson, C. M. and M. S. Strawderman. 2003. Gestational weight gain and postpartum behaviors associated with weight change from early pregnancy to 1 y postpartum. *International Journal of Obesity and Related Metabolic Disorders* 27 (1):117–127.

Olson, C. M. and M. S. Strawderman. 2008. The relationship between food insecurity and obesity in rural childbearing women. *Journal of Rural Health* 24 (1):60–66.

Osei, A., P. Pandey, D. Spiro, J. Nielson, R. Shrestha, Z. Talukder, and N. Haselow. 2010. Household food insecurity and nutritional status of children aged 6 to 23 months in Kailali District of Nepal. *Food & Nutrition Bulletin* 31 (4):483–494.

Oyefara, J. L. 2007. Food insecurity, HIV/AIDS pandemic and sexual behaviour of female commercial sex workers in Lagos metropolis, Nigeria. *SAHARA J* 4 (2):626–635.

Peterman, J. N., P. E. Wilde, L. Silka, O. I. Bermudez, and B. L. Rogers. 2013. Food insecurity among Cambodian refugee women two decades post resettlement. *Journal of Immigrant and Minority Health* 15 (2):372–380.

Piwoz, E. 2004. *Nutrition and HIV/AIDS: Evidence, Gaps and Priority Actions.* Washington, DC: Academy for Educational Development.

Richter, L. 2004. The importance of caregiver-child interactions for the survival and healthy development of young children. A review. Department of Child and Adolescent Health and Development. World Health Organization. Accessed September 10, 2014. http://whqlibdoc.who.int/publications/2004/924159134X.pdf.

Ringold, S., A. Burke, and R. M. Glass. 2005. Refugee mental health. *JAMA* 294 (5):646–646.

Rose, D. and V. Oliveira. 1997. Nutrient intakes of individuals from food-insufficient households in the United States. *American Journal of Public Health* 87 (12):1956–1961.

Saha, K. K., E. A. Frongillo, D. S. Alam, S. E. Arifeen, L. A. Persson, and K. M. Rasmussen. 2009. Household food security is associated with growth of infants and young children in rural Bangladesh. *Public Health Nutrition* 12 (9):1556.

Salaam-Blyther, T. and C. E. Hanrahan. 2009. The Impact of Food Insecurity and Hunger on Global Health: Issues for Congress. Congressional Research Service. Accessed September 10, 2014.

Schlüssel, M. M., A. A. Silva, R. Perez-Escamilla, and G. Kac. 2013. Household food insecurity and excess weight/obesity among Brazilian women and children: A life-course approach. *Cad Saude Publica* 29 (2):219–226.

Seubsman, S. A., L. L. Lim, C. Banwell, N. Sripaiboonkit, M. Kelly, C. Bain, and A. C. Sleigh. 2010. Socioeconomic status, sex, and obesity in a large national cohort of 15–87-year-old open university students in Thailand. *Journal of Epidemiology* 20 (1):13–20.

Shah, D. and H. P. Sachdev. 2001. Effect of gestational zinc deficiency on pregnancy outcomes: Summary of observation studies and zinc supplementation trials. *British Journal of Nutrition* 85 (S2):S101–S108.

Shariff, Z. M. and G. L. Khor. 2005. Obesity and household food insecurity: Evidence from a sample of rural households in Malaysia. *European Journal of Clinical Nutrition* 59 (9):1049–1058.

Singh, A., A. Singh, and F. Ram. 2014. Household food insecurity and nutritional status of children and women in Nepal. *Food & Nutrition Bulletin* 35 (1):3–11.

Sorkin, D., A. L. Tan, R. D. Hays, C. M. Mangione, and Q. Ngo-Metzger. 2008. Self-reported health status of Vietnamese and non-Hispanic White older adults in California. *Journal of the American Geriatrics Society* 56 (8):1543–1548.

Tarasuk, V. S. and G. H. Beaton. 1999. Women's dietary intakes in the context of household food insecurity. *Journal of Nutrition* 129:672–679.

Tayie, F. A. and C. A. Zizza. 2009. Height differences and the associations between food insecurity, percentage body fat and BMI among men and women. *Public Health Nutrition* 12 (10):1855–1861.

Tessema, M., T. Belachew, and G. Ersino. 2013. Feeding patterns and stunting during early childhood in rural communities of Sidama, South Ethiopia. *Pan African Medical Journal* 14:75.

Townsend, M. S., J. Peerson, B. Love, C. Achterberg, and S. P. Murphy. 2001. Food insecurity is positively related to overweight in women. *Journal of Nutrition* 131 (6):1738–1745.

Tsai, A. C., K. J. Hung, and S. D. Weiser. 2012a. Is food insecurity associated with HIV risk? Cross-sectional evidence from sexually active women in Brazil. *PLOS Medicine* 9 (4):e1001203. doi: 10.1371/journal.pmed.1001203.

Tsai, A. C., D. R. Bangsberg, E. A. Frongillo, P. W. Hunt, C. Muzoora, J. N. Martin, and S. D. Weiser. 2012b. Food insecurity, depression and the modifying role of social support among people living with HIV/AIDS in rural Uganda. *Social Science & Medicine* 74 (12):2012–2019.

United Nations Development Fund for Women. 2010. Women, poverty & economics. Accessed November 29. http://www.unifem.org/gender_issues/women_poverty_economics/.

United Nations World Food Programme, and United Nations High Commissioner for Refugees. 2009. Micronutrient Powder (MixMe TM) use in Kakuma Refugee Camp in Kenya (AFRICA). United Nations World Food Programme.

Velasquez-Melendez, G., M. M. Schlussel, A. S. Brito, A. A. M. Silva, J. D. Lopes-Filho, and G. Kac. 2011. Mild but not light or severe food insecurity is associated with obesity among Brazilian women. *Journal of Nutrition* 141 (5):898–902.

Ver Ploeg, M., L. Mancino, B.-H. Lin, and C.-Y. Wang. 2007. The vanishing weight gap: Trends in obesity among adult food stamp participants (US)(1976–2002). *Economics & Human Biology* 5 (1):20–36.

Wang, Z. P., X. X. Shang, and Z. T. Zhao. 2012. Low maternal vitamin B(12) is a risk factor for neural tube defects: A meta-analysis. *Journal of Maternal-Fetal and Neonatal Medicine* 25 (4):389–394. doi: 10.3109/14767058.2011.580800.

Webb, A. L., A. Schiff, D. Currivan, and E. Villamor. 2008. Food Stamp Program participation but not food insecurity is associated with higher adult BMI in Massachusetts residents living in low-income neighbourhoods. *Public Health Nutrition* 11 (12):1248–1255.

Wehler, C., L. F. Weinreb, N. Huntington, R. Scott, D. Hosmer, K. Fletcher, and C. Gundersen. 2004. Risk and protective factors for adult and child hunger among low-income housed and homeless female-headed families. *American Journal of Public Health* 94 (1):109–115.

Weiser, S. D., K. Leiter, D. R. Bangsberg, L. M. Butler, F. Percy-de Korte, Z. Hlanze, and M. Heisler. 2007. Food insufficiency is associated with high-risk sexual behavior among women in Botswana and Swaziland. *PLOS Medicine* 4 (10):1589–1597; discussion 1598. doi: 10.1371/journal.pmed.0040260.

Weiser, S. D., D. M. Tuller, E. A. Frongillo, J. Senkungu, N. Mukiibi, and D. R. Bangsberg. 2010. Food insecurity as a barrier to sustained antiretroviral therapy adherence in Uganda. *PLOS ONE* 5 (4):e10340. doi: 10.1371/journal.pone.0010340.

Whitaker, R. C., S. M. Phillips, and S. M. Orzol. 2006. Food insecurity and the risks of depression and anxiety in mothers and behavior problems in their preschool-aged children. *Pediatrics* 118 (3):e859–e868. doi: 10.1542/peds.2006–0239.

Whitaker, R. C. and A. Sarin. 2007. Change in food security status and change in weight are not associated in urban women with preschool children. *Journal of Nutrition* 137 (9):2134–2139.

Young, S., A. C. Wheeler, S. I. McCoy, and S. D. Weiser. 2014. A review of the role of food insecurity in adherence to care and treatment among adult and pediatric populations living with HIV and AIDS. *AIDS and Behavior* 18 (suppl. 5): S505–S515.

Zagorsky, J. L. and P. K. Smith. 2009. Does the US Food Stamp Program contribute to adult weight gain? *Economics & Human Biology* 7 (2):246–258.

8 Understanding Food Insecurity in Navajo Nation through the Community Lens

Dana Eldridge, Robyn Jackson, Shruthi Rajashekara, Emily Piltch, Mae-Gilene Begay, Joan VanWassenhove, Jacque Jim, Jonathan Abeita, LaJuanna Daye, Leroy Joe, Martha Williams, Maxine Castillo, Meria Miller-Castillo, Sherry Begaye, Vangie Tully, and Sonya Shin

CONTENTS

INTRODUCTION

Marginalized communities that struggle with food insecurity have been traditionally excluded from academic discourse. Therefore, describing food insecurity in such affected populations requires a critical appraisal of the historical, economic, and political factors that have shaped these communities. Furthermore, many minority groups have deep traditional ties with food within their cultures. Understanding food insecurity within this myriad of dynamic and interrelated issues is crucial to informing interventions that can address food insecurity at its root causes and have lasting impact across a spectrum of objectives. This understanding can only be

155

gained through insight into the wisdom and perspectives of community members themselves.

This chapter describes the historical roots, extent, and current impact of food insecurity within the context of Navajo Nation. Community-based participatory methods and a cross-disciplinary approach were used to understand the underlying issues related to food insecurity and inform food security initiatives.

FOOD INSECURITY IN THE UNITED STATES

Food insecurity is a profound issue that drives a number of health disparities within the United States, particularly those linked to obesity-related diseases. According to the United States Department of Agriculture (USDA), in 2012, an estimated 14.5% of American households—49 million people—were food insecure (Coleman-Jenson et al. 2013).

Food insecurity is acknowledged to be the result of underlying social, economic, and institutional factors (Cohen et al. 2002, Jernigan et al. 2012, Vasquez et al. 2007). Thus, it follows that those experiencing the highest rates of food insecurity are households with incomes near or below the federal poverty line,* households with children headed by a single parent, and non-White households. Over 40% of households with incomes below the poverty line were food insecure, compared to 6.8% of those with incomes above 185% of the poverty line. Further, food insecurity is found to be most prevalent in large cities and rural areas, compared to suburban and exurban areas (Coleman-Jenson et al. 2013). Rural households are particularly vulnerable, as they face more limited access to affordable food than urban households (Huddleston-Casas et al. 2009).

Food insecurity is associated with low food expenditure, low fruit and vegetable consumption, and a less healthy diet (Drewnowski and Specter 2004, Pan et al. 2012). Numerous studies have demonstrated the association of food insecurity with adverse child and adult health outcomes in U.S. populations, including low nutrient intake, hypertension, diabetes, depression, and other mental health problems (Cook et al. 2013, 2006, Gunderson et al. 2011, Seligman et al. 2007, 2010). Research suggests that food-insecure women are more likely to be overweight or obese, while research on the relationship between food insecurity and obesity among men has produced mixed results (Pan et al. 2012).

In addition to the health implications of food insecurity, the topic of food access interfaces with a multitude of disciplines, ranging from social justice (e.g., food security as a human right) to community sovereignty, and economic development to the fundamental role of food in the survival of traditions and cultures among minority communities within the United States. Furthermore, food access and dietary habits in different communities—particularly those most vulnerable to food insecurity and health disparities—can be characterized at a given moment in time, but in

---

* The Federal poverty line was $23,283 for a family of two adults and two children in 2012. Percentage multiples of federal poverty lines, such as 125%, 150%, 185%, are used as eligibility criteria for a number of federal programs.

reality, they are a dynamic evolution of historical and ongoing forces, both internal and external to the community itself. Thus, food access must be understood and addressed within a socioecological framework, recognizing that disease risk and outcome are influenced by embedded, dynamic, and interconnected social spheres, from individual and household factors to broad historical, cultural, and economic determinants (Bronfenbrenner 1979).

COMMUNITY-BASED UNDERSTANDING OF FOOD INSECURITY IN NAVAJO NATION

The Diné, or Navajo People, are a Native American tribe indigenous to the American Southwest. They are the largest tribe in the United States in both population and land base, with approximately 300,000 members and a reservation the size of West Virginia located in what is today Utah, New Mexico, and Arizona (Figure 8.1). The boundaries of the traditional homeland (Diné Bikéyah) of the Diné are marked by four mountains, considered sacred, *Sisnaajiní* (Mount Blanca in Alamosa, CO), *Tsoodził* (Mt. Taylor near Grants, NM), *Dook'o'oosłííd* (San Francisco Peak in Flagstaff, AZ), and *Dibé Ntsaa* (Hesperus Peak in Hesperus, CO).

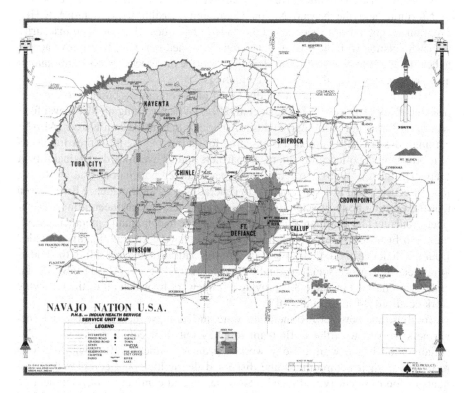

FIGURE 8.1 Map of Navajo Nation.

Diné Bikéyah
The names of the mountains are:

Sisnaajiní
Tsoodził
Dook'o'oosłííd
Dibé Ntsaa

Starting in 2011, the Diné Policy Institute (DPI) embarked on an in-depth assessment on Diné Food Systems, Food Sovereignty and Food Policy, based on a critical review of the literature and community-based interviews and surveys. The Diné Policy Institute was established within Diné College as a research institute to "mesh" Western research practices with traditional Navajo values; Natural, Traditional, Customary, and Common laws (Stokols 1996). DPI sought to analyze how traditional and sustainable food practices can be supported and revitalized to address the high rates of nutrition-related illnesses in Navajo Nation, as well as to rebuild local food economies. Evaluation included research on the historical roots of food insecurity, qualitative interviews and surveys with community members to understand the current food system, and an analysis of how current and past policy shapes food access in Navajo Nation.

Simultaneously, a collaborative effort involving Harvard University, Tufts School of Nutrition, and the Navajo Nation Community Health Representative (CHR) Program sought to better understand the underlying issues related to food insecurity in Navajo Nation with the goal of developing informed strategies to improve access to healthy foods in Navajo Nation. Here, we describe the process of both community assessments, as well as the synthesized findings.

Both initiatives were fundamentally based on a community-based participatory research (CBPR) approach (Jernigan et al. 2012). When working on local-level food security efforts, and particularly within American Indian/Alaskan Native (AI/AN) communities, a CBPR approach is essential for addressing the most pressing needs of residents with co-learning among all partners and an eye toward sustainability at each step (Stokols 1996). Particularly for marginalized populations that are facing food insecurity, CBPR is fundamental to generating a "critical evidence base," given that the existing body of scientific and historical literature has been almost exclusively generated by dominant culture. Giving a voice to community members as cultural and historical informants—individuals who have been traditionally excluded from the dialogue about their own societies—is critical to understanding the underlying determinants of social inequalities, such as food access. The 11 CBPR principles, summarized in Table 8.1, provide a framework by which all of the following work occurred (Minkler et al. 2012).

To illustrate how CBPR methods were utilized, we describe how external partners worked with the CHR team to carry out their collaborative work. The collaboration began with a 2-day workshop during which CHRs identified food resources in their communities and discussed the multiple and complex determinants of food insecurity and its effects on health and community development on the Nation. Following the identification of these determinants, nutrition and food

TABLE 8.1

Principles for Community-Based Participatory Research

Effective, authentic community-based participatory research aspires to the following qualities:

1. Recognizes community as a unit of identity.[a]
2. Builds on strengths and resources within the community.[a]
3. Facilitates a collaborative, equitable partnership in all phases of research, involving an empowering and power-sharing process that attends to social inequalities.[a]
4. Fosters co-learning and capacity building among all partners.[a]
5. Integrates and achieves a balance between knowledge generation and intervention for the mutual benefit of all partners.[a]
6. Focuses on the local relevance of public health problems and on ecological perspectives that attend to the multiple determinants of health.[a]
7. Involves systems development using a cyclical and iterative process.[a]
8. Disseminates results to all partners and involves them in the wider dissemination of results.[a]
9. Involves a long-term process and commitment to sustainability.[a]
10. Openly addresses issues of race, ethnicity, racism, and social class, and embodies "cultural humility."[b]
11. Works to ensure research rigor and validity but also seeks to "broaden the bandwidth of validity" with respect to research relevance.[b]

Source: Minkler, M. et al. 2012. Community-Based Participatory Research: A Strategy for Building Healthy Communities and Promoting Health Through Policy Change: A Report to the California Endowment.

[a] Coles, C.L. et al. 2005. *American Journal of Epidemiology* 162 (10):999–1007; Israel, B.A. et al. 1998. *Annual Reviews in Public Health* 19:173–202.

[b] Wilson, N. et al. 2008. *Health Promotion and Practice* 9 (4):395–403.

experts presented existing food surveys that had been used in the region to the team of CHRs (Bell-Sheeter 2004, USDA 2008), who then developed a food access survey specifically for their communities. In addition to identifying the areas of inquiry that were most important to understanding their communities, CHRs were also instrumental in their local knowledge of language and culture, providing critical feedback to contextualize each question to specific cultural and regional aspects of their communities. A total of 253 surveys were completed by 13 CHRs between July 2012 and April 2013. CHRs used convenience sampling to interview heads of households in the Eastern Navajo region, referred to as Crownpoint Service Unit. The same collaborative team held a subsequent 1-day workshop to review the findings and elaborate a plan to conduct in-depth qualitative interviews with key stakeholders in their respective communities (community members, local government officials, and CHRs themselves).

These findings were presented back to CHRs, community members, and Navajo Nation leadership through an iterative process. At the completion of each stage, data were compiled, presented to the CHRs, and summarized using plain language. Before written documents were finalized, CHRs' feedback on format and language choice was incorporated. Additionally, CHRs presented findings back to their communities at stakeholder meetings and at conferences. Engaging community partners to formulate the questions for inquiry and relying heavily on indigenous knowledge was a crucial aspect of "broadening the bandwidth of validity" of the findings.

The collective findings of DPI and the Harvard, Tufts, and CHR collaboration provide insight into the "root causes" of food insecurity and the current influence of food insecurity on the daily choices that individuals must make. In other words, these findings as a whole provide evidence that broad historical, political, and environmental factors are strong determinants on individual health behavior, such as dietary intake. Here, we present the findings of the groups' collective work: historical research including oral history, as well as a critical review of published literature, survey findings among community members, and qualitative findings based on in-depth interviews with key stakeholders.

HISTORICAL ROOTS OF FOOD INSECURITY IN NAVAJO NATION

According to Diné emergence stories, corn, squash, beans, and tobacco (a spiritual food) were gifts from the Diyin Diné'e (Holy People) at the time of emergence into this world, and these foods formed the backbone of the diet of the people. Diyin Diné'e also informed the Diné that everything that they needed to lead good lives and reach old age could be found within Diné Bikéyah and the boundaries of the four sacred mountains. Outside of the cultivated crops, this diet included wild animals such as elk, deer, antelope, prairie dogs, rabbits, and excluded fish, birds, bear, cougars, and coyotes, which were culturally restricted. Diné also relied on wild plants, including yucca fruit, sumac berries, wild spinach, Navajo tea, piñons, and wild onions. So extensive was the knowledge of wild plants that a preliminary attempt to document Diné ethnobotany found that Navajo informants were able to identify over 500 plants for food, beverage, medicine, and ceremonial usage (Kopp 1986). Other foods were obtained by Diné through trade with other tribes, including peaches, plums, and cherries from Hopi orchards.

With the arrival of the Spanish to the Americas in the late fifteenth century and to the Southwest in the sixteenth century, the Diné gained access to new food sources. Wheat was adopted into Diné agriculture, while coffee and sugar were obtained through trade. The Spanish also brought to the Americas horses, cattle, goats, and most notably, the Churro sheep, which would become synonymous with Navajo life and diet in the following centuries. The integration of livestock into the Diné life marked not only a significant dietary shift, but also major lifestyle and economic shifts, as Diné shifted from game as the primary meat source to domesticated animals through communally managed subsistence herds. While the Spanish, and later Mexican, influences to the Navajo diet are significant, it is important to note that Navajo people still actively managed their food system by continuing to produce their food during this time period.

Diné food sovereignty ceased with the next major shift in diet, which came with the arrival of the Americans into the Southwest some 200 years later.

In the 1800s, the United States carried out aggressive and violent Western expansion under the premise of Manifest Destiny, a belief that White Americans had a divinely sanctioned right to claim lands not only claimed by Mexico but also inhabited by Native peoples. This expansion gave way to the Mexican–American War, ended by the Treaty of Guadalupe Hidalgo in 1848. This treaty gave the United States legal claim to occupy what is now the southwestern United States, including the territories of the Diné. The presence of American military forces added to the existing tensions in the region among the Diné, neighboring tribes, and New Mexican settlers.

By the 1850s, the U.S. military declared war on the Diné, and instituted a series of aggressive campaigns including the deliberate use of "scorched earth" tactics (Frink 1968). The American military commander of New Mexico, General James H. Carlton, resolved to eradicate the Diné from their lands, with the express intent of opening Diné lands to American settlers and mining interests (Carleton 1863). General Carlton employed Kit Carson to carry out a campaign of terror and force the people to relocate to a "reservation," a concentration camp in eastern New Mexico. Carson oversaw the most aggressive and systematic attack on the Diné and their food system. Carson's scorched earth campaign included the slaughtering of livestock, burning of fields and orchards, and the destruction of water sources. The extensive peach orchards of Canyon de Chelly were a particular focus of this destruction. Under the command of Carson, Captain John Thompson cut and burned down over 4000 peach trees throughout the canyon, in addition to cornfields, during a week-long campaign in the late summer of 1864 (Jett 1977). An account by Diné informant, Howard W. Gorman, describes:

> Unexpectedly, *Bi'éé' Łichíí'í* ... (Red Clothes' [Kit Carson] Soldiers) arrived, destroying water wells – contaminating them, breaking the rocks edging the waterholes, or filling up the holes with dirt so that they became useless. They also burned cornfields and the orchards of peaches. That is what they did to us unexpectedly and unreasonably, because most of us were not harming anybody. In the open fields, we planted squash and corn. We lived peacefully, not expecting a conflict. We naturally were a peaceful people (Gorman 1973, pp. 23–24.).

This scorched earth policy effectively starved many Diné into surrender. Word reached those who had not been captured that food was being distributed at Fort Defiance. Many families chose to go to the fort to alleviate their hunger and discuss peace, unaware of Carlton's plans for relocation (Wheeler 1973). Upon arrival at the fort, the Diné found they could not return back to their homes and were captives of the U.S. military.

Beginning in the fall of 1863, Diné captives made the first of many forced marches to Fort Sumner, known as "The Long Walk" (Iverson 2002). The Long Walk and period of internment at Fort Sumner is called Hwéeldi (time and place of great suffering). Along the way, the people suffered from cold, starvation, slave raids, rape, and brutality from the soldiers. Numerous oral histories tell of pregnant women and elderly being shot because they were unable to keep up with the pace set by soldiers (Iverson 2002). Upon arriving to Fort Sumner, the people found that the site that Carlton had selected was inadequate to provide for the people. The soil was arid and high in alkali content, not suited to farming, and did not yield enough crops to sustain the nearly ten thousand Navajos now living there.

... the Diné tried to plant corn, but it was no use. It didn't grow. They were told to plant it in the way of the Bilagáana (White Men). But still it didn't grow. So they were given corn from somewhere else to survive on. (Gorman 1973, p. 35.)

Owing to failure of crops, restrictions on hunting, and the unavailability of familiar native plants, the Diné had to depend on the U.S. military to feed them, marking a major turning point in the history of Diné food. Food rations were inadequate and extremely poor in nutritional content, consisting primarily of salted pork cattle, flour, salt, sugar, coffee, and lard (Iverson 2002). Narratives of hunger and starvation are prominent in oral histories passed down to younger generations:

They were not used to the food that was offered to them as rations. You had white flour; beans, green coffee beans, rancid bacon... They got diarrhea and dysentery and died from the food as well. They also tell stories about how the food had just been destroyed and they would have to resort to having to eat coyote and crow to discover that they were just utterly inedible... And so this was a very, very traumatic time for my people, and we still haven't forgotten. It's still very much a part of our memories. (Denetdale)

Over 2000 people died while held in captivity at Fort Sumner, largely due to starvation. Fort Sumner was deemed a failure, and General Carlton was relieved of his command. While the U.S. government had planned to relocate the Diné people to a territory in Oklahoma, Barboncito—the Diné spokesperson elected to advocate on behalf of his people—successfully negotiated their return to a portion of their original homeland.

While successful in this respect, the Treaty of 1868 also established several policies that would have profound, long-term impacts on the Diné food system. First, the Federal Government committed to distributing food on the Navajos' return to their homeland, inaugurating the federal food assistance programs that would play a major role in dietary shifts among the Diné a century later. Second, the treaty gave the United States regulatory authority of agricultural land use within the newly established reservation through a certification to be administered by an Indian agent (1868). This process outlawed communal land use, disregarding the existing Diné views of agricultural land management, undermining the matrilineal tradition in Navajo society, and putting land disputes under the jurisdiction of the United States rather than families and communities.

Finally, the Treaty of 1868 also stipulated that the government would distribute livestock to the Diné upon their return in order to allow them to rebuild their herds (Henderson 1989). This support allowed the Diné economy to recover (Weisiger 2009), generating income for many households.

Diné women wove blankets for a commercial market, and families bartered wool, pelts, and blankets for goods at trading posts. (Weisiger 2009)

Recognizing that the Diné could contribute economically through sheep products, the Bureau of Indian Affairs encouraged the expansion of Navajo herds. Yet for Navajo people, sheep and livestock had greater significance than as means of wage income. Many Diné described their livestock as their mother. Sheep and livestock were their "means of subsistence, their years of labor invested in building herds, their legacy to their children," and very much interwoven into their culture (Weisiger 2009).

During this time, sheep became a dietary staple. Several nutrition surveys in the early 1900s provide a more detailed understanding of the Diné diet in that era. Other staples included mutton, goat, goat's milk, coffee, flour, corn, squash, beans, potatoes, canned vegetables (no doubt obtained from the trading posts that came onto Diné land after the reservation had been established), as well as continued consumption of wild plants and game meats (Carpenter and Steggerda 1939, Kopp 1986). The 1930s, however, saw another major disruption to Diné life, and thereby the Diné diet.

In the 1930s, numerous economic relief programs and agencies were created under the New Deal. In response to the drought across the Western states and concerns over another "dust bowl," the government enacted the Emergency Conservation Work Act, which authorized the Civilian Conservation Corps to focus on conservation efforts of federal lands, including Indian reservations (Weisiger 2009). The Bureau of Indian Affairs (BIA) ordered a series of Diné stock reductions from 1933 through 1945, with the goal of reducing the livestock herd size from an estimated 1.3 million to below 560,000 (Frink 1968). While New Dealers cited concerns that overgrazing from Diné livestock herds was contributing to the soil erosion, some historians have suggested that the underlying motive for the livestock reduction was less about land conservation and more about the very real fact that Diné herds clashed with American expansionism (Carpenter and Steggerda 1939). At first, reduction was voluntary but then became mandatory (Chamberlain 2000).

Implementing a reservation-wide stock reduction had harsh and traumatic results. Most agree that under the direction of BIA Commissioner John Collier, the livestock reduction was poorly conceived and implemented, and did not consider a replacement for the Diné economy that the livestock represented. In some areas, reduction was carried out more humanely and meat was shipped back to families, but in many instances, herds were slaughtered senselessly and inhumanely (Weisiger 2009). Many Diné families were horrified at witnessing the mass killing of their herds, livelihood, and source of nourishment and life. In the end, New Dealers reduced Diné livestock to well below the set out carrying capacity figure. Furthermore, livestock reduction had little effect on slowing soil erosion on Diné lands (Weisiger 2009).

The reduction crippled the Diné economy. Many families lost their means of providing for themselves, and as a result, became dependent on government food assistance (Kopp 1986). While federal food distribution programs had existed in one form or another since the establishment of the reservation in 1868, the 1950s saw the formal introduction of the Federal Food Distribution Program in Navajo Nation, also known as the "commodity food" program.

> The surplus commodity program was introduced on the [Diné] reservation in 1958 with four foods—flour, corn meal, rice, and dry milk. In 1965, the number of foods was increased from nine to 12 depending on whether the family lived in the New Mexico, Arizona, or Utah section of the reservation, and in 1971, when the Donated Food Program replaced the commodity program, 20 items were included. Additional foods included sugar, syrup, lard, peanut butter, dried beans, rolled wheat, and in some areas butter and cheese … canned products—fruits, juices, meat or chicken, and vegetables—and macaroni, cereals, and dehydrated products. (Kopp 1986)

Thus, the 1950s and 1960s marked a major shift in the diet of Diné people, moving away from their traditional diet (Darby et al. 1956), consuming fewer "home-produced" foods, such as beans, melons, and squash, and relying more on processed foods from trading posts (Darby et al. 1956). The growing reliance on commodity foods of low nutritional value contributed to a shift in nutritional status from adequate to poor. By the 1960s, nutritional deficiencies were documented among the Diné (Ballew et al. 1997).

A number of additional factors contributed to this dietary shift from traditional foods to a more Westernized diet. The enrollment of Diné children into boarding schools as well as relocation programs—placing Diné children with non-native foster families out of state—created a generation of children who were alienated from traditional diets. When school children and adults returned to their Diné homes, they brought new dietary preferences back with them, often along with rhetoric that valued Western over traditional Diné foods (Kopp 1986). The separation of Diné youth from their families and their inculcation with the values of the dominant culture had profound implications on the Diné's spiritual connection with food as well, as the younger generation lost the opportunity to receive the inter generational knowledge of Diné food practices, including how food was traditionally grown, prepared, and used for ceremonial purposes.

This period also saw the emergence of several other Federal supplemental food assistance programs. In the 1960s, the federal government created the Women, Infants and Children program (WIC) and re-enacted the Food Stamp program (Haering and Syed 2009), the latter of which reached the Navajo reservation in 1977 (Van Duzen et al. 1976). Finally, the uptake of Western foods was escalated by the emergence of grocery stores within the reservation in the late 1960s and 1970s.

By the 1980s, soda and sweetened drinks, store-bought bread, and milk were growing components of the Diné diet. At the same time, fry bread and tortillas, potatoes, mutton, and coffee continued as staples (Wolfe and Sanjur 1988). Although many Navajo families still farmed (with corn, squash, and melon reported as the most cultivated crops), gardens were generally small and "no longer appeared to be a major source of food for many families" (Wolfe and Sanjur 1988, p. 824). While corn was still commonly consumed, blue corn mush being the most popular, nutritional studies of this era noted that the use of traditional foods had declined substantially while the consumption of store-bought, nutritionally inferior foods was increasing; according to one study, "many of the traditional foods were rarely if ever consumed" (Wolfe et al. 1985, p. 343). This transition away from sheepherding and agriculture as primary food sources further reinforced the Diné dietary shift from lean meats, corn, and homegrown fruits and vegetables to increasingly processed meats, sugar sweetened beverages, and fried potato dishes (Darby et al. 1956).

The lesson that emerges from this critical historical review is that the dietary changes in the Diné population did not occur by chance, but were fostered by a series of foreign interventions and food policies imposed by the U.S. government; namely forced removal, repeated destruction of food sources, boarding schools, relocation, and food distribution programs. Aside from the profound health implications of this dietary shift, the value shift that accompanied the uptake of Western foods had a disruptive impact on traditional teachings and practices associated with food in the Diné culture. So profound is this disconnect that many Diné consider fry bread and sheep to be "Native" traditional foods, despite the fact that these foods were introduced through European and American contact and mainstreamed into Diné culture by the same American policies that instituted reservation life. This historical trajectory is perpetuated in the current relationship between Navajo Nation and the U.S. government, and is very much embodied in the current situation of food insecurity in Navajo Nation.

STATE OF THE NAVAJO FOOD SYSTEM, DIET, AND NUTRITION TODAY

Currently, 56% of the Navajo Nation lives below the federal poverty level (Phase II Housing Needs Assessment and Demographic Analysis 2011), and the USDA classifies the Navajo Nation as a "food desert" (USDA). Along with the vast geography and limited infrastructure (with 78% of public roads still unpaved), low incomes and a low population density discourage retail food sources on the reservation (Smith and Morton 2009). The few stores that sell food—such as trading posts, convenience stores, and gas stations—typically sell processed foods with virtually no options for fresh produce or meats, all at higher costs compared with larger, off-reservation grocery stores.

Faced with limited access to local food sources, most families are forced to travel off the reservation to purchase their food and rely on food assistance programs. Over 80% of Diné get their groceries off the reservation (Lu et al. 2008, Navajo Nation Division of Economic Development 2012), diverting money away from the tribe. Our survey findings from the Crownpoint Service Unit demonstrate that most community members in that region shop two to three times a month, and a small proportion of individuals (3%) shop less than once a month. Half of respondents travel more than 1 hour to get to nearest grocery store. Food purchasing decisions were most heavily influenced by price (81%) and availability (62%), while family preferences (55%) and health and nutritional needs (31%) also figured into purchasing choices. Of note, 21% felt that they had no choice at all in what they ate.

In the 2012 Crownpoint survey (Figure 8.2), while the vast majority of families (94%) shopped at a grocery store, only 11% relied on stores as their sole food

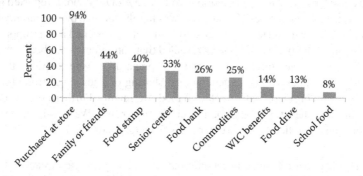

FIGURE 8.2   Sources of food within the past month, N = 253.

source. Most households (60%) obtained food from at least three sources in the past month, most commonly from family and friends (44%), food stamps (40%), senior centers (33%), food pantries or food banks (26%), and the commodities program (25%). Because qualifying individuals must choose to receive either commodity foods or Food Stamps but not both (Landers 2007), many Diné households factor a number of considerations into which program they choose to utilize. For instance, the Food Stamp Program allows consumers to pick which foods they want, but requires access to transportation and resources to get to the stores that accept Food Stamps. Food Stamps can also be bartered for gas and cash (Gittelsohn et al. 2009). On the other hand, households that receive commodity foods typically report that they sacrifice choice for larger quantities of food. Commodities are distributed monthly, often at local chapter houses (community centers). While this facilitates food access, monthly distribution also poses a challenge for many families without refrigeration who cannot store food for the entire month. The Navajo Food Distribution Program has responded to consumer demand to distribute healthier foods (such as frozen meat rather than processed meat, and vegetable fats instead of lard); nonetheless, the program is also mindful of the constraints of many households lacking electricity and refrigeration; thus, the mainstay of commodity foods is selected for long shelf-life.

In addition to limited retail sources, food production in Navajo Nation has also declined (Adams and Ruffing 1977). Farming is increasingly difficult due to low yields and high costs, mostly related to irrigation, although many who do continue to farm are motivated by a responsibility to preserve Diné culture and tradition, particularly dry-land farming techniques. The few farms in operation have been in families for decades (Setala et al. 2011) but have grown smaller as help is harder to find, in part because children move away from the reservation in search of work opportunities (Setala et al. 2012). While many farmers continue to grow traditional crops, such as corn and squash, they are often unable to sell them due to varying crop yields, low selling prices, and difficulty in transporting crops (Setala et al. 2011). Successful sellers tend to have more resources and support. Another barrier to selling, however, is that it is not a traditional practice: farms were historically maintained to feed the family, rather than for commercial purposes.

In Crownpoint, CHR surveys and interviews revealed that agriculture was declining but still considered vital to Diné traditions. While 23% of households reported growing fruits or vegetables in the past 5 years, this was highly variable by community (Figure 8.3). Lack of water (or distance and cost to haul water) was cited as an important barrier to farming. Qualitative interviews revealed that community members strongly felt that traditions in agriculture, herding, and food preparation were central to their communities' cultural survival. Intergenerational sharing of knowledge around food and agriculture was considered vital to Navajo food sovereignty. Furthermore, respondents were aware that their traditional foods were healthier than Western-influenced diets. These insights are reflected in several quotes from respondents:

> The people of our tribe used to eat only vegetables and meat before commodity and food stamps and it seemed like there were no diabetics then and people lived longer
> Community member.

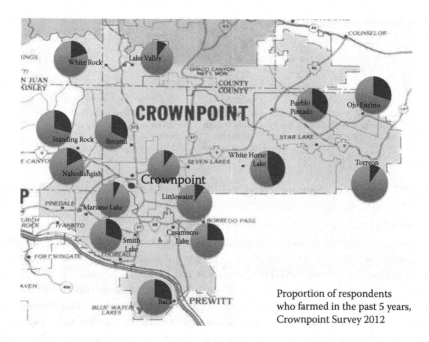

Proportion of respondents who farmed in the past 5 years, Crownpoint Survey 2012

FIGURE 8.3 Farming in the past 5 years by chapters (communities), N = 253.

Learn how to cook and keep the tradition alive by teaching them what our elders consumed and just make it an important part of our teaching for our young adults Community member.

Respect your traditions your elders and the food their parents set out for them. Some children are not that fortunate Community member.

These complex challenges have resulted in pervasive food insecurity characterized by a lack of nutritionally adequate foods and excess intake of high-calorie, low-nutritional foods. The Navajo Health and Nutrition Survey conducted in early 1990s found minimal consumption of traditional foods, such as blue corn mush, squash, and melons. Fruits and vegetables were reportedly consumed less than once per day (Ballew et al. 1997), markedly lower than average consumption in the United States (Setala et al. 2012). While mutton is still consumed, it no longer serves as a major source of daily caloric intake. Instead, the primary sources of calories are fried potatoes, fry bread and tortillas, sugary drinks, and processed meats (Sharma et al. 2010). In Crownpoint, two-thirds of surveyed households felt that healthy foods were unaffordable; not surprisingly, 60% felt they did not get enough fresh fruits and vegetables for their household. Among those who felt that healthy food was unaffordable, food insecurity was common (Figure 8.4): 61% of households shopped for the least expensive food, 58% limited meal sizes, and 28% skipped meals due to lack of money.

It is not surprising that the health trends in Navajo Nation parallel these dietary changes. The first case of diabetes in Navajo Nation was documented in the 1930s

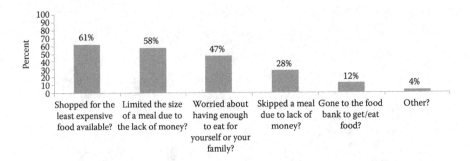

FIGURE 8.4 Food insecurity among those reporting healthy food to be unaffordable, N = 153.

(Sugarman et al. 1990). In fact, diabetes and heart disease were relatively uncommon until the 1960s when rates of obesity-driven disease began to soar (Sugarman et al. 1990). The Navajo EARTH (Education and Research Towards Health) Study conducted from 2004 to 2007 found that only 17% of adults have a BMI that is considered normal. One-third of participants were overweight and one-half were obese (Slattery et al. 2010). The rate of obesity among Diné children is also high: data from 1997 indicate that the prevalence of overweight and obesity in Navajo children aged 6–12 years old was 41% (Eisenmann et al. 2000). Health consequences of poor diet are high; recent data indicates a high rate of diabetes in Navajo youth aged 15–19 at 2.78 per 1000 (Dabelea et al. 2009). Although more recent published data are absent, in 1997, 23% of Diné aged 20 and older, and 40% aged 45 and older were confirmed to have diabetes based on oral glucose tolerance testing (Will et al. 1997), and a community-based survey in 1991–1992 revealed hypertension in 19% of adults (Percy et al. 1997). Among Diné, heart disease is the second leading cause of death after unintentional injuries (Leavitt et al. 2003).

TOWARD COMMUNITY SOLUTIONS

CBPR is based on the premise that community members themselves are best poised to narrate their own history, describe the issues that most impact their well-being, and identify the best solutions to meet their needs. In Navajo Nation, many community members are exquisitely aware of how often their culture, history, and health have been described by others. The Diné people are also critical to external solutions that may address food insecurity, but in a way that fails to promote food sovereignty and community development.

When presented with a "picture menu" of interventions that could improve access to healthy foods (Figure 8.5), community members in Crownpoint strongly endorsed making fresh produce available at chapter houses (78%), a mobile grocery truck (53%), and reduced prices for healthy foods at places where they usually shopped (47%). While local farming and livestock was endorsed by only 22% of community members in the survey, qualitative interviews highlighted the importance of passing on Navajo traditions to youth through farming and other food activities:

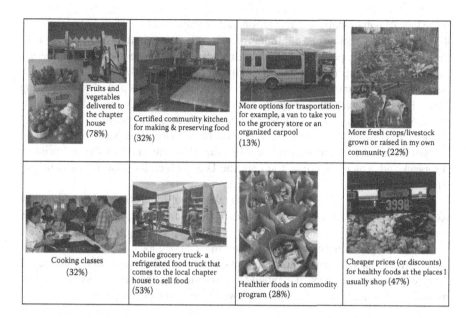

FIGURE 8.5 Community preferences for food access strategies (% endorsed), N = 253.

Summer students… [could be hired] at the local chapters to learn healthy cooking and to learn how to plant. These are not offered during the summer. It's all part of learning Community member.

Teach our youth about traditional food and culture … And clans-wise it is very important for our youth [to know] where they are coming from and know their relatives Community member.

Other investigators have identified growing interest among Diné farmers to engage in programs, such as Farm to Table that could connect producers to local retail venues and schools (Setala et al. 2012).

This input is consistent with the survey findings that suggest that food insecurity is driven by lack of access to food sources within these remote rural communities, as well as the higher cost of buying fruits and vegetables, particularly when factoring in the cost of travel. Although community members recognized that revitalizing agricultural traditions was fundamental to maintaining Diné food traditions, local production was not consistently viewed as a sole solution to overcome the lack of access to healthy food, perhaps due to the constraints of limited water and seasonal availability.

CONCLUSION

At the global level, many communities struggle with food insecurity in terms of hunger and malnutrition. In settings characterized by lower rates of absolute poverty but steep gradients of inequality, the challenge of food insecurity may be characterized by the lack of nutritionally adequate food, rather than food as a whole. These aspects of food insecurity represent a continuum, as "developing countries" that have transitioned from absolute poverty to growing prosperity have witnessed a rise in obesity, particularly affecting poor women (Tanumihardjo et al. 2007, Wells et al. 2012). Even in wealthy countries such as the United States, obesity is a marker of growing health disparities, perhaps most poignantly illustrated by American Indian communities. As illustrated in this chapter, the current Diné food system is the result of U.S. policies toward American Indians, particularly within the past century. These changes have led to a nutritionally inferior diet than the one that existed prior to European and American contact among the Diné, which has also resulted in epidemic levels of nutrition-related illnesses.

As with any community, however marginalized, collective knowledge and agency exist. To understand and address food insecurity, a deep understanding of the issues from the perspective of community members is critical to adopting solutions that address the priorities of the community itself. Partnerships among local and external organizers, experts, and nongovernmental organizations, along with infusion of resources, can catalyze the momentum needed to rebuild a food system that addresses widespread food insecurity, while maintaining indigenous sovereignty and food traditions.

ACKNOWLEDGMENTS

The authors would like to acknowledge the entire team of Crownpoint Service Unit Community Health Representative Program who carried out this work, as well as those who participated in community surveys. Research carried out by the Diné Policy Institute was funded by the First Nations Institute.

REFERENCES

1868. Treaty between the United States of America and the Navajo Tribe of Indians.
2011. Phase II Housing Needs Assessment and Demographic Analysis. Accessed September 18, 2013. http://hooghan.org/index.php?option=com_banners&task=click&bid=11.
Adams, W.Y. and L.T. Ruffing. 1977. Shonto revisited: Measures of social and economic change in Navajo community, 1955–1971. *American Anthropologist* 79 (1):58–83.
Ballew, C., L.L. White, K.F. Strauss, L.J. Benson, J.M. Mendlein, and A. Mokdad. 1997. Intake of nutrients and food sources of nutrients among the Navajo: Findings from the Navajo Health and Nutrition Survey. *Journal of Nutrition* 127:2085S–2093S.
Bell-Sheeter, A. 2004. *Food Sovereignty Assessment Tool.* Fredericksburg, VA: First Nations Development Institute. 2004. http://www.indigenousfoodsystems.org/sites/default/files/tools/FNDIFSATFinal.pdf
Bronfenbrenner, U. 1979. *The Ecology of Human Development: Experiments by Nature and Design.* Cambridge: Harvard University Press.
Carleton, J.H. 1863. Letter to Major General Harry Halleck. In *Select Navajo Historical Occurrences, 1850–1923,* edited by R.A. Roussel, Jr. Tsaile, AZ: Navajo Community College Press.
Carpenter, T.M. and M. Steggerda. 1939. The food of the present-day Navajo Indians of New Mexico and Arizona. *Journal of Nutrition* 18 (3):297–305.
Chamberlain, K.P. 2000. *Under Sacred Ground: A History of Navajo Oil, 1922–1982.* Albuquerque: University of New Mexico Press.

Cohen, B., M. Andrews, and L.S. Kantor. 2002. Community Food Security Assessment Toolkit. *Economic Research Service*. Report no. (EFAN-02-013), and 166pp. Accessed September 10, 2014. http://www.ers.usda.gov/media/327699/efan02013_1_.pdf.

Coleman-Jenson, A., M. Nord, and A. Singh. 2013. Household Food Security in the United States in 2012. [Economic Research Report No. (ERR-155) 41] http://www.ers.usda.gov/publications/err-economic-research-report/err155.aspx#.UjnnXeCc9UQ.

Coles, C.L., D. Fraser, N. Givon-Lavi, D. Greenberg, R. Gorodischer, J. Bar-Ziv, and R. Dagan. 2005. Nutritional status and diarrheal illness as independent risk factors for alveolar pneumonia. *American Journal of Epidemiology* 162 (10):999–1007. doi: 10.1093/aje/kwi312.

Cook, J.T., M. Black, M. Chilton, D. Cutts, S. Ettinger de Cuba, T.C. Heeren, and D.A. Frank. 2013. Are food insecurity's health impacts underestimated in the U.S. population? Marginal food security also predicts adverse health outcomes in young U.S. children and mothers. *Advances in Nutrition* 4 (1):51–61. doi: 10.3945/an.112.003228.

Cook, J.T., D.A. Frank, S.M. Levenson, N.B. Neault, T.C. Heeren, M.M. Black, and M. Chilton. 2006. Child food insecurity increases risks posed by household food insecurity to young children's health. *Journal of Nutrition* 136 (4):1073–6.

Dabelea, D., J. DeGroat, C. Sorrelman, M. Glass, C.A. Percy, C. Avery, and R.F. Hamman. 2009. Diabetes in Navajo Youth: Prevalence, incidence, and clinical characteristics: The SEARCH for diabetes in youth study. *Diabetes Care* 32 (Suppl 2):S141–7. doi: 10.2337/dc09-S206.

Darby, W.J., W.J. McGanity, and E.B. Bridgforth. 1956. A study of the dietary background and nutriture of the Navajo Indian: V. Interpretation. *Journal of Nutrition* 60 (2S):75–79.

Darby, W.J., C.G. Salsbury, W.J. McGanity, H.F. Johnson, E.B. Bridgforth, and H.R. Sandstead. 1956. A study of the dietary background and nutriture of the Navajo Indian: I. Background and food production. *Journal of Nutrition* 60 (S2):3–18.

Denetdale, J.N. Interview. Accessed August 29, 2013. http://www.kued.org/productions/thelongwalk/film/interviews/jenniferNezDenetdale.php.

Drewnowski, A. and S.E. Specter. 2004. Poverty and obesity: The role of energy density and energy costs. *American Journal of Clinical Nutrition* 79 (1):6–16.

Economic Research Service, 2012. US Adult Food Security Survey Module: Three-Stage Design, with Screeners. Economic Research Service, USDA http://www.ers.usda.gov/topics/food-nutrition-assistance/food-security-in-the-us/survey-tools.aspx#adult.

Eisenmann, J.C., P.T. Katzmarzyk, D.A. Arnall, V. Kanuho, C. Interpreter, and R.M. Malina. 2000. Growth and overweight of Navajo youth: Secular changes from 1955 to 1997. *International Journal of Obesity and Related Metabolic Disorders* 24 (2):211–8.

Frink, M. 1968. *Fort Defiance & The Navajos*. Boulder, CO: Pruett Press.

Gittelsohn, J. M. Qi, M. Pardilla, and S. Suratkar. 2009. *Understanding the Impact of Food Assistance Program Usage on Diet among American Indians*. Johns Hopkins School of Public Health. http://www.nptao.arizona.edu/RIDGE_UPDATE/Johns%20Hopkins%20Year%202%202%20Report.pdf

Gorman, H. 1973. *Navajo Stories of the Long Walk Period*, edited by R. Roessel and B. Johnson. Tsaile, AZ: Navajo Community College, 23–24.

Gunderson, C., B. Krieider, and J. Pepper. 2011. The economics of food insecurity in the United States. *Applied Economics Perspectives and Policy* 33 (3):281–303.

Haering, S.A. and S.B. Syed. 2009. *Community Food Security in United States Cities: A Survey of the Relevant Scientific Literature*. Johns Hopkins School of Public Health. http://www.jhsph.edu/research/centers-and-institutes/johns-hopkins-center-for-a-livable-future/research/clf_publications/pub_rep_desc/CFS_USA.html.

Henderson, E. 1989. Navajo livestock wealth and the effects of the Stock Reduction Program of the 1930s. *Journal of Anthro Research* 45 (4):379–403.

Huddleston-Casas, C., R. Charnigo, and L.A. Simmons. 2009. Food insecurity and maternal depression in rural, low-income families: A longitudinal investigation. *Public Health Nutrition* 12 (8):1133–40. doi: 10.1017/S1368980008003650.

Israel, B.A., A.J. Schulz, E.A. Parker, and A.B. Becker. 1998. Review of community-based research: Assessing partnership approaches to improve public health. *Annual Reviews in Public Health* 19:173–202. doi: 10.1146/annurev.publhealth.19.1.173.

Iverson, P. 2002. *Dine: A History of the Navajos.* Albuquerque, NM: University of New Mexico Press.

Jernigan, V.B., A.L. Salvatore, D.M. Styne, and M. Winkleby. 2012. Addressing food insecurity in a native American reservation using community-based participatory research. *Health Education Research* 27 (4):645–55. doi: 10.1093/her/cyr089.

Jett, S.C. 1977. History of fruit tree raising among the Navajo. *Agricultural History* 51 (4):681–701.

Kopp, J. 1986. Crosscultural contacts: Changes in the diet and nutrition of the Navajo Indians. *American Indian Culture Research Journal* 10 (4):1–30.

Landers, P.S. 2007. The Food Stamp Program: History, nutrition education, and impact. *American Diet Association* 107:1945–1951.

Leavitt, M.O., R.G. McSwain, R.M. Church, and E.L. Paisano. 2003. Regional differences in Indian Health: 2002–2003 edition. Indian Health Services, U.S. Department of Health and Human Services. Accessed September 10, 2014. http://www.ihs.gov/dps/files/RD_entirebook.pdf.

Lu, Z., J. Fassett, X. Xu, X. Hu, G. Zhu, J. French, and Y. Chen. 2008. Adenosine A3 receptor deficiency exerts unanticipated protective effects on the pressure-overloaded left ventricle. *Circulation* 118 (17):1713–21. doi: 10.1161/CIRCULATIONAHA.108.788307.

Minkler, M., A. Garcia, V. Rubin, and N. Wallerstein. 2012. *Community-Based Participatory Research: A Strategy for Building Healthy Communities and Promoting Health through Policy Change: A Report to the California Endowment.*

Navajo Nation Division of Economic Development. 2012. *Navajo Economic Data Bulletin* 001-0212. Accessed September 10, 2014. http://navajobusiness.com/pdf/Ads/NavEconomicDataBulletinFinal_030212.pdf.

Pan, L., B. Sherry, R. Njai, and H.M. Blanck. 2012. Food insecurity is associated with obesity among US adults in 12 states. *Journal of the Academy of Nutrition and Dietetics* 112 (9):1403–9. doi: 10.1016/j.jand.2012.06.011.

Percy, C., D.S. Freedman, T.J. Gilbert, L. White, C. Ballew, and A. Mokdad. 1997. Prevalence of hypertension among Navajo Indians: Findings from the Navajo Health and Nutrition Survey. *Journal of Nutrition* 127 (10 Suppl):2114S–2119S.

Seligman, H.K., A.B. Bindman, E. Vittinghoff, A.M. Kanaya, and M.B. Kushel. 2007. Food insecurity is associated with diabetes mellitus: Results from the National Health Examination and Nutrition Examination Survey (NHANES) 1999–2002. *Journal of General Internal Medicine* 22 (7):1018–23. doi: 10.1007/s11606-007-0192-6.

Seligman, H.K., B.A. Laraia, and M.B. Kushel. 2010. Food insecurity is associated with chronic disease among low-income NHANES participants. *Journal of Nutrition* 140 (2):304–10. doi: 10.3945/jn.109.112573.

Setala, A., S.N. Bleich, K. Speakman, J. Oski, T. Martin, R. Moore, and J. Gittelsohn. 2012. The potential of local farming on the Navajo Nation to improve fruit and vegetable intake: Barriers and opportunities. *Ecology of Food and Nutrition* 50 (5):393–409.

Setala, A., J. Gittelsohn, K. Speakman, J. Oski, T. Martin, R. Moore, and S.N. Bleich. 2011. Linking farmers to community stores to increase consumption of local produce: A case study of the Navajo Nation. *Public Health Nutrition* 14 (9):1658–1662.

Sharma, S., M. Yacavone, X. Cao, M. Pardilla, M. Qi, and J. Gittelsohn. 2010. Dietary intake and development of a quantitative FFQ for a nutritional intervention to reduce the risk of chronic disease in the Navajo Nation. *Public Health Nutrition* 13 (3):350–9. doi: 10.1017/S1368980009005266.

Slattery, M.L., E.D. Ferucci, M.A. Murtaugh, S. Edwards, K.N. Ma, R.A. Etzel, and A.P. Lanier. 2010. Associations among body mass index, waist circumference, and health indicators in American Indian and Alaska Native Adults. *American Journal of Health Promotion* 24 (4):246–54. doi: 10.4278/ajhp.080528-QUAN-72.

Smith, C. and L.W. Morton. 2009. Rural food deserts: Low-income perspectives on food access in Minnesota and Iowa. *Journal of Nutrition Education and Behavior* 41 (3):176–187.

Stokols, D. 1996. Translating social ecological theory into guidelines for community health promotion. *American Journal of Health Promotion* 10 (4):282–98.

Sugarman, J.R., M. Hickey, T. Hall, and D. Gohdes. 1990. The changing epidemiology of diabetes mellitus among Navajo Indians. *Western Journal of Medicine* 153 (2):140–5.

Tanumihardjo, S.A., C. Anderson, M. Kaufer-Horwitz, L. Bode, N.J. Emenaker, A.M. Haqq, and D.D. Stadler. 2007. Poverty, obesity, and malnutrition: An international perspective recognizing the paradox. *Journal of the American Dietetic Association* 107 (11):1966–72. doi: 10.1016/j.jada.2007.08.007.

United States Department of Agriculture 2014. "Food Desert Locator." http://www.ers.usda. gov/data-products/food-access-research-atlas/go-to-the-atlas.aspx. Accessed December 15, 2014.

Van Duzen, J., J.P. Carter, and R.Vander Zwagg. 1976. Protein and calorie malnutrition among preschool Navajo Indian children, a follow-up. *American Journal of Clinical Nutrition* 97 (1):657–662.

Vasquez, V.B., D. Lanza, S. Hennessey-Lavery, S. Facente, H.A. Halpin, and M. Minkler. 2007. Addressing food security through public policy action in a community-based participatory research partnership. *Health Promotion Practice* 8 (4):342–9. doi: 10.1177/1524839906298501.

Weisiger, M. 2009. *Dreaming of Sheep in Navajo Country*. Seattle, WA: University of Washington Press.

Wells, J.C., A.A. Marphatia, T.J. Cole, and D. McCoy. 2012. Associations of economic and gender inequality with global obesity prevalence: Understanding the female excess. *Social Science & Medicine* 75 (3):482–90. doi: 10.1016/j.socscimed.2012.03.029.

Wheeler, R. 1973. *Navajo Stories of the Long Walk Period*, edited by R. Roessel and B. Johnson. Tsaile, AZ: Navajo Community College Press, 82.

Will, J.C., K.F. Strauss, J.M. Mendlein, C. Ballew, L.L. White, and D.G. Peter. 1997. Diabetes mellitus among Navajo Indians: Findings from the Navajo Health and Nutrition Survey. *Journal of Nutrition* 127 (10 Suppl):2106S–2113S.

Wilson, N., M. Minkler, S. Dasho, N. Wallerstein, and A.C. Martin. 2008. Getting to social action: The Youth Empowerment Strategies (YES!) Project. *Health Promotion and Practice* 9 (4):395–403. doi: 10.1177/1524839906289072.

Wolfe, W.S. and D. Sanjur. 1988. Contemporary diet and body weight of Navajo women receiving food assistance: An ethnographic and nutritional investigation. *Journal of the American Dietetic Association* 88 (7):822–7.

Wolfe, W.S., C.W. Weber, and K.D. Arviso. 1985. Use and nutrient composition of traditional Navajo foods. *Ecology of Food and Nutrition* 17 (4):323–244.

9 Overview of the Cost of Hunger in Africa— Executive Summary

Social and Economic Impact of Child Undernutrition in Egypt, Ethiopia, Swaziland, and Uganda[*]

UN Economic Commission for Africa; New Partnership of Africa's Development Planning and Coordinating Agency (NEPAD); Regional Integration Division (NRID)

CONTENTS

---

[*] This executive summary was first published in the report, "The Cost of Hunger in Africa: Social and Economic Impact of Child Undernutrition in Egypt, Ethiopia, Swaziland, and Uganda," and is reproduced with permission (African Union Commission, NEPAD Planning and Coordinating Agency, UN Economic Commission for Africa, and UN World Food Programme. The Cost of Hunger in Africa: Social and Economic Impact of Child Undernutrition in Egypt, Ethiopia, Swaziland and Uganda. Report. Addis Ababa: UNECA, 2014).

INTRODUCTION

The Cost of Hunger in Africa (COHA) Study is a project led by the African Union Commission (AUC) and the New Partnership of Africa's Development (NEPAD) Planning and Coordinating Agency, and supported by the UN Economic Commission for Africa (ECA) and the UN World Food Programme (WFP). COHA is a multi-country study aimed at estimating the economic and social impacts of child undernutrition in Africa (Table 9.1).

TABLE 9.1

Effects of Child Undernourishment through Life

0–5 years	Undernourished children are at higher risk of anemia, diarrhea, fever, and respiratory infections. These additional cases of illness are costly to the health system and to families. Undernourished children are at a higher risk of dying.
6–18 years	Stunted children are at a higher risk of repeating grades in school and dropping out of school. Grade repetitions are costly to the education system and to families.
15–64 years	If a child has dropped out of school early and has entered the workforce, he or she may be less productive, particularly in the non manual labor market. If engaged in manual labor, he or she is likely to have reduced physical capacity and will tend to be less productive. People who are absent from the workforce as a result of undernutrition-related child mortality represent lost economic productivity.

This continent-wide initiative is being led by the Department of Social Affairs, AUC, within the framework of the Revised African Regional Nutrition Strategy (2005–2015), the objectives of the African Task Force on Food and Nutrition Development (ATFFND), and the principles of the AU/NEPAD's Comprehensive Africa Agriculture Development Programme (CAADP) Pillar 3.

In March 2012, the COHA study was presented to African Ministers of Finance, Planning, and Economic Development, who met in Addis Ababa, Ethiopia. The ministers issued Resolution 898, confirming the importance of the study, and recommending that it continue beyond the initial stage.

The core implementers of the study are national teams organized in each participating country, drawn from relevant governmental institutions, such as the Ministry of Health, Ministry of Education, Ministry of Social Development, Ministry of Planning, Ministry of Finance, and the National Statistics Institution.

The COHA study is a watershed initiative that highlights a new understanding by African governments of child undernutrition as not only a health or social issue, but also as an economic issue. The initiative also highlights the African Union's strong leadership in addressing development issues, as well as the collaboration among governments and agencies within the continent.

The COHA study is being carried out in 12 countries, namely Botswana, Burkina Faso, Cameroon, Egypt, Ethiopia, Ghana, Kenya, Malawi, Mauritania, Rwanda, Swaziland, and Uganda. The data in this document are the results collected from the COHA initiative in the four first-phase countries: Egypt, Ethiopia, Swaziland, and Uganda.

BACKGROUND

Africa has experienced a recent period of economic growth that has positioned the continent as a key area for global investment and trade. The pace of real gross domestic product (GDP) growth on the continent has doubled in the last decade, and six of the world's fastest growing economies are in Africa. All of this has occurred despite some of the highest rates of child undernutrition in the world.

The vast and rising numbers of food-insecure and undernourished people continue to pose very serious concerns in Africa. Over the past 2 years, global food price increases, followed by economic and financial crises, have pushed more people into poverty and hunger. Globally, as many as 868 million people are affected by food insecurity, with Africa contributing to nearly one-third of the world's hungry people (Food and Agriculture Organization 2012).

Child undernutrition is one of the most critical negative effects of hunger. When a child is undernourished before the age of 5, his or her body and brain cannot develop at its potential, and they are at risk of cognitive delays. Seventeen countries on the continent have stunting rates above 40%, and 36 countries have rates above 30% (United Nations Children's Fund, World Health Organization, and The World Bank 2012).

COHA also provides a useful opportunity to compare the nutritional situations of several countries across the continent. The countries were selected based on availability of data, geographic distribution, and socio economic diversity. These differences allow stakeholders to consider the contextual factors that impact the economic burden of child undernutrition.

BRIEF DESCRIPTION OF THE METHODOLOGY

COHA is based on a model originally developed in Latin America by the Economic Commission for Latin America and the Caribbean (ECLAC). With support from ECLAC and the African Task Force for Food and Nutrition Security, the model has been adapted for use on the African continent. The COHA model is used to estimate the additional cases of morbidities, mortalities, school repetitions, school dropouts, and reduced physical capacity that can be directly associated to a person's undernutrition before the age of 5.

To estimate social impacts for a single year, the model focuses on the current population, identifies the proportion of that population that were undernourished before the age of 5, and then estimates the associated negative impacts experienced by the population in the current year. Estimates on health, education, and productivity are based on the concept of the relative (or differential) risk experienced by individuals who suffer from undernutrition.

Using these risk factors, alongside economic, demographic, nutritional, health, and educational data provided by each country team, the model then estimates the associated economic losses incurred by the economy in health, education, and potential productivity in a single year.

With the support of experts and representatives from the National Implementation Teams (NITs) of the participating countries, a conceptual framework was adapted to the context of Africa. This framework establishes clear linkages between the direct consequences of undernutrition, taking into account the particular structures of the labor market on the continent, as well as the limitations in available data. The result allows the model to clearly define boundaries in the cost analysis, both from public and individual perspectives, as well as to define a clear differentiation between direct costs and opportunity costs in the results.

The COHA model utilizes a two-dimensional analysis to estimate the costs arising from the consequences of child undernutrition in health, education, and productivity. The incidental retrospective dimension analyzes the history of child undernutrition in the country in order to estimate the current economic and social consequences. To complement this analysis, a prospective dimension is used to project and generate scenarios for analysis.

SOCIAL AND ECONOMIC IMPACT OF CHILD UNDERNUTRITION IN FOUR COUNTRIES

According to the initial results generated by the COHA study, the equivalent losses shown in Table 9.2 are incurred by each studied country annually as a result of child undernutrition. These losses summarize costs to health, education, and productivity, as discussed in more detail below.

TABLE 9.2

Summary of Costs of Child Undernutrition

Country	Losses in Local Currency	Losses in USD	Equivalent% of GDP
Egypt	EGP20.3 billion	3.7 billion	1.9
Ethiopia	ETB55.5 billion	4.7 billion	16.5
Swaziland	SZL783 million	92 million	3.1
Uganda	UGX1.8 trillion	899 million	5.6

Source: COHA Study.

SOCIAL AND ECONOMIC IMPACT OF CHILD UNDERNUTRITION ON HEALTH

When a child is undernourished, he or she will have an increased chance of experiencing specific health problems (DHS). Research shows that undernourished children under 5 are more likely to experience cases of anemia, acute diarrheal syndrome (ADS), acute respiratory infection (ARI), and fever. The treatment of undernutrition and related illnesses is a critical, recurrent cost for the health system. For example, treating a severely underweight child requires a comprehensive protocol that is often more costly than the monetary value and effort needed to prevent undernutrition, especially when other diseases are present in parallel. Table 9.3 summarizes the total costs incurred by each country as a result of additional morbidities.

Research shows that undernourished children under 5 have an increased risk of dying (Rice et al. 2000). In this case, the costs associated with mortality are identified in losses to national productivity. If these children were able to reach adulthood, they could have contributed to the economy. Table 9.4 highlights the number of children who died from causes associated with undernutrition and the percent of child mortalities that can be attributed to undernutrition.

TABLE 9.3

Economic Impact of Child Undernutrition on Health

Country	Underweight Children	Annual Additional Morbidity Episodes	Economic Cost National Currency	Economic Cost USD (millions)	Proportion Covered by the Families
Egypt	658,516	901,440	EGP1.1 billion	213	73
Ethiopia	3.0 million	4.4 million	ETB1.8 billion	155	90
Swaziland	9645	25,446	SZL60.7 million	7	88
Uganda	975,450	1.6 million	UGX525.8 billion	254	87

Source: COHA Study.

TABLE 9.4
Child Mortalities Associated with Undernutrition

	Number of Mortalities Associated with Undernutrition (last 5 years)	% Total Child Mortalities Associated with Undernutrition
Egypt	28,102	11
Ethiopia	378,591	28
Swaziland	1351	8
Uganda	110,220	15

Source: COHA Study.

SOCIAL AND ECONOMIC IMPACT OF CHILD UNDERNUTRITION IN EDUCATION

IMPACT OF UNDERNUTRITION ON REPETITION

There is no single cause for students to repeat grades and dropout of school; however, there is substantive research that shows that students who were stunted before the age of 5 will have reduced cognitive capacity and are more likely to underperform in school and to repeat grades (Daniels and Adair 2004). Figure 9.1 illustrates the repetition rates for stunted children as compared to non stunted children in each of the countries.

Repetitions are costly, both to the family of the student and to the education system, as both need to invest resources for an additional year of schooling. Table 9.5 highlights the economic costs of additional repetitions associated with students' childhood undernutrition. A more detailed analysis shows that the cost of a repetition in secondary school is significantly higher than in primary school; however, the majority of repetitions occur during primary school years.

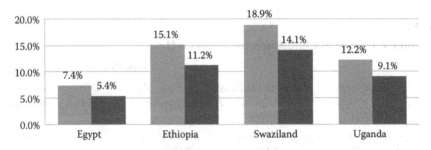

FIGURE 9.1   Repetition rates by nutritional status.

TABLE 9.5

Economic Costs of Grade Repetitions Associated with Child Undernutrition

Country	Number of Stunted Children of School Age	% of Repetitions Associated with Stunting	Economic Cost Local Currency	Economic Cost USD	Proportion Covered by the Education System (%)
Egypt	7.9 million	10	EGP271 million	49 million	61
Ethiopia	17.5 million	15.8	ETB93 million[a]	8 million[a]	36
Swaziland	168,228	10.1	SZL6 million	0.7 million	70
Uganda	5.8 million	7.3	UGX20 billion	9.5 million	46

Source: COHA Study.

[a] Only considers primary school.

IMPACT OF UNDERNUTRITION ON RETENTION

Students who are undernourished are also more likely to drop out of school than those who experience healthy childhoods. The data from the first-phase countries indicate that the expected number of schooling years achieved by a student who was stunted is as much as 1.2 years lower than the expected schooling for a student who was never undernourished. The graph in Figure 9.2 illustrates these levels of expected schooling achievement. As shown, countries with low overall schooling achievement also illustrate a higher differential achievement between children who were stunted and those who were never undernourished.

The economic impact of school dropout does not, however, incur while a person is of school age. Rather, the economic costs are incurred when the population is of working age, as people may be less productive and earn less income as a result of fewer years of schooling achieved.[*] Thus, considerations of losses associated to lower schooling are described in the following section.

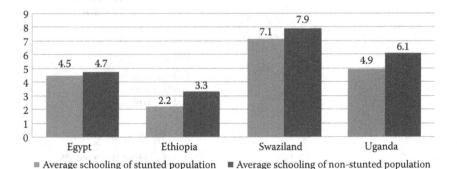

FIGURE 9.2   Expected schooling years by nutritional status.

[*] Based on income data from NITs.

SOCIAL AND ECONOMIC IMPACT OF CHILD UNDERNUTRITION IN PRODUCTIVITY

Losses in Potential Productivity

The COHA model estimated that between 40% and 67% of the working-age population in the four countries were stunted as children (Figure 9.3). Research shows that adults who suffered from stunting as children are less productive than non stunted workers and are less able to contribute to the economy (Alderman et al. 2006).

The impact of this lower productivity varies depending on the particular labor structure of the country and the type of economic achievement in which the individual is engaged. For people engaged in non manual sectors, the lower educational levels achieved by those affected by stunting is reflected in a lower income (Daniels

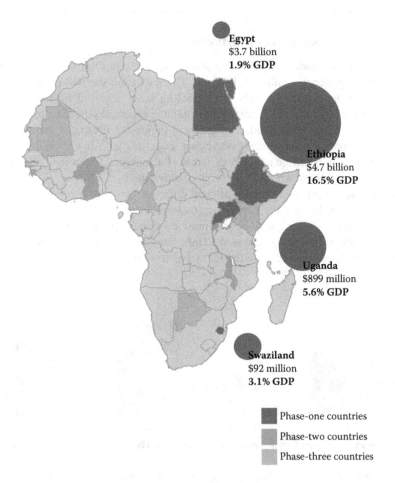

Egypt
$3.7 billion
1.9% GDP

Ethiopia
$4.7 billion
16.5% GDP

Uganda
$899 million
5.6% GDP

Swaziland
$92 million
3.1% GDP

Phase-one countries

Phase-two countries

Phase-three countries

FIGURE 9.3   COHA countries and 1st phase results—Social and Economic Impact of Child Undernutrition. According to the initial results generated by the COHA study, the equivalent losses above are incurred by each country annually as a result of child undernutrition.

TABLE 9.6

Losses in Productivity Associated with Child Undernutrition

	Stunted Population of Working Age (15–64)		Lost Productivity in Manual Activities		Lost Productivity in Non-manual Activities	
Country	Number	Estimated Prevalence (%)	National Currency	USD	National Currency	USD
Egypt	21 million	41	EGP10.7 billion	2.0 billion	EGP2.7 billion	484 million
Ethiopia	26 million	67	ETB12.9 billion	1.1 billion	ETB625 million	53 million
Swaziland	283,618	40	SZL126 million	15 million	SZL251 million	30 million
Uganda	8 million	54	UGX417 billion	201.5 million	UGX241 billion	116.5 million

Source: COHA Study.

and Adair 2004). As for stunted workers engaged in manual activities, research shows that they tend to have less lean body mass (Martins et al. 2004) and are more likely to be less productive in manual activities than those who were never affected by growth retardation (Haddad and Bouis 1991). As a result, losses in productivity are classified as losses in potential productivity in manual and non-manual activities, which are summarized in Table 9.6.

LOSSES IN PRODUCTIVITY DUE TO WORKING HOURS LOST AS A RESULT OF MORTALITY

As mentioned in the health section of this report, undernourished children have a higher risk of dying compared to children who are not underweight. In addition to the clear social problems associated with increased mortality, there is also a related economic cost. The COHA model estimates the proportion of child mortalities that is associated with undernutrition and then estimates the potential productivity of those individuals, had they lived and been part of the workforce (aged 15–64) in 2009. The model uses current income data to estimate this lost productivity in terms of both lost income and lost working hours. According to these estimates, the working hours lost are equivalent to between 0.7% and 8.3% of the current workforce as a result of undernutrition-related mortalities. Considering the present value of these working hours lost, in many countries, this is the most significant productivity cost associated with undernutrition (Table 9.7).

SCENARIOS

The model generates a baseline, to be compared to the nutritional goals established in each country. These scenarios are constructed based on the estimated costs of the children born in each year, from 2009 to 2025 (net present value). While the previous sections calculated the costs incurred in a single year by historical undernutrition,

TABLE 9.7

Losses in Productivity Due to Mortality Associated with Child Undernutrition

	Total Annual Working Hours Lost	Percentage of Current Workforce (%)	Cost in National Currency	Cost in USD
Egypt	857 million	0.7	EGP5.4 billion	988 million
Ethiopia	4.7 billion	8.3	ETB40.1 billion	3.4 billion
Swaziland	37 million	2.4	SZL340 million	40 million
Uganda	943 million	3.8	UGX657billion	317 million

Source: COHA Study.

these values represent the projected costs and savings generated by children born during and after 2009.

> *Baseline Scenario. The Cost of Inaction: Progress in reduction of stunting and underweight child stops.* In this scenario, the progress of reduction of the prevalence of undernutrition stops at the level achieved in 2009. Although highly unlikely, it serves as a basis for estimating the saving for other scenarios.
> *Scenario #1. Cutting by Half the Prevalence of Child Undernutrition by 2025.* In this scenario, the prevalence of underweight and stunted children would be reduced to half of the value of the reference year of 2009.
> *Scenario #2. The Goal Scenario: Reduce Stunting to 10% and Underweight Children to 5%, by 2025.* In this scenario, the prevalence of stunted children would be reduced to 10% and underweight children with less than 5 years to 5%.

As presented in Table 9.8, the potential economic benefits illustrate an opportunity to help build a case for increased investment in nutrition. With this information countries can have a benchmark for increasing investment, while at the same time, being able to compare this with the potential economic gains of reduced stunting rates.

CONCLUSIONS

The COHA study is an important step forward to better understand the role that child nutrition and human development can play as a catalyzer, or as a constraint, in the social and economic transformation of Africa.

HEALTH SECTOR

Child undernutrition generates health costs equivalent to between 1% and 11% of the total public budget allocated to health. These costs are due to episodes directly associated with the incremental quantity and intensity of illnesses that affect underweight children, and the protocols necessary for their treatment.

TABLE 9.8

Comparison of Projected Costs and Savings of Reduced Stunting Rates in Two Scenarios

	Scenario #1: Halving the Prevalence of Child Undernutrition by 2025			Scenario #2: The Goal Scenario: 10 and 5 by 2025		
Country	% Annual Reduction of Stunting Required[a]	Total Savings to be Achieved	Average Annual Savings	% Annual Reduction of Stunting Required[a]	Total Savings to be Achieved	Average Annual Savings
Egypt	0.9%	EGP11.7 billion	EGP732 million (USD133 million)	1.2%	EGP14.5 billion	EGP907 million (USD165 million)
Ethiopia	1.5%	ETB71 billion	ETB4.4 billion (USD376 million)	2.3%	ETB148 billion	ETB9.2 billion (USD784 million)
Swaziland	0.9%	SZL402 million	SZL25 million (USD3 million)	1.2%	SZL511 million	SZL32 million (USD4 million)
Uganda	1.1%	UGX2.8 trillion	UGX179 billion (USD88 million)	1.6%	UGX4.3 trillion	UGX267 billion (USD132 million)

Source: COHA Study.
[a] Percentage points.

In the larger proportion of these episodes, 69%–82%, do not seek medical attention, or are treated at home, increasing the risk for complications and evidencing an unmet demand for health care.

Eliminating the inequality in access to health care is a key element of the social transformation agenda in Africa, which requires, as a precondition, a reduction of the rural/urban coverage gap. As health coverage expands to rural areas, there will be an increase of people seeking medical attention; this can potentially affect the efficiency of the system to provide proper care services. This study illustrates that a reduction of child undernutrition could facilitate the effectiveness of this expansion by reducing the incremental burden generated by the health requirements of underweight children.

EDUCATION SECTOR

Children who were stunted experienced higher repetition rates in school ranging from 2% to 4.9%.

Moreover, 7%–16% of all grade repetitions in school are associated with the higher incidence of repetition among stunted children, the majority (90%) of which occurs in primary school.

These numbers suggest that a reduction in stunting prevalence could support an improvement in school quality, as it would reduce preventable burdens to the education system.

Increasing the educational levels of a population, and maximizing the productive capacity of Africa's population dividend, is a key element in increasing competitiveness and innovation on the continent. This represents a particular opportunity in sub-Saharan Africa, where the population under 15 years is estimated to be 40% of the total population. Children and youth must be equipped with the skills necessary for competitive labor. Thus, underlying causes for low school performance and early dropout must be addressed. As there is no single cause for this phenomenon, a comprehensive strategy must be put in place that considers improving the quality of education and the conditions required for school attendance. This study demonstrates that stunting is one barrier to attendance and retention that must be removed to effectively elevate educational levels and improve individuals' labor opportunities in the future.

LABOR PRODUCTIVITY

Fifty-two percent of the working-age population in the analyzed countries is currently stunted. This population has achieved, on average, lower school levels than those who did not experience growth retardation, ranging from 0.2 to 1.2 years of less schooling.

The working-age population has been diminished by 1%–8% due to child mortality associated with undernutrition.

On the continent, more than half of the population is expected to live in cities by 2035 (Program 2011). An important component to prepare for this shift is to ensure that the workforce is ready to make a transition toward a more skilled labor, and economies are able to produce new jobs to reduce youth unemployment. By preventing child stunting, thus avoiding the associated loss in physical and cognitive capacity that hinders individual productivity, people can be provided with a more equal opportunity for success.

POTENTIAL ECONOMIC BENEFITS

The model estimated that a reduction of the prevalence of undernutrition to half of the 2009 level by the year 2025 can generate annual average savings from USD3 million to USD376 million for the analyzed countries.

This economic benefit, which would result from a decrease in morbidities, lower repetition rates, and an increase in manual and non manual productivity, presents an important economic argument for the incremental investments in child nutrition. This does not only impact those people affected by undernutrition, but the society as a whole.

EVIDENCE-BASED POLICY

COHA is an important example of how South–South collaboration can work to implement cost-effective activities in development and knowledge sharing. It demonstrated that developing and implementing tools that are sensitive to the particular conditions of the continent is feasible.

It illustrates the valuable role that data and government-endorsed research can play in shedding light on pertinent issues on the continent. Although the availability of uniform and readily available data in Africa is limited, the COHA results have shown that analysis has the potential to bring the issue of child nutrition to the forefront of the development arena.

POLICY RECOMMENDATIONS

STUNTING IS A USEFUL INDICATOR TO EVALUATE EFFECTIVE SOCIAL POLICIES

The causes of and solutions for chronic hunger are linked to social policies across numerous sectors. As such, stunting reduction will require interventions from the health, education, social protection, and social infrastructure perspectives. Stunting can be an effective indicator of success in larger social programs.

STRONG POLITICAL WILL CAN BE REFLECTED IN AGGRESSIVE GOALS

This study encourages countries not to be content with "acceptable" levels of stunting; equal opportunity should be the aspiration of the continent. In this sense, it is recommended that aggressive targets are set in Africa for the reduction of stunting that go beyond proportional reduction, to establish an absolute value as the goal for the region at 10%. Countries with high and very high levels of stunting, of over 35%, might pursue an interim goal of reduction to 20%, but for countries that have been able to achieve progress enough to reduce stunting to below 35%, the establishment this target would be acceptable and desirable.

A MULTI-CAUSAL PROBLEM REQUIRES A MULTI-SECTORAL RESPONSE

The achievement of this aggressive goal cannot be reached from just the health sector. To have a decisive impact on improving child nutrition, a comprehensive, multi-sectorial policy must be put in place, with strong political commitment and allocation of adequate resources for its implementation.

EFFICIENT RURAL ECONOMIES AND EFFECTIVE SOCIAL PROTECTION SCHEMES ARE KEY DRIVERS FOR THE SUSTAINED REDUCTION OF CHILD UNDERNUTRITION

Fostering rural economies, by enhancing the productivity of agricultural activities and expanding the non agricultural activities, is a key element in accelerating the reduction rate of malnutrition. Efforts carried out by CAADP and the development of value chains of strategic agricultural commodities can be key elements to focus efforts on in the coming years. Additionally, it is important to consider the role of social protection programs in reducing hunger and malnutrition, in order to achieve the appropriate combination of transfers and services that is adequate for each context.

SUSTAINABILITY REQUIRES STRONG NATIONAL CAPACITY

To ensure sustainability of these actions, whenever possible, the role of international aid must be complementary to nationally led investments, and further efforts have to be made in ensuring the strengthening of national capacity to address child undernutrition.

MONITORING IS NEEDED FOR PROGRESS

To measure short-term results in the prevention of stunting, a more systematic approach with shorter periodicity is recommended, such as 2 years between each assessment. As prevention of child undernutrition should target children before 2 years of age, these results would provide information to policy makers and practitioners on effectiveness of social protection and nutrition programs.

LONG-TERM COMMITMENT IS NECESSARY TO ACHIEVE RESULTS

The COHA initiative represents a valuable opportunity to place nutrition within a strategy to ensure Africa's sustainable development. As the deadline for Millennium Development Goals nears, new priorities and targets will be set that will serve as a guide for development policies in years to come. It is recommended that the prioritization of the elimination of stunting be not only presented in the traditional forums, but also included in the wider discussions of development, as a concern for the economic transformation of Africa.

PENDING QUESTIONS AND RESEARCH OPPORTUNITIES

The COHA represents an important step forward in shedding light on the importance of nutritional investments, as a fundamental basis for human development. Nevertheless, the process also served as an important exercise to identify gaps in knowledge that can help increase the dimensions of the analysis, that include:

- *Sub national differences in the social and economic impacts of child undernutrition.* There is an opportunity to raise the advocacy on sub regional and local actions by developing a model to distribute the cost of hunger by region and further engage local governments and communities in the implementation of local actions to improve nutrition.
- *The impact of early child malnutrition on women's contributions to the household.* As most women in Africa are responsible for household chores and caring activities, their contributions are not accurately measured by proxy of labor productivity, rather, by their capacity to provide well-being in the household. Nevertheless, the intensity in which this capacity is affected as a consequence of child malnutrition in not comprehensibly addressed in the current literature.

- *There are still gaps of region-specific risk analysis in Africa, particularly in educational outcomes and labor productivity.* A comprehensive analysis of a longitudinal study in Africa, can also serve as an important source of information to update further the relative risks faced by undernourished children, in different aspects of their lives.
- Complementary analysis could be carried out to further understand the sectoral consequences of undernutrition. Additional multi-variable analysis could also help to explain variations across countries.

"Cutting hunger and thereby achieving food and nutrition security in Africa is not only one of the most urgent means of reducing the vulnerability and enhancing the resilience of national economies, but also one of those which produces the highest returns for broader social and economic development."

5th African Union Conference of Ministers of Finance, Planning and Economic Development Resolution 898 (United Nations Economic and Social Council and African Union Commission 2012).

REFERENCES

Alderman, H., J. Hoddinott, and B. Kinsey. 2006. Long term consequences of early childhood malnutrition. *Oxford Economic Papers, Oxford University Press* 58 (3):450–474.

Daniels, M. C. and L. S. Adair. 2004. Growth in young Filipino children predicts schooling trajectories through high school. *Journal of Nutrition* 134 (6):1439–1446.

DHS, MEASURE. Quality information to plan, monitor and improve population, health, and nutrition programs. Accessed March 14, 2013. http://www.measuredhs.com.

Food and Agriculture Organization. 2012. The State of Food Insecurity in the World 2012 http://www.fao.org/publications/sofi/en/. Rome: FAO.

Haddad, L. and H. E. Bouis. 1991. The impact of nutritional status on agricultural productivity: Wage evidence from the Philippines. *Oxford Bulletin of Economics and Statistics* 53 (1).

Martins, P. A., D. J. Hoffman, M. T. Fernandes, C. R. Nascimento, S. B. Roberts, R. Sesso, and A. L. Sawaya. 2004. Stunted children gain less lean body mass and more fat mass than their non-stunted counterparts: A prospective study. *British Journal of Nutrition* 92 (5):819–25.

Program, United Nations Development. 2011. World Urbanization Prospects: The 2011 Revision.

Rice, A. L., L. Sacco, A. Hyder, and R. E. Black. 2000. Malnutrition as an underlying cause of childhood deaths associated with infectious diseases in developing countries. *Bulletin of the World Health Organization* 78 (10):1207–1221.

United Nations Children's Fund, World Health Organization, and The World Bank. 2012. UNICEF-WHO-World Bank Joint Child Malnutrition Estimates. UNICEF, New York; WHO, Geneva; The World Bank, Washington, DC.

United Nations Economic and Social Council, and African Union Commission. 2012. Resolution 898: The Cost of Hunger in Africa: Social and Economic Impacts of Child Undernutrition, in Report of the Committee of Experts of The Fifth Joint Annual Meetings of the AU Conference of Ministers of Economy and Finance and ECA Conference of African Ministers of Finance, Planning And Economic Development. Addis Ababa, Ethiopia: United Nations Economic And Social Council: Economic Commission For Africa, African Union Commission.

10 Integrating Nutrition Support for Food-Insecure Patients and Their Dependents into an HIV Care and Treatment Program in Western Kenya[*]

Joseph Mamlin, Sylvester Kimaiyo, Stephen Lewis, Hannah Tadayo, Fanice Komen Jerop, Catherine Gichunge, Tomeka Petersen, Yuehwern Yih, Paula Braitstein, Robert Einterz, and Cleophas Wanyonyi Chesoli[†]

CONTENTS

---

[*] This paper was first published in the *American Journal of Public Health*, and is reproduced with permission (Mamlin et al. 2009).

[†] Author contributed contents of Box 10.1.

ABSTRACT

The Academic Model Providing Access to Healthcare (AMPATH) is a partnership between Moi Teaching and Referral Hospital, Moi University School of
Medicine, and a consortium of universities led by Indiana University. AMPATH
has over 50,000 patients in active care in 17 main clinics around western Kenya.

Despite antiretroviral therapy, many patients were not recovering their
health because of food insecurity. AMPATH therefore established partnerships
with the World Food Program and U.S. Agency for International Development
and began high-production farms to complement food support.

Today, nutritionists assess all AMPATH patients and dependents for food
security and refer those in need to the food program. We describe the implementation, challenges, and successes of this program.

There is a compelling monotony to the maps of sub-Saharan Africa that delineate
high-prevalence areas of HIV, poverty, and food insecurity—each map might liter-
ally be superimposed on the others. This overlap is not a coincidence. The interplay
between HIV, poverty, and food insecurity is increasingly recognized as a major con-
tributor to the devastation now challenging much of sub-Saharan Africa (Kadiyala
and Gillespie 2004, Anabwani and Navario 2005, Wanke 2005). It is unlikely that
any scientific evidence can depict the actual human and economic costs to societies
burdened by the disability and death of young adults, endless numbers of widows,
unparalleled numbers of orphans, and falling school attendance by an expanding
number of malnourished, vulnerable children. Responses targeting only the rapid
scale up of antiretroviral therapy are unlikely to meet the needs of many of the
patients they serve. To those on the front lines of HIV care in sub-Saharan Africa, it
is clear that food security and poverty reduction are essential components of a mean-
ingful response to the havoc wrought by the HIV pandemic (Kadiyala and Gillespie
2004, Chopra and Darnton-Hill 2006, Au et al. 2006). Medical care is necessary but
insufficient, whereas health care attends to all these sectors.

In 2001, Kenya's second national referral hospital, Moi Teaching and Referral
Hospital, its second medical school, Moi University School of Medicine, and a consortium of medical schools from the United States led by Indiana University School
of Medicine initiated a bold response to the HIV pandemic in western Kenya. They
launched the Academic Model for the Prevention and Treatment of HIV/AIDS now
known as the Academic Model Providing Access to Healthcare (AMPATH), which
has grown into one of Africa's largest and most rapidly growing HIV care programs
(Mamlin et al. 2004, Einterz et al. 2007). AMPATH is currently working in a network of 17 Ministry of Health facilities in western Kenya, including a national referral hospital, several district hospitals, subdistrict hospitals, and many rural health
centers (Figure 10.1, Table 10.1). AMPATH is currently serving over 50,000 HIV-
infected patients, half of whom are receiving combination antiretroviral treatment.

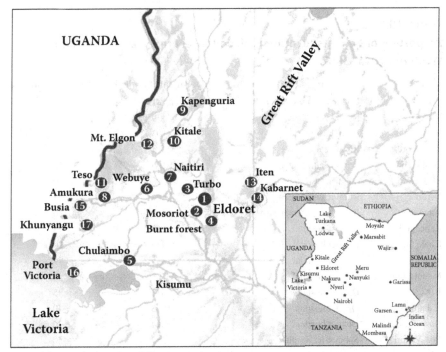

Note: Eldoret is the location of the program headquarters.

FIGURE 10.1 Map of western Kenya showing locations of Academic Model Providing Access to Healthcare (AMPATH) clinics.

Each month, approximately 2000 new patients are enrolled, roughly 40%–50% of whom begin antiretroviral treatment.

Early on, AMPATH care providers became acutely aware of the impact hunger and poverty were having on patients presenting for care and on the vulnerable members of their households, most notably children. AMPATH leaders decided to provide nutritional support for all food-insecure patients and dependents within their homes. That decision alone initiated a series of challenges for AMPATH that have proven just as complex as scaling up Kenya's largest antiretroviral delivery program. AMPATH is one of the first HIV care programs in sub-Saharan Africa to roll out comprehensive HIV treatment combined with extensive nutritional support for food-insecure patients and their dependents. We provide an overview of the program, including challenges, successes, and lessons learned, so others might be assisted in building their own food support programs.

AMPATH NUTRITION PROGRAM

ELIGIBILITY

A qualified nutritionist completes a standardized initial encounter form for all newly registered patients at each AMPATH site. The interview focuses on level of immune

TABLE 10.1

Proportion of Patients Identified as Food Insecure by AMPATH Clinics, Western Kenya, 2007

Clinic Site	Type of Center	No. of Patients Enrolled[a]	Food Insecure (%)
MTRH	National referral hospital	17,781	39
Mosoriot	Rural health center	5329	40
Turbo	Rural health center	4103	30
Burnt Forest	Rural health center	2654	20
Chulaimbo	Rural health center	8105	40
Webuye	Subdistrict hospital	4508	20
Naitiri	Rural health center	1447	25
Amukura	Rural health center	1769	30
Kapenguria	District hospital	1168	44
Kitale	District hospital	5943	20
Teso	District hospital	1855	29
Mount Elgon	District hospital	708	28
Iten	District hospital	683	35
Kabarnet	District hospital	1083	40
Busia	District hospital	5814	30
Port Victoria	Subdistrict hospital	2257	50
Khunyangu	Subdistrict hospital	1831	50
Total		67,038	33.5[b]

Note: Academic Model Providing Access to Healthcare = AMPATH; MTRH = Moi Teaching and Referral Hospital.

[a] As of January 1, 2008.

[b] Mean percentage.

suppression, body mass index (or equivalent for children), socioeconomic status and circumstances, and patient's access to food in terms of both quantity and quality, using a version of the Household Food Insecurity Access Scale specifically adapted by the U.S. Agency for International Development (USAID) Food and Nutrition Technical Assistance project for use in developing countries (Coates et al. 2006). The determination of whether a patient and his or her dependents are food secure ultimately rests with the clinical judgment of the nutritionist. After considering all related variables, if the nutritionist feels that the patient or dependents are unlikely to meet minimal daily nutritional requirements, that family is judged food insecure. Once food insecurity is determined, the patient and all dependents in the home automatically qualify for food support for 6 months.

Careful assessment of individual homes showed that food insecurity extended beyond the food-insecure patient. AMPATH decided that it was unethical to offer food to only the index patient while children in the home lacked access to food. The decision was consistent with existing policies of the World Food Program.

The nutritionist writes a "food prescription" that entitles the patient and dependents to a 1-month supply of food. The patient must return to the nutritionist monthly for a new prescription until 6 months are completed. At each monthly visit, the nutritionist reminds the patient how much time is left on the food prescription. Depending on the needs of the patient and family and the food supply, the nutritionist will provide up to 100% of caloric needs for the patient and dependents.

The proportion of patients eligible for food support varies widely among AMPATH sites (Table 10.1), but, in general, there is more food insecurity in rural areas. Rural populations in the far western part of the catchment area tend to have high poverty levels, small plots of land per family, and poor soil quality. In addition, these western sites have a higher proportion of widows entering care than the overall average within AMPATH of 25%. In Khunyangu, for example, 68% of women who have ever been married are widows at the time of their first visit, as are 46% in Port Victoria and 43% in Busia.

FOOD DEMAND

For a given day, week, or month, the total demand for food is defined as the sum of the food prescribed by nutritionists for all patients and their dependents throughout AMPATH for that period. Each food prescription records the quantity and type of food required for each household along with the day and location of anticipated pickup of food. As summarized in Table 10.2, AMPATH nutritionists, during 2007, assessed over 130,000 patients and their dependents for food insecurity (75% female, 85% aged 19 years or older), counseled 61,535 of them about nutrition, and enrolled 9623 new patients (plus an average of 4 dependents per patient) into the food program.

FOOD SUPPLY

To meet the major challenge of supplying sufficient food to meet patients' needs, AMPATH uses a combination of production, donation, and purchase.

A key component of the AMPATH nutrition program is food production. AMPATH currently manages six farms; four are high-production, continuous-irrigation farms and two are teaching and demonstration farms that aim to demonstrate ways of increasing the yield in small plots owned by AMPATH patients. With a continuous source of water, these farms are able to produce a reliable, year-round supply of fresh vegetables. The combined monthly output of the continuous-irrigation farms is in excess of 20 metric tons of fresh produce (Figure 10.2). As orchards become more productive by mid-2009, it is hoped that these same farms will add an additional 4 metric tons of fresh fruit each month.

The major donors of donated food are the World Food Program and USAID. The World Food Program currently provides pulses (legumes), corn, corn–soy blends, and cooking oil for up to 30,000 recipients and recently committed to supporting

TABLE 10.2

Summary of AMPATH Nutrition Program Activities, by Selected Demographics, Western Kenya, 2007

	Patients and Their Dependents Assessed for Food Insecurity, No. (%)	Patients and Their Dependents Counseled about Nutrition, No. (%)	Patients Enrolled to Receive Food, No. (%)	Patients Discharged From Food Program, No. (%)
Total	133,792	61,535	9623	1805
Gender				
Male	33,784 (25)	17,573 (29)	2584 (27)	499 (28)
Female	100,008 (75)	43,962 (71)	7039 (73)	1306 (72)
Age, years				
≤5	12,562 (9)	4553 (7)	852 (9)	157 (9)
6–18	8181 (6)	4981 (8)	1,232 (13)	152 (8)
≥19	113,049 (85)	52,001 (85)	7539 (78)	1496 (83)

Source: Western Kenya, 2007.

Note: Academic Model Providing Access to Healthcare = AMPATH.

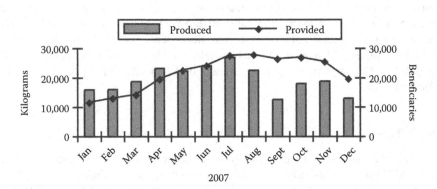

FIGURE 10.2 Kilograms of food produced by the Academic Model Providing Access to Healthcare (AMPATH) nutrition program and the numbers of its beneficiaries: Western Kenya, 2007. *Note:* A serious hailstorm negatively affected food production in October; Christmas and the lead-up to national elections affected it in December.

up to 1500 orphans and vulnerable children through AMPATH. USAID provides vitamin-enriched corn–soy blends for an additional 2000 recipients.

AMPATH purchases up to 3000 eggs per day from a network of chicken houses managed by its own patients. Packets of fermented milk are purchased from a local dairy farm. Fermented milk is preferred because it has a shelf life of approximately 10 days in the absence of refrigeration.

The supply of food now available from all these sources provides a culturally acceptable food basket consisting of fresh vegetables, fruit, eggs, milk products, an occasional chicken, corn, pulses, corn–soy blends, and cooking oil.

FOOD DISTRIBUTION AND COST

The daily balance of supply and demand within the AMPATH service area must be supported by a delivery system capable of getting the right food at the right time to the right location for individual patients who live throughout much of western Kenya in an area in excess of 30,000 square kilometers. In response to this challenge, industrial engineers from Purdue University joined AMPATH to create a computerized nutrition information system.

Each day, the food prescription for each patient is entered in the nutrition information system along with an estimate of the total supply of food available. The nutrition information system then creates daily work logs detailing the amount, type, and location of food that needs to be moved. In addition, the nutrition information system lists individual patients scheduled to pick up food by day and site. Moving the food requires a transportation system and access to appropriate storage and packing centers. Distribution at the sites requires adequate space and distribution workers. Most distribution workers are specially trained AMPATH patients.

The cost of the food provided to beneficiaries includes the value of donations from the World Food Program and USAID, food purchased, and the total cost of production of food on the AMPATH high-production farms. In addition, the fixed costs of transport, nutritionist, distributors, and data management were totaled for the entire program. Once the program reached its target of 30,000 beneficiaries, this combination of food and fixed costs resulted in a cost per patient of US$0.27 per day.

TRANSITION TO FOOD SECURITY

The designers of the AMPATH nutrition system anticipated that 6 months of food support, coupled with restoration of the immune system through antiretroviral therapy, would enable many patients to return to an adequate level of food security. Table 10.2 shows the number of beneficiaries successfully discontinued from food support in 2007. When it appears that additional nutrition support will be needed beyond 6 months, the patient is evaluated by an AMPATH social worker. If the social worker feels that continued food support is warranted, food will be continued while the patient is referred to another important arm of AMPATH, the Family Preservation Initiative.

This initiative provides an array of programs aimed at enhancing income security for AMPATH patients. For urban patients, this may take the form of microenterprise training with or without the assistance of microfinancing. For rural patients, it often involves linkage with AMPATH agriculture extension workers for consideration of improved farming techniques, planting new crops, or participation in cooperatives with other rural patients to grow high-value produce. The agriculture arm of the initiative is extending its services to all AMPATH sites, offering food and income security rather than dependency for thousands of AMPATH patients and their dependents.

DISCUSSION

Early in the history of the AMPATH program, food insecurity was identified as a pervasive and pernicious companion of HIV-infected patients in western Kenya. Patients who had walked miles to present themselves to AMPATH sites for evaluation and were offered antiretroviral therapy were known to decline therapy and walk back home when they learned that no food was available to allay their hunger. In spite of the challenges of scaling up an expensive and complex nutritional support system, AMPATH proceeded on the assumption that food is necessary for food-insecure patients and their dependents if antiretroviral therapy is to be of any benefit.

Having made the commitment to feed all food-insecure patients and their dependents, AMPATH fully understood the gap between goals and practice in sub-Saharan Africa. Even with adequate funding in hand, scaling up robust antiretroviral therapy of large populations proved to be a formidable challenge. Many of the same barriers to rapid scale up of antiretroviral therapy in sub-Saharan Africa are equally capable of frustrating the best-intended nutrition program. In this report, however, we clearly document that the demand for food by individual patients and their dependents can be determined and, most importantly, that demand can be met by a combination of food production, food donations, and an effective food distribution infrastructure. Our experience suggests that the addition of food to combination antiretroviral therapy has a synergistic clinical and immunological benefit; proving that benefit will be an important next step.

CHALLENGES

Food support is an expensive addition to HIV care, and currently there are no funding sources that explicitly target food security for HIV-infected patients and their dependents. Beyond the costs of growing food, there are additional costs in managing large food donations. Significant investments were necessary for computer support systems, physical facilities, vehicles, and dedicated program management and food distribution staff. AMPATH has been able to support its nutrition program with a combination of funding sources. The U.S. President's Emergency Plan for AIDS Relief was the first to provide partial support of AMPATH's effort to establish a pilot model of nutrition support as a component of comprehensive HIV treatment. The World Food Program joined with AMPATH in a commitment to provide its basic food basket for up to 30,000 food-insecure patients and their dependents. USAID followed by contributing its corn–soy blend for an additional 2000 persons.

Remarkably, all of the land for continuously irrigated high-production farms used by AMPATH has been made available without cost. The initial farm used land made available by a nearby high school. Subsequently, land was provided at no cost to AMPATH by churches, the Ministry of Health, the Moi Teaching and Referral Hospital, Moi University, and local nongovernmental organizations. In addition, philanthropic donations have added critical funding every step of the way.

An immediate concern that arises when food support is provided to poor populations is the prospect of long-term dependency. It is unrealistic to think that one can feed patients until they have regained their health and then expect all of them to return to their previous means of securing food for themselves and their dependents. In our experience, some of the patients on antiretroviral therapy are able to return directly to self-sufficiency; for others, however, food security remains elusive even when their clinical and immune status has returned to normal. Too many jobs have been lost, too many spouses have died, and too many assets have been eroded for many patients who were food insecure even before HIV entered their lives. AMPATH will rely on the increasing strength of its social services program and the expanding capability of the Family Preservation Initiative to assist with those families for whom food security seems like an unattainable goal. Fortunately, additional funds now available will support a more rapid scale up of the Family Preservation Initiative in the years ahead. It is too early to determine the true proportion of patients capable of returning to food security until AMPATH gains more experience with the expanded initiative programs now being made available at all sites.

SUCCESSES

The fact that almost 2000 beneficiaries have been able to come off—and stay off—of food support since January 2007 is encouraging. The simultaneous rapid scale up of AMPATH's clinical services and nutritional support program means that most beneficiaries began receiving food support early in 2007 and, therefore, have not reached the time for discontinuation at the time of writing. As the Family Preservation Initiative continues to expand and make its services available to additional AMPATH sites, we expect most patients to eventually become income—and hence food—secure.

It is unlikely that any program in sub-Saharan Africa can fully eliminate food insecurity and dependency in all patients. However, a successful program blending food support with economic development will probably avoid adding to the ranks of the food dependent and, we hope, can reduce the number destined to need food support indefinitely (Marston and De Cock 2004). Other successes include the extensive infrastructure developed for the nutrition and food programs, the total number of beneficiaries, the fact that food is provided to the family and not just the individual patient, and the linking of the food program with agricultural or business training through the Family Preservation Initiative.

SUSTAINABILITY

Sustainability of food support on a scale now operational in AMPATH remains an additional concern. Every facet of the AMPATH nutrition program is vulnerable. Funds supporting the high production farms are from private donations and the President's Emergency Plan for AIDS Relief. Continuing donations from the World Food Program compete with endless pressure on an organization constantly facing some of this world's most daunting challenges. And the infrastructure and staff so essential to the distribution of food depend on a patchwork of contributions from many supporters of AMPATH. It is difficult to envision the sustainability of the AMPATH nutrition program or replication to other programs unless new commitments from the national government and the international donor community emerge. These commitments will need to support food security with the same vigor as those currently targeting universal access to antiretroviral therapy in sub-Saharan Africa.

CONCLUSIONS

At the time of writing, every food-insecure patient within AMPATH, and every child within that patient's family, has access to food. If nothing else, AMPATH has demonstrated that providing food security to food-insecure families can be done.

AMPATH proceeded with food support for its patients with the full conviction that impoverished HIV-infected patients and their dependents who are hungry require food as an integral component of care. Although improved monitoring and evaluation of the effectiveness of this program are required, further delay in replicating elsewhere the food security programs that AMPATH has implemented means that hundreds of thousands of patients and their dependents will remain hungry in sub-Saharan Africa and in other resource-constrained settings. Having demonstrated that food security can be provided, AMPATH's task now is to find the most cost-effective delivery systems, better understand the path toward sustainability, and welcome the efforts of those interventions that can prevent food insecurity in the first place.

CONTRIBUTION

J. Mamlin led the writing of the chapter. Y. Yih led the development of the nutrition information system. P. Braitstein led the analysis of the data. All other authors participated in the conception of the nutrition program and its implementation and reviewed drafts.

ACKNOWLEDGMENTS

This research was supported in part by a grant to the USAID–AMPATH Partnership from the U.S. Agency for International Development as part of the President's Emergency Plan for AIDS Relief (grant 623-A-00-08-00003-00).

We thank the many nutritionists who devote their time and energy toward helping patients maintain or recover their food security, and Johnson Kimeu and Max Riana, who ensure that accurate and timely records are maintained. We also thank the World Food Program, the Moore Foundation, and the many individual donors who have made this work possible.

BOX 10.1 "WE CAN DO THIS OURSELVES"

ADDRESSING FOOD SECURITY AND WEALTH CREATION IN KENYA: AN UPDATE ON THE AMPATH CASE, 2014

CLEOPHAS WANYONYI CHESOLI

The Academic Model Providing Access to Healthcare—AMPATH—is an alliance of Moi University, Moi Teaching and Referral Hospital, and a consortium of North American academic institutions led by Indiana University. In 2001, AMPATH joined with Kenya's Ministry of Health to tackle the devastating HIV pandemic. The results have far exceeded any initial expectations. AMPATH has grown into one of Africa's largest and most comprehensive HIV prevention and treatment programs. In recent years, AMPATH has broadened its services to include primary health care and noncommunicable chronic disease services to combat cancer, cardiovascular disease, diabetes, and mental illnesses. The services go far beyond standard hospitals and clinics and extend into every village and home served by AMPATH. But as many know, in sub-Saharan Africa, disease is just part of the problem and no amount of purely medical intervention can claim victory.

Those who live and work in sub-Saharan Africa (SSA) realize fully that disease is intimately enmeshed with its dreaded twins, poverty and hunger. The three heads of this monster (disease, poverty, and hunger) feed off of each other and no medical care system can by itself expect to break the vicious downward cycle that drains so many in SSA of their last thread of hope. For this reason, AMPATH from its beginning has struggled to move beyond disease management and attempt to enhance opportunities for income and food security for the families it serves.

WORLD FOOD PROGRAM/AMPATH PARTNERSHIP

AMPATH fed its first patient in 2002 and watched her double her weight over the next 6 months. The power of combining nutritional support with HIV drugs for food-insecure patients was obvious. This was followed by a series of high-production AMPATH farms capable of providing fresh produce to thousands of food-insecure patients and members of their household. In 2005, AMPATH partnered with the World Food Program and in no time the WFP/AMPATH partnership became the largest healthcare-affiliated food program in the World, feeding over 33,000 persons each day. WFP complemented AMPATH's fresh produce with maize, beans, corn–soy blends, and vegetable oil. The WFP donation consistently provided more than 250 metric tons of food commodities each month for the last 5 years.

The WFP/AMPATH food program was guided by a specific nutritionist prescription for each index patient along with all household members. Beneficiaries received the WFP/AMPATH food basket for up to 8 months.

Feeding the entire household in addition to the index patient was a decision unique to WFP and AMPATH. To AMPATH and the WFP, a food-insecure patient could not be given successful food support without caring for the children and others at risk in that same home.

The WFP/AMPATH food program successfully supported the vast majority of food-insecure AMPATH patients while they got back on their feet. The number of beneficiaries reached a peak of approximately 33,000 in 2011. And between 2011 and 2012, over 15,000 beneficiaries had been weaned off food. It was in the context of this successful food support program that WFP and AMPATH leadership began to explore ways food support could simultaneously have some impact on income security for individual clients and communities served by AMPATH.

MOVING THE WFP/AMPATH FOOD PROGRAM TO THE VILLAGE

The major shortcoming of the WFP/AMPATH food support program became increasingly clear. It was providing vital support to food-insecure families but failing to address their parallel problem of income insecurity. Two key initiatives provided hope for linking food support to income generation for the very communities AMPATH served.

The first initiative was the WFP Purchase for Progress (P4P) program. This creative initiative was supported by the Gates and H.G. Buffett Foundations along with a host of countries. P4P sought to encourage groups of low-income farmers to sell their produce at commercial prices to WFP. As a result an increasing proportion of the food provided to AMPATH by WFP was food WFP had purchased from AMPATH-affiliated farmer associations. AMPATH moved as quickly as possible as a P4P participant. The initial target was to create fairly large groups of farmers since each P4P contract mandated at least 56 metric tons. Nine large groups were initially formed with each consisting of up to 100 farmers. By May 2013, 36 farmer groups were participating in the initiative in Uasin Gishu, Nandi North, Trans-Nzoia, and Bungoma Districts. This represents about 3600 smallholder farmers. AMPATH-affiliated farmer associations have to date provided over half of the commodities purchased by WFP/P4P in Kenya.

The P4P initiative stimulated financial institutions to redefine their engagement with farmers. Farmers' groups that could not previously access credit for lack of collateral now had access to financial support from banks. One group, for example, was able to access over KES 40 million (almost USD 500,000) within 2 years.

Given the fact that Africa loses much of its produce to poor post-harvest management especially due to lack of storage facilities, AMPATH and the World Food Program initiated a campaign to support groups to set up storage facilities on a cost sharing basis (the farmer group contributes its resources to building the walls of the facility and the WFP funds the cost of the roof). With over 10 groups putting up their own storage facilities, loss of produce has been reduced and some groups are now contributing their surplus produce to local community food banks in order to support vulnerable individuals and families.

The second major new initiative was a pilot program funded by the H. G. Buffett Foundation called the AMPATH green initiative. In this initiative, patients were given vouchers that allow them to buy produce from participating local farms in lieu of receiving food hand-outs from AMPATH farms. This initiative promoted locally grown, fresh produce with emphasis on African Indigenous Vegetables (AIVs). AIVs are particularly appealing because of their low cost, hardy stock, nutritional value, and ease of production. This initiative spurs patients themselves to grow fresh produce utilizing a combination of sack gardens and kitchen gardens. Each sack garden can be created for less than $1 and two sacks are capable of providing all of the fresh produce needed by five to seven persons. Sack gardens are particularly appealing to individuals who do not own a plot of land. To date, over 1000 patients have initiated their own sack gardens. Landless AMPATH patients who reside in Kenya's second largest slum. They have learned to provide fresh produce for themselves, and to sell excess produce to neighbors. To date, more than 6000 farmers have participated in the AMPATH Green Initiative.

In addition to P4P and the AMPATH green initiative, AMPATH partnered with the Ministry of Agriculture and other stakeholders to encourage agribusiness and market development. In the Value Initiative Project (VIP), AMPATH partnered with the Export Promotion Council, Kenya Agricultural Research Institute, Ministry of Agriculture, and the Small Enterprise Education Programme (SEEP) Network to promote the passion fruit value chain. As a result, several farmers formed an export company that now helps many passion fruit farmers in the region to sell their produce in structured markets. This initiative formed the foundation for many more initiatives around the passion fruit crop and has been duplicated in other crops.

REFERENCES

Anabwani, G. and P. Navario. 2005. Nutrition and HIV/AIDS in sub-Saharan Africa: An overview. *Nutrition* 21 (1):96–9. doi: 10.1016/j.nut.2004.09.013.

Au, J. T., K. Kayitenkore, E. Shutes, E. Karita, P. J. Peters, A. Tichacek, and S. A. Allen. 2006. Access to adequate nutrition is a major potential obstacle to antiretroviral adherence among HIV-infected individuals in Rwanda. *AIDS* 20 (16):2116–8. doi: 10.1097/01. aids.0000247580.16073.1b.

Chopra, M. and I. Darnton-Hill. 2006. Responding to the crisis in sub-Saharan Africa: The role of nutrition. *Public Health Nutr* 9 (5):544–50.

Coates, J., A. Swindale, and P. Bilinsky. 2006. *Household Food Insecurity Access Scale (HFIAS) for Measurement of Household Food Access: Indicator Guide.* Washington, DC: Food and Nutrition Technical Assistance Project, Academy for Educational Development.

Einterz, R. M., S. Kimaiyo, H. N. Mengech, B. O. Khwa-Otsyula, F. Esamai, F. Quigley, and J. J. Mamlin. 2007. Responding to the HIV pandemic: The power of an academic medical partnership. *Acad Med* 82 (8):812–8. doi: 10.1097/ACM.0b013e3180cc29f1.

Kadiyala, S. and S. Gillespie. 2004. Rethinking food aid to fight AIDS. *Food Nutr Bull* 25 (3):271–82.

Mamlin, J., S. Kimaiyo, S. Lewis, H. Tadayo, F. K. Jerop, C. Gichunge, T. Peterson, Y. Yih, P. Braitstein, and R. Einterz. 2009. Integrating nutrition support for food-insecure patients and their dependents into an HIV care and treatment program in western Kenya. *Am J Public Health* 99 (2):215–21.

Mamlin, J., S. Kimaiyo, W. Nyandiko, W. Tierney, and R. Einterz. 2004. *Academic Institutions Linking Access to Treatment and Prevention: Case Study.* Geneva, Switzerland: World Health Organization.

Marston, B. and K. M. De Cock. 2004. Multivitamins, nutrition, and antiretroviral therapy for HIV disease in Africa. *N Engl J Med* 351 (1):78–80. doi: 10.1056/NEJMe048134.

Wanke, C. 2005. Nutrition and HIV in the international setting. *Nutr Clin Care* 8 (1):44–8.

Index

A

Academic Model Providing Access to
    Healthcare (AMPATH), 192
  eligibility, 193–195
  food demand, 195
  food distribution and cost, 197
  food security, transition to, 197–198
  food supply, 195–197
  kilograms of food production, 196
  map of western Kenya, 193
  nutrition program, 193–198
  proportion of patients, 194, 195
  sustainability, 199–200
Acute diarrheal syndrome (ADS), 179
Acute respiratory infection (ARI), 179
Adjusted Hazard Ratio (AHR), 33
ADS, *see* Acute diarrheal syndrome (ADS)
Aflatoxin, 123–124
African Indigenous Vegetables (AIVs), 203
African Task Force on Food and Nutrition
    Development (ATFFND), 177
African Union Commission (AUC), 176, 177
AHR, *see* Adjusted Hazard Ratio (AHR)
AI, *see* American Indian (AI)
AIVs, *see* African Indigenous Vegetables
    (AIVs)
Alaskan Native (AN), 158
American Indian (AI), 158
AMPATH, *see* Academic Model Providing
    Access to Healthcare (AMPATH)
AN, *see* Alaskan Native (AN)
Anthropometric indicators, 58
Antiretroviral therapy (ART), 32, 70, 86, 140,
    192
  food and nutrition support for PLHIV, 82–84
  malnourished PLHIV nutritional status,
    81–82
  nutritional needs during malnutrition,
    80–81
  nutrition and, 79
  nutritious foods requiring to restore health,
    81–82
  PLHIV nutritional needs, 82
ARI, *see* Acute respiratory infection (ARI)
ART, *see* Antiretroviral therapy (ART)
ATFFND, *see* African Task Force on Food and
    Nutrition Development (ATFFND)
AUC, *see* African Union Commission
    (AUC)

B

Bacillus Calmette-Guérin vaccine (BCG vaccine),
    93, 101
Barker hypothesis, 118–119
Behavioral pathway, 27–28, 39; *see also* Mental
    health pathway; Nutritional pathway
  diabetes and cardiovascular risk, food
    insecurity to, 31
  HIV acquisition and disease progression,
    food insecurity to, 35–36
Body mass index (BMI), 33, 94, 120, 136
Bureau of Indian Affairs (BIA), 163

C

CAADP, *see* Comprehensive Africa Agriculture
    Development Programme (CAADP)
Cardiovascular disease; *see also*
    Noncommunicable disease (NCD);
    Obesity
  food insecurity and, 29
  immunologic pathways, 36–37
  pathways linking food insecurity, 28–31
Cash-for-work program, 146–147
CBPR approach, *see* Community-based
    participatory research approach
    (CBPR approach)
CCHIP, *see* Community Childhood Hunger
    Identification Project (CCHIP)
Child(ren), 104–105
  health, 86–87, 143
  malnutrition, 1
  undernourishment effects, 176
Child undernutrition, 177
  child mortalities association, 180
  economic costs of grade repetitions, 181
  in education, 180–181
  in four countries, 178
  on health, 179–180
  in productivity, 182–183
  on repetition, 180
  repetition rates by nutritional status, 180
  on retention, 181
  social and economic impact of, 178
  summary of costs, 179
CHR Program, *see* Community Health
    Representative Program (CHR
    Program)
Churro sheep, 160

Printed in the United States
by Baker & Taylor Publisher Services